Women Physicians
in Leadership Roles

Women Physicians in Leadership Roles

Edited by

Leah J. Dickstein, M.D.

and

Carol C. Nadelson, M.D.

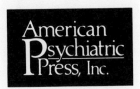

American Psychiatric Press, Inc.

1400 K Street, N.W.
Washington, DC 20005

Library of Congress Cataloging in Publication Data

Women physicians in leadership roles.

   Based on a symposium held at the 1984 Annual Meeting of the American Psychiatric Association in Los Angeles, Calif.
   Includes bibliographies.
   1. Women psychiatrists--Congresses. 2. Women psychiatrists--United States--Biography--Congresses. 4. Leadership--Congresses. I. Dickstein, Leah J., 1934-   . II. Nadelson, Carol C., 1936-   . III. American Psychiatric Association. Meeting (137th : 1984 : Los Angeles, Calif.) [DNLM: 1. Leadership--congresses. 2. Physicians, Women--history--congresses. 3. Psychiatry--history--congresses. WZ 80.5.W5 / W8725 1984]
RC440.82.W66 1986   616.89'008042   86-3574
ISBN 0-88048-203-6 (pbk.)

Dedication

We dedicate this book to future women physician leaders in the hope that what has been shared by others will assist them in reaching their goals.

We also dedicate this book to our husbands, Herbert Dickstein, M.D., and Theodore Nadelson, M.D., who share our involvements with our families and with our dual careers.

To our children, Stuart, Daniel, and Steven Dickstein and Robert and Jennifer Nadelson: we thank them for their understanding when we work and for their help in some of our projects. We hope they also choose future lifestyles and careers which will enable them to achieve personal satisfaction as they contribute to a larger society.

Contents

Introduction

This volume, probably the first of its kind, is a unique compilation of personal and general histories of women physicians as leaders in medicine, primarily from the field of psychiatry, in the United States, Canada and Australia.

It is an outgrowth of a symposium, entitled "Women in Leadership Roles," which took place quite successfully during the 1984 American Psychiatric Association annual meeting in Los Angeles. The participants included Leah J. Dickstein, M.D., chair, Carol C. Nadelson, M.D., co-chair, Patti Tighe, M.D., Jeanne Spurlock, M.D., Nancy J. Chodorow, Ph.D., Jean Baker Miller, M.D., Elissa P. Benedek, M.D., and Nancy C. A. Roeske, M.D., discussant. With the recommendation of the APA Scientific Program Committee and by invitation of the American Psychiatric Press, Inc., this edited volume is based on that symposium.

Though women were known to be physicians from earliest recorded history, their roles, except in rare instances, did not involve formal leadership positions.[1] Even in the fifth century A.D. women who had been leaders in health and hospital administration were forbidden to continue in these roles after the Council of Trent (1545-1563).

Although formal higher education and the professions were closed to women until the mid-nineteenth century, there was occasional evidence of interest in and support for women's scientific development. In the early years of the fifteenth century, an Italian woman, Christine de Pisan, wrote *The City of Women* which in fiction described women rulers, scientists and inventors.[2] In the early Middle Ages when convents were important intellectual as well as educational centers, a German nun, Hildegarde of Bingen (1098-1178), wrote two major treatises on medicine.[3] In the usual circumstance women served as midwives and herbalists and practiced household medicine. Through the mid-nineteenth century in the United States women not only were barred from attending most regular medical schools but even with formal medical training they were refused admission to medical societies and hospital staffs.

The reasons included a repetitively held belief in women's inadequacy for intellectual pursuits and for leadership in particular.

Since the second women's movement for equality, begun in 1963 with Betty Freidan's book, *The Feminine Mystique*,[4] many women and an increasing number of men have investigated and discovered much of the unrecognized history of women in America regarding their educational, work and lifestyle opportunities and experiences.

Certainly since Mary Roth Walsh's book in 1977, *Doctors Wanted: No Women Need Apply*,[5] many thousands of women have entered medical school, received their degrees, gone on to residencies and entered all specialty areas in greater numbers than before.

The number of women physicians in the United States remained at the low stable rate of 4-6 percent between 1910 and 1960, but changed dramatically beginning in the 1970's to reach the current national average of medical school classes which consist of at least one third women.

What has unfortunately not shown a similar dramatic increase is the number of women faculty whose numbers remain low, whose senior academic titles take longer to reach and whose leadership roles are fewer. Women are proportionally underrepresented in administration and other leadership positions and few women serve on specialty boards or are heads of departments.

This disproportionate underrepresentation of women in positions of leadership is partially expected as the increasing numbers of women only recently entering these fields have not yet had the opportunity to attain these positions. At the same time, however, we must understand our historical lessons if permanent cultural change is to occur. Where women have had a significant influence in health fields, external factors have often been influential, including wars, physician shortages and major cultural reorganization. Only then have attitudinal changes followed. The changes brought about by expedience or pragmatics invariably gave way to reversion to previous patterns of gender role differentiation when circumstances allowed.

Currently the number of women in psychiatry has increased to at least 50 percent in many residency programs. Approximately 6 of 32 thousand members of the American Psychiatric Association are women. Although a number are entering academic, administrative and organizational spheres, an historical perspective of individual women physicians in leadership roles particularly in psychiatry has not been written before.

The women in this book developed strong personal goals to become physicians, whenever and wherever they were born and however they were raised. They do not appear to have been angry women consumed with negative feelings and attitudes. Rather, their singlemindedness appears to have come from within and, fortunately for many, to have been reinforced by friends, teachers, family and significant others. They experienced all types of rejections and stumbling blocks along the way yet were not thwarted from their goals, at least not permanently.

Most evidenced a sense of humor, a strong work ethic, adaptability, optimism, selflessness, intellectual curiosity and creativity, a faith in themselves and the ability to tolerate frustration, and at times, ongoing isolation, and loneliness or at least aloneness whether at home, in school or in their professional roles.

Experiences of frustration and rejection pervade all of the women's personal accounts. Many were not included but were recounted in initial informal contacts with the first editor. But bitterness is absent. In its place are humor and partial acceptance of the frustrations, as well as confession that at the time the rejection was not seen as such. The women were not aware that the rejection was a phenomenon based on sex-role socialization and socio-cultural mores of the time.

In part, this book is about women physicians and the opportunities they found and made for themselves to use their abilities to pursue power for the good of their patients, peers, staff, residents and students as well as for the general good of humanity. It is obvious that these women physicians also enjoyed the satisfactions of using power constructively and competently.

What is clear is that these women have often worked under cultural limitations and duress. Often they have had to choose whether to accommodate to our culture's definition of women's proper role, place and behavior. They have often adopted stereotypically male defined characteristics of stamina, courage, independence of thought and action, competency, steadfastness, and creative leadership while retaining their sex-role assigned characteristics of caring for others. Many have also functioned under the pressures of dual roles, as wife (or significant other) and professional, or triple roles of wife (or significant other), professional and mother. Dual career relationships have only added to the pressures of choices to make and time to be apportioned. Overall these women appear satisfied with their choices and with their roles and lifestyles.

The growth of this book is itself a paradigm of how many women leaders function. Early authors suggested others, first authors chose to invite co-authors to work with them. Obviously all of these women developed unique leadership styles that worked for them, but that also allowed and ensured that their leadership experiences, particularly in research, permitted and permits others, men as well as women, to follow in their footsteps if they so choose.

It appears that these able women lead others constructively for rational and pragmatic reasons. Their "cooperative leadership" styles, rather than the single person "command style" attributed to men, was also used by the majority of women physician administrators in the national survey described in Chapter 26.

For ease of access and interest the book is divided into nine sections. Section 1 includes episodes from the unique struggles women experienced in American medicine from three different historical perspectives, the city of Boston, the state of Kentucky and one woman's personal odyssey.

In Section 2 the history of women in psychiatry is unveiled and one immediately realizes that a large portion of psychiatry's history has heretofore been missing. As is often the case, these women physicians functioned with little recognition of their value and their contributions. In a more circumspect vein the leadership styles among early women psychoanalysts offers more of an understanding of the personal and culturally accepted feminine modes of functioning as leaders through nurturance and teaching even in their professional roles.

Section 3 narrows our historical focus to the eight individual universally accepted early leaders in psychiatry. What is important and unique is that we are allowed to meet them as human beings and observe their personal as well as professional development in the context of their time, their culture, their families, their problems and their support systems. The glimpses offered of their mutual interactions not only with each other but with their contemporary male mentors and colleagues are fascinating as well as enlightening.

In Section 4, three current women, not surprisingly, two in child psychiatry, offer their personal and professional paths to leadership roles in academic and organizational arenas.

In Section 5, eight areas in psychiatry are detailed in which women have chosen to be leaders. Their experiences as competent physicians and as women should encourage all readers to rethink past and current work roles and situations for similar experiences and for ways to cope constructively with what has recently become more subtle differentiation and discrimination.

Section 6 includes a national survey of women physician administrators from five medical specialties which presents statistical evidence that women physicians enjoy functioning as administrators and feel competent to do so though their styles may vary. More personal administrative and leadership issues are discussed in the second two papers. In Section 7, women psychiatrists in academia are highlighted from an historical and general as well as from a personal perspective. Section 8 includes interesting overviews of women's experiences in medicine and in psychiatry in Canada and Australia. Finally, Section 9 deals with women physicians as leaders in the area of politics, both in organized medicine and in comparison with women political leaders in general.

As editors, it is our dream that readers of this book, professionals and non-professionals, young and old, male and female, will extract from the numerous unique and general histories included about named and nameless women, that women are competent and ready to be leaders now and in the future. We hope the message is clear: leadership styles can vary but opportunities must be made available to all who are competent and desire to expend their creative talents in this sphere. Certainly, our patients, our communities and we, as professionals, will benefit personally from offering access to all who seek enhanced leadership paths, particularly the increasing

number of women physicians today.

Carol chose *Unity Amidst Diversity: Future Challenges* as her theme for the 139th Annual Meeting of the American Psychiatric Association, held in Washington D.C., in May 1986, to encourage psychiatrists with diverse interests to work together for the common welfare of our patients. This theme can be applied to our book as well. The women leaders described in the pages to follow came from diverse backgrounds, engaged in various activities yet all progressed to the book's theme, leadership roles. They or their forebears probably immigrated at different times throughout Europe, the Middle East and Africa earlier, and from the seventeenth to the twentieth century, to North America and Australia. Their ethnic, racial, religious and personal lifestyle choices may differ, but their desire to become physicians and leaders is an expression of their creative abilities. This unites them and allows them to serve as much needed historical and current female role models of competent leaders for our youth today and for those, regardless of age, who still seek challenge and opportunity in leadership roles in the future.

Leah J. Dickstein, M.D.
Louisville, KY

Carol C. Nadelson, M.D.
Boston, MA

References

[1]Nadelson C: The Woman Physician: Past Present and Future, in The Physician: A Professional Under Stress. Edited by Callan JP. Englewood Cliffs, NJ, Appleton-Century-Crofts, 1983, p. 261.
[2]Harris BJ: The power of the past, in In the Shadow of the Past: Psychology Portrays the Sexes. Edited by Lewin M. New York: Columbia University Press, 1984, pp 6-7.
[3]See note 2.
[4]Friedan B: The Feminine Mystique. New York: W. W. Norton, 1963.
[5]Walsh MR: Doctors Wanted: No Women Need Apply: Sexual Barriers in the Medical Profession. New Haven: Yale University Press, 1977.

Acknowledgments

To Ron McMillen, General Manager of the American Psychiatric Press, and to Tim Clancy, Managing Editor, we offer gratitude for their guidance, assistance, and support throughout the process of completing this book.

We want to acknowledge the help of many secretaries and assistants to all the authors. However, we especially want to recognize three women at the University of Louisville, Jayne Zickafoose, who typed and retyped with skill and good cheer and organized the incoming chapters, Kathy Garvin, who contacted all of the contributors for numerous reasons over the past year and a half, and Lillian Jones who edited tirelessly. Finally, on behalf of all who read this book, we want to acknowledge and express our sincere appreciation for the extraordinary efforts expended by our colleagues who made time to research and share their special talents and knowledge in these chapters.

*Only people who give themselves without pretensions just as they
are, who cannot do otherwise than they do, have a beneficient
influence on others.*

--Karen Horney

The Adolescent Diaries of Karen Horney
(New York, Basic Books, 1980, p. 252)

1

Women Doctors and the Quest
for Professional Power: 1881-1926

Virginia G. Drachman, Ph.D.

*Associate Professor of History,
Tufts University,
Boston, Massachusetts*

I would like to thank Douglas L. Jones for his help throughout the writing of this paper. An earlier version of this paper was presented at the 55th Annual Meeting of the American Association for the History of Medicine, held on 30 April 1982, in Bethesda, Maryland.

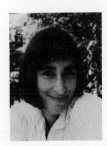

Virginia G. Drachman, Ph.D.

1

Women Doctors and the Quest
for Professional Power: 1881-1926

In 1904 Dr. Bertha Van Hoosen was a leader among women doctors of her day. She was an accomplished and highly respected physician whose career thrived as she practiced alongside men physicians. Her specialty was surgery, an area dominated almost exclusively by male physicians, and she was a professor of gynecology at the College of Physicians and Surgeons in Chicago which was run by men. Despite her status as a woman doctor, Van Hoosen held far less favor among her male colleagues. Regardless of her accomplishments alongside male physicians, as a woman she was still isolated from them. Her attendance at the annual meeting of the American Medical Association in 1904 underscored her separateness. "It was a dreary experience," she recalled, "for I met no one whom I knew and was too timid to make any new acquaintances."[1]

The loneliness and disappointment which Van Hoosen experienced at that meeting in 1904 indicates the position of women doctors--leaders as well as rank-and-file--in the late nineteenth and early twentieth centuries. Van Hoosen's attendance at the meeting was part of a larger trend toward integrating women into institutions previously for men only. This shift represented a break with the tradition of separatism--the foundation of women's lives in nineteenth century America. Barred from male institutions, women founded their own, including schools, clubs and reform societies where they gathered apart from men.[2] Women doctors participated in this development of female institutions. Excluded from male medical establishments, they built their own medical schools and hospitals, therefore making their professional journey apart from men.

As the century drew to a close, the male medical institutions began to open their doors to women. In 1894, women comprised at least 10 percent of the enrollment at eighteen medical schools run by men in various parts of the country. Accelerating this process of integration was the fact that all but two of the fourteen regular women's medical schools founded in the second half of the nineteenth century closed or merged with other schools by the first decade of the twentieth.[3] By the turn of the century, coeducation was a viable option for the aspiring woman doctor and appeared to be on the threshold of replacing separate medical school training for women.

This trend toward sexual integration permeated other areas of the medical profession as well. Women joined formerly male-only medical societies, gained internships at major urban hospitals and entered male medical specialties.

As women doctors entered the twentieth century, many were convinced that separatism in medicine would hinder their careers and that working alongside men was the key to their professional success and power. While many placed their faith in integration with their medical brethren, most women doctors in the first quarter of the twentieth century found that separation continued to define their professional lives. Indeed, separation persisted--though in new forms--within the newly integrated medical profession of the early twentieth century.

The experience of the accomplished Dr. Bertha Van Hoosen at the American Medical Association meeting revealed not only the limits of her own power and influence, but also the limits of integration for women doctors in the late nineteenth and early twentieth centuries. Precisely during this period in American history, women doctors became more self-conscious about their professional status in American society. The discovery of a professional identity among women doctors led to the first systematic surveys of women in medicine. Between 1881 and 1926, women doctors conducted three surveys to define the boundaries of their colleagues' working lives and to chart their progress.[4] Taken together, these surveys demonstrated women doctors' accomplishments over the course of a half-century, indicating their gradual integration into the male-dominated medical profession. At the same time, the surveys showed that separatism did indeed continue to affect the careers of women doctors throughout the first quarter of the twentieth century.

In 1881, two of the leading American women's medical institutions simultaneously sponsored the first and second of these studies. Dr. Rachel Bodley, dean of the Woman's Medical College of Pennsylvania, analyzed the careers of 189 graduates of her college. In Boston, Drs. Emma Call and Emily and Augusta Pope from the New England Hospital for Women and Children published a broader survey of 390 women doctors from various parts of the country.[5] Following the best scientific methods of the day, Bodley, Call and the Popes gathered data to demonstrate women's professional success in medicine. In particular, they shared an interest in four general topics: the nature of women doctors' professional practice, the extent of their professional affiliations, their financial success and their marital status.

From the answers to these questions, the Bodley and Pope studies drew remarkably similar profiles of women doctors in 1881. The emerging picture was one of professionally active and successful women--working apart from men. In fact, separatism shaped every aspect of women doctors' working lives. Most women physicians lived in New York, Boston or Philadelphia, the cities where the first women's medical schools and hospitals were established. They trained at one or

more of these women's medical institutions for slightly more than four years and began to practice medicine, on the average, at the age of thirty-one. They had been in active practice for up to ten years, working almost entirely among women--doctors as well as patients. Their private practice consisted of either general medicine or a combination of general medicine, obstetrics and gynecology. Those who worked in institutional settings did so in separate women's institutions such as hospitals, dispensaries, asylums and schools. Finally, at a time when most medical societies did not admit women, almost two-thirds had no medical society affiliation.

Separatism defined the private lives of most women doctors as well. The majority were single while they were medical students and interns, and they remained single in professional practice. Only 20 to 30 percent married at some point after completing their training. Among women doctors, a few admitted that balancing both career and family was difficult. Most, however, claimed it was not and continued to practice even after they had children. Unique among women of their day, they successfully defied the separation of marriage and professional work for nineteenth-century women.

Most women doctors, married or single, considered themselves professionally successful. Satisfied with their average annual earnings of $1000 to $3000, they claimed they received "cordial social recognition" from male peers and the public. Moreover, they forged careers without sacrificing their health. This was an important finding because it contradicted the prevailing wisdom about the impact of work on women's health. Only eight years earlier in 1883, the highly respected Harvard physician, Dr. Edward H. Clarke, published his book, *Sex in Education; or A Fair Chance for the Girls*, warning about the dangers of excessive physical and mental exertion to women's health.[6] *Sex in Education* was a widely read book which left its mark on a whole generation of young women. Despite its dire warnings and popular appeal, it did not describe the experiences of the women in the Bodley and Pope studies. Instead, most women doctors claimed that they were healthy throughout their training and during their professional practice. Only a handful of women doctors reported that they stopped practicing because of poor health. In sum, the Bodley and Pope surveys proclaimed women doctors' professional accomplishments and promised their continued progress in the future. At the same time the surveys uncovered, though perhaps unintentionally, the strong foundation of separatism upon which women doctors in 1881 built their professional lives. They studied in women's medical schools, trained in women's hospitals, cared almost exclusively for female patients and remained single.

Forty-five years later, in 1926, Dr. Martha Tracy, dean of the Woman's Medical College of Pennsylvania, published a survey of women doctors in the early twentieth century. Her findings revealed both the change and the continuity in women doctors' professional lives since 1881. Based on the responses of 471 women who had received their medical degrees between 1905 and 1921, Tracy's survey suggested that the optimism of the 1881 studies had not been misplaced. Moreover, it pointed to an important new trend: the professional changes women doctors had made since the Bodley and Pope studies, indicating a decline of separatism and a new emphasis on integration with men into the mainstream of the medical profession.[7]

This development was part of larger changes in the history of medicine and of women since the Bodley and Pope studies of 1881. Scientific advances, professional consolidation and educational reform had changed the shape of the medical profession. The Flexner Report on medical schools in 1910 set higher standards in medical education while hospital internships, postgraduate training and even specialization became part of medicine.[8]

These changes in medicine coincided with significant changes in women's lives in the late nineteenth and early twentieth centuries. Within the halls of academe, women social scientists challenged the notion of sexual differences between men and women, the backbone of nineteenth century separatism.[9] Meanwhile, more women began to develop public lives as college and career became an acceptable path for middle-class women to follow. In 1920, women won their long-fought battle for suffrage and entered the political arena as equals with men. In 1921, they won another major legislative victory, the passage of the Sheppard-Towner Act, which provided federal funds to instruct women in maternal and infant hygiene.[10] Against the background of this political activity and social change, the numbers of women in medicine reached a peak of 9,015 in 1910, and

women doctors began to claim with confidence that their struggle to achieve professional success was over.[11]

During this period of substantial progress for women, Tracy sought to establish the new boundaries of women doctors' financial success and the relationship between their careers and marriage. Yet the Tracy study had unique characteristics which reflected the changed status of women doctors since the nineteenth century. Because the Bodley and Pope studies were conducted in an era of debate over women's physical limitations, they sought to demonstrate that women could be doctors and were, indeed, successful in their practice. Tracy, on the other hand, conducted her survey at a time when the notion of female inferiority had begun to give way to the idea of sexual equality. As a result, she was unconcerned about the late nineteenth-century debate over the physical dangers of higher education for women and did not seek information on the condition of women doctors' health. Instead, Tracy sought to prove that women doctors were successfully keeping up with rising professional standards. With this in mind, she focused on women doctors' educational background and professional training. Despite the apparent trend toward sexual integration in the medical profession since the Bodley and Pope studies, Tracy, consciously or not, still treated women doctors as a separate group and did not compare them with men. Still, in focusing on medical education and training, Tracy's survey provided an implicit comparison, for it was male physicians' professional standards which provided the measure of achievement for women doctors.

Tracy's findings verified that women doctors who received medical degrees between 1912 and 1921 had indeed kept up with the rising professional standards in medicine. They were college graduates with a bachelor of arts or science degree. They pursued further professional training after medical school, usually completing a hospital internship and often planning to undertake further postgraduate medical study. Most women doctors kept up with new standards in professional training and kept pace with changes in professional practice as well. They earned annual incomes ranging between $2000 and $5000, an increase of at least a third over the typical income of $1000 to $3000 earned by women in 1881. Moreover, in keeping with the trend away from general practice, 53 percent were specialists.

Most significantly, Tracy's study demonstrated the shift away from the nineteenth century pattern of professional separation of men and women doctors. The women doctors who graduated between 1912 and 1921 were integrated into the predominately male medical profession. Almost four-fifths of the women in Tracy's study graduated from coeducational medical schools. While most still entered the traditional female specialties of internal medicine, pediatrics, obstetrics and gynecology, some entered a range of traditionally male specialties, including otolaryngology, ophthalmology, dermatology and anesthesiology.

Complementing the integration in their professional lives, fewer women doctors in the 1910's remained single. Some 43 percent chose to marry, with most claiming that marriage did not interfere with their careers. In fact, almost 80 percent of those married continued to practice after marriage.[12]

Looked at together, the Bodley, Pope, and Tracy surveys offer an optimistic picture of the developments in the lives and careers of women doctors in the second half of the nineteenth century and the first quarter of the twentieth. Moreover, the Tracy survey depicted women doctors in 1926 as substantially different from their predecessors in 1881. They were more educated, better trained, moving into specialties, financially secure, often balancing career and marriage--and they were working among, rather than apart from, their male colleagues.

While the Tracy survey proved important changes had occurred in women doctors' professional lives since the Bodley and Pope surveys, a clearer understanding of the evolution of these changes is possible by looking at other sources. An examination of turn-of-the-century women doctors in the midst of their medical training at the New England Hospital for Women and Children provides a more detailed record of women doctors in this period of transition from the 1880's through the first quarter of the twentieth century.

Founded in Boston in 1862, the New England Hospital was one of the most important women's medical institutions in nineteenth-century America.[13] The applications of the women seeking internships at the hospital between 1880 and 1925 expose both the tenacity of separatism and the trend toward integration. Despite growing opportunities for women at hospitals run by men, women increasingly applied for internships at the New England Hospital around the turn of the century. From 1891 through 1895, sixty-two women applied. From 1900 through 1904, there were ninety-six applicants.[14]

Most of those who applied for internships at the New England Hospital in the last decade of the nineteenth century were in their twenties. A smaller group of women was in their early thirties, and an even smaller group was in their late thirties. The picture was roughly the same in the early years of the twentieth century as well, although more applicants were in their late twenties and fewer were in their early twenties. Throughout these years, only a handful of applicants was in their forties.[15] (See Table 1.)

Almost all of the intern applicants to the New England Hospital were single. Applications from a married woman or even a widow were unusual. From 1891 through 1895 and from 1900 through 1904, only three married women and five widows sought internships.[16] Two-thirds of the women who applied to the New England Hospital between 1891 and 1895 went to women's medical schools. Nineteen were graduates of the Woman's Medical College of the New York Infirmary, while another twenty-three graduated from the Woman's Medical College of Pennsylvania. A few others attended either the Ontario Medical College for Women in Toronto or the Woman's Medical College in Chicago. Only five applicants graduated from the coeducational University of Michigan.

This picture changed in the early years of the twentieth century, reflecting women's increasing opportunities for medical study with men and their shrinking opportunities for study at the rapidly closing women's medical schools. Only the women's medical colleges in Pennsylvania and Baltimore remained open by 1903. As a result,

Table 1. Ages of the Applicants for Internships at the New England Hospital

Age	1891–1895		1900–1904	
	Percent	Number	Percent	Number
20–24	36	21	27	25
25–29	38	22	52	48
30–34	17	10	15	14
35–40	9	5	6	5
Total	100	58	100	92

Source: Intern applications, Boxes 10–13, NEH Collection.

fewer women came to the New England Hospital from the women's medical schools. While graduates of the Woman's Medical College of Pennsylvania continued to comprise the hospital's largest group of applicants, they represented just over a quarter of the applicants from 1900 through 1904 rather than a third as in the late 1890's. With the closing of the Woman's Medical College of the New York Infirmary in 1899, its graduates who made up almost a third of the intern applicants in the 1890's comprised less than 10 percent of the applicants from 1900 through 1904. At the same time, there was a significant increase in the number of applicants from coeducational medical schools. Ten percent graduated from Tufts University alone, while another 20 percent earned degrees from the medical schools at Johns Hopkins, the University of Michigan, the University of Buffalo and Syracuse University. (See Table 2.)

An applicant's prior work experience also mirrored this era of transition. Between 1891 and 1895, slightly over one-half the applicants had worked in another job at some time before they applied to the New England Hospital. Of this group, most had been teachers, the profession women entered most frequently throughout the nineteenth century. A much smaller number had been nurses, and several had been office workers. The rest of the applicants, slightly less than one-half of the group, had followed a direct career path, never working before entering medical school. In marked contrast, the typical applicant

in the early years of the twentieth century had no prior work experience or career. Of the minority who had worked, teaching was again the most common occupation. This shifting pattern forecast the greater ease with which women could become doctors at the beginning of the twentieth century, and, as the century progressed, the more direct career path which women followed into medicine. (See Table 3.)

The selection of interns was the responsibility of a group of attending doctors comprising the hospital's board of physicians. In their choice of interns, these doctors helped to forward the trend toward integration in the early twentieth century. They initially reinforced the single status of women doctors by refusing to accept a married woman intern through the first decade of the twentieth century. In 1910, however, they admitted their first married intern, Myrtle Jack. But for her marital status, little distinguished Mrs. Jack from other intern applicants. She was a 35-year-old former teacher and a graduate of the medical school of Western University in Pittsburgh. Two letters on Jack's behalf convinced the board members that her candidacy was an exception. "We need your help for our women," wrote one woman doctor from Pittsburgh, "for Pittsburgh does not grant many favors to women." Another woman doctor echoed the same plea: "The Western University . . . has excluded women and would like to annihilate every institution in the city that women are connected with . . . ," she

Table 2. Applications and Acceptances for Internships at the New England Hospital, by Medical School of the Applicants

Medical School	1891–1895		1900–1904	
	Applied	Accepted	Applied	Accepted
Woman's Medical College of Pennsylvania	23	11	26	11
Woman's Medical College of the New York Infirmary	19	9	9	4
University of Michigan	5	3	6	4
University of Buffalo and Syracuse University	1	0	5	2
Medical Schools in Chicago	6	1	11	4
Johns Hopkins	0	0	7	7
Tufts University	0	0	10	5
University of Minnesota	2	0	3	0
Schools in Canada	1	0	10	4
Schools in Europe	1	1	0	0
Other	3	1	7	3
Total	61	26	94	44

Source: Intern applications, Boxes 10–13, NEH Collection.

explained. "The girls here need hospital instruction," she continued, "and I, therefore, urge you to do all you can to help . . ."[17] Persuaded of the importance of Jack's candidacy, the doctors accepted her for 1911.

The physicians at the New England Hospital helped to accelerate the professional integration of women doctors in other ways as well. While more than 75 percent of the interns they accepted between 1881 and 1895 were graduates of women's medical schools, 41 percent of the interns accepted from 1900 through 1904 were graduates of coeducational medical schools. In choosing these applicants, the doctors displayed an overt preference for any graduate of Johns Hopkins, the most prestigious medical school in the country. From 1900 through 1904, they accepted all seven of the women who applied from there. The doctors looked also for the brightest candidates from other schools who showed promise of being able to keep up with male physicians.[18] Finally, most of the interns the doctors accepted between 1900 and 1904 followed a direct career path into medicine, whereas 60 percent of the interns they accepted in the earliest years of the twentieth century had not.

The data on the lives of the interns after they left the New England Hospital add depth to Tracy's profile of women doctors in the early twentieth century. While the information is not complete, data are available on six of the interns accepted between 1900 and 1904.[19] In the first group, three of the six married sometime after their training. One left the New England Hospital in 1886 at the age of thirty-three. Later she married, had four children and returned to her home state of New Hampshire. Marriage and motherhood did not deter her from her professional work, at least at the beginning, for she

practiced until 1911, retiring at the age of forty-eight.

The three externs who remained single were still in practice in 1934. One, Alice Hamilton, became a leader in the field of industrial medicine and was the first woman to join the Harvard Medical School faculty.[20] The other two had less spectacular professional records. One left the New England Hospital in 1896 when she was thirty-one. Though the details of her medical career are unknown, in 1934, at the age of sixty-nine, she was living in her hometown of New Wilmington, Pennsylvania, where she was the physician in charge of a sanitarium. The other took a similar professional path. She completed her internship in 1895 at the age of twenty-six. Though she had a strong interest in surgery as an intern, by 1908 she was running her own sanitarium for "mild and nervous cases," and was still doing so in 1934 at age sixty-five. Given that less than 3 percent of all women doctors were surgeons between 1905 and 1910, her failure to go into surgery despite her early ambitions in that direction was typical of women doctors of her day.[21] Moreover, despite the apparent trend toward professional integration, surgery remained a special enclave of male physicians which was particularly hard for women to enter.

The interns at the New England Hospital in the early twentieth century present a somewhat different picture. Of the twenty about whose lives information is available, nine married sometime after their internship. At least two successfully managed both marriage and career. One completed her internship at the New England Hospital at age twenty-seven. She married in 1913 at age thirty-five, subsequently giving birth to one child. In 1934 she was still in active practice as the chief physician at the Pennsylvania State Tuberculosis

Table 3. Applicants for Internships at the New England Hospital by Prior Work Experience and Acceptance

Prior Work Experience	1891–1895		1900–1904	
	Applied	Accepted	Applied	Accepted
None	25	7	51	23
Teacher	20	10	31	13
Other	11	1	8	4
Total	56	18	90	40

Source: Intern applications, Boxes 10–13, NEH Collection.

Dispensary in Erie, Pennsylvania, and served as a staff physician at another Erie hospital.

The career of the other, Dr. Margaret Noyes Kleinert, symbolized more clearly the impact of integration. Kleinert completed her internship in 1905 at age twenty-four. By 1910 she opened a private practice in Boston, specializing in "Ears, Nose and Throat," and was a visiting physician at the New England Hospital. In 1916, at age thirty-five, she married and subsequently gave birth to a daughter. In 1934 she was the chief surgeon of otolaryngology at the New England Hospital and an assistant surgeon of otolaryngology at Massachusetts General Hospital. Though chief of surgery at New England Hospital, Kleinert never achieved that position of leadership at Massachusetts General.

Overall, balancing marriage and career was a major challenge for most women doctors in the early twentieth century. Some, such as Elsie Miller, Rebecca Clark and Anna Cook, gave up their careers after they married. Miller married at some time after she left the New England Hospital in 1905. By 1934 she was the mother of two children and had retired from practice. Clark and Cook left the New England Hospital in 1905 and 1907 respectively and then married. Though neither had children, neither was in practice in 1934.

The remaining eleven ex-interns from the New England Hospital covered the spectrum of professional practice characteristic of women doctors in the early decades of the twentieth century. Three served as medical missionaries in China or India, and one of them became sick and was forced to retire. One ran her own school for "mentally deficient children," two were involved in public health work and three worked in educational institutions. Only one was in private practice, and she and one other ex-intern also had hospital practices.

The experiences of interns at the New England Hospital add more than depth to the picture of successful women doctors which the Bodley, Pope and Tracy surveys provide. The interns' experiences suggest, instead, more obstacles were in the path of integration and power for women doctors than appeared on the surface, and that the optimism, particularly of the Tracy study, was premature. For the women who trained at the New England Hospital, balancing marriage and medical practice, for example, was more problematic than the surveys suggested. Even with the

trend toward specialization and the acceptance of women into the previously men-only medical schools, many New England Hospital interns carved out their careers in typically "female" areas of medical practice such as schools, public health work and missionary activity.

A closer look at the Tracy study verified that the women at the New England Hospital were not unique. While more women doctors specialized from 1910-1920 than in the first decade of the century, the percentage of women in typically "male" laboratory specialties declined in that short period of time. The percentage of women doctors in otolaryngology and ophthalmology dropped from 8 percent to 6 percent and from 13 percent to 4 percent respectively, while in surgery, a symbol of male medical practice, the percentage of women doctors dropped from 3 percent to 0. At the same time, women doctors increasingly congregated in typically "female" specialties and in the service areas of medicine. The percentage of women doctors in internal medicine increased from 3 percent to 11 percent, in pediatrics from 1 percent to 10 percent and in gynecology from 8 percent to 10 percent. Similarly, the percentage of women doctors working in colleges and teaching in medical schools increased from 4 to 8 percent and from 0 to 6 percent respectively, while general practitioners with special interest in venereal diseases, infant and children's health and tuberculosis more than doubled from 14 to 30 percent.[22] The tendency of the women in the Tracy survey as well as those from the New England Hospital to cluster in "female" specialties and in social medical services reflected the expanding opportunities for women doctors in these particular areas. As one woman explained in 1921, the "medical profession today offers . . . increasingly varied opportunities for women, especially in connection with promotion of the health of children, of girls and women in industry, of the community and of the home."[23]

In the final analysis, the changes in women doctors' career patterns in the first quarter of the twentieth century did not signal a trend toward full and permanent integration. Rather, women doctors' career paths showed that after a temporary foray into high-status laboratory specialties, women congregated instead into low-status "female" specialties and in social medical service. At the same time, most women doctors continued to lead single lives, while balancing marriage and career continued to present a major challenge to those who tried to have both. Despite the apparent shift toward integration with men in education and practice, women doctors did not achieve the professional success and power they had expected. Instead, a new version of separatism accompanied the integration of women doctors into male-dominated medicine. As one woman doctor astutely observed: "A generation earlier, women doctors were on the outside standing together. Now they were on the inside sitting alone."[24]

Some women doctors made active attempts to accommodate this new version of separatism. Van Hoosen's lonely experience at the American Medical Association meeting in 1904 inspired her in 1908 to initiate the custom at subsequent American Medical Association meetings of holding an annual banquet for women doctors only. More important, in 1915, the same year that the American Medical Association accepted women as members, Van Hoosen founded and became the first president of the American Medical Women's Association. Thereafter, women doctors who chose to join both organizations could enjoy the benefits of integration as well as those of separation. Some early twentieth century women doctors, however, strove instead to replace separatism with integration and denounced any attempts to organize women doctors as a backward "move to segregation."[25] Opportunity for integration did represent a major step toward professional power for women doctors. In the long run, however, the integration of women into the medical profession with men was more elusive than it appeared. While some women doctors did forge truly integrated professional lives, most early twentieth century women doctors worked within the mainstream of American medicine, but remained isolated from men and from the center of power as well.

Notes

[1] Bertha Van Hoosen's autobiography is Petticoat Surgeon (Chicago: Pellegrini and Cudahy, 1947). For quote, see p. 201. Parts of this paper appear in the author's book Hospital with a Heart: Women Doctors and the Paradox of Separatism at the New England Hospital, 1862-1969 (Ithaca: Cornell University Press, 1984).
[2] On the impact of the doctrine of separate

spheres on the lives of women in nineteenth-century America see Nancy F. Cott, The Bonds of Womanhood: "Woman's Sphere" in New England, 1780-1835 (New Haven: Yale University Press, 1977) and Carroll Smith-Rosenberg, "The female world of love and ritual: relations between women in nineteenth-century America," Signs, 1975, 1:1-30. For an analysis of the phenomenon of women's institution building, see Estelle Freedman, "Separatism as strategy: female institution building and American feminism, 1870-1930," Feminist Studies, 1979, 5:512-29. There have been several important studies of the women's movement in the late nineteenth century. See, for example, Karen J. Blair, The Clubwoman as Feminist: True Womanhood Redefined, 1868-1914 (New York: Holmes and Meier, 1980); Ruth Bordin, Woman and Temperance: The Quest for Power and Liberty, 1873-1920 (Philadelphia: Temple University Press, 1981) and MariJo Buhle, Women and American Socialism, 1870-1920 (Urbana: University of Illinois Press, 1981). For a detailed study of the quest for integration among professional women, see Rosalind Rosenberg, Beyond Separate Spheres: Intellectual Roots of Feminism (New Haven: Yale University Press, 1982).
[3] Mary Roth Walsh, "Doctors Wanted: No Women Need Apply": Sexual Barriers in the Medical Profession, 1835-1975 (New Haven: Yale University Press, 1977), pp. 193, 204.
[4] Rachel L. Bodley, The College Story: Valedictory Address to the Twenty-Ninth Graduating Class of the Woman's Medical College of Pennsylvania (Philadelphia: Grant, Faires, and Rodgers, 1881); Emily F. Pope, Emma L. Call, and C. Augusta Pope, The Practice of Medicine in the United States (Boston: Wright and Potter, 1881); and Martha Tracy, "Women graduates in medicine," Bull. Amer. Assoc. Med. Coll., 1927, 2:21-28. Several historians have relied on the data in these surveys to describe women doctors' professional progress. They have not, however, interpreted the meaning of these surveys to show the change and continuity in women doctors' professional lives. See Walsh, "Doctors Wanted: No Women Need Apply," and Patricia M. Hummer, The Decade of Elusive Promise: Professional Women in the United States, 1920-1930 (Champaign, Illinois: Research Press, 1979).

[5]Bodley sought to survey the graduates of the Woman's Medical College of Pennsylvania from its founding in 1850 through 1880. Of the total 276 graduates, 244 were still alive. Her survey is based on the 189 graduates who responded to her questionnaire. Pope, Call, and Pope sent out 470 questionnaires to female graduates of regular medical schools nationwide. While the exact number of respondents is unclear, they explain that they received "a little over three hundred answers" and "partial information" from 130 others.

[6]Edward H. Clarke, Sex in Education; or, A Fair Chance for the Girls (Boston: James R. Osgood, 1873).

[7]Tracy sent questionnaires to 1,833 women who graduated from medical schools in the years 1905 through 1910 and 1912 through 1921. Her survey was based on the responses of 471 women doctors, 200 from the earlier group and 271 from the later group. The analysis in this paper focuses on the responses of the 271 women who graduated in the years from 1912 through 1921.

[8]For a discussion of changes in the medical profession, see Morris J. Vogel, The Invention of the Modern Hospital: Boston 1870-1930 (Chicago: University of Chicago Press, 1980); Charles E. Rosenberg, "The Therapeutic Revolution: Medicine, Meaning and Social Change in Ninteenth-Century America," in Morris J. Vogel and Charles E. Rosenberg, eds., The Therapeutic Revolution: Essays in the Social History of American Medicine (Philadelphia: University of Pennsylvania Press, 1979), pp. 3-26; and Charles E. Rosenberg, "Inward vision and outward glance: the shaping of the American hospital, 1880-1914," Bull. His. Med., 1979, 53:346-91.

[9]Rosenberg, Beyond Separate Spheres.

[10]For a discussion of women's changing social position see William Chafe, The American Woman: Her Changing Social, Economic, and Political Roles, 1920-1970. New York: Oxford University Press, 1972); Blair, Clubwoman as Feminist; and R. Rosenberg, Beyond Separate Spheres.

[11]Walsh, "Doctors Wanted: No Women Need Apply," p. 186. For an analysis of the problems this professional progress produced for women doctors, see Virginia Drachman, Hospital with a Heart, and idem, "Female solidarity and profes-

sional success: the dilemma of women doctors in late nineteenth-century America," J. Soc., Hist., 1982, 15:607-619.

[12]Walsh confirms the trend among women to study in coeducational medical schools in "Doctors Wanted: No Women Need Apply," p. 240. For an analysis of women doctors' choices of specialty in the late nineteenth and early twentieth centuries, see Edna Manzer, "Women Doctors' Choices of Specialty: The Vanishing Woman 'Woman's Doctor,' " unpublished paper presented at the Fifth Berkshire Conference on the History of Women, Vassar College, Poughkeepsie, New York, 18 June 1981.

[13]For a history of the New England Hospital, see Virginia G. Drachman, Hospital with a Heart. See also Walsh, "Doctors Wanted: No Women Need Apply," ch. 3.

[14]Intern applications, Boxes 10 through 13, the New England Hospital Collection, Sophia Smith Collection, Smith College, Northampton, Mass., hereafter cited as NEH Collection. Intern applications were unavailable for the period 1896 through 1899. Otherwise all 158 available intern applications from 1891 through 1904 have been examined.

[15]For example, Louise Husted, application for internship to the New England Hospital, 23 January, 1894, Box 11, Folder 7, NEH Collection. Intern data were calculated from the 158 intern applications in 1891 through 1895 and 1900 through 1904, in Boxes 10-13, NEH Collection. Tables one through three are tabulated from the intern applications. The grand total of applications in each table varies depending on the availability of data.

[16]For example, Annie R. Baker, application for internship, 9 January 1903, Box 13, Folder 28, NEH collection.

[17]Myrtle Jack, application for internship, 17 September 1910, Box 16, Folder 57, NEH Collection; Amelia Dranga to Stella Taylor, 16 September 1910; and Mary Naylor to Taylor, 16 September 1910, Box 16, Folder 37, NEH Collection.

[18]George Lockwood, to the New England Hospital, 16 January, 1894, Box 11, Folder 7, NEH Collection; E. Channing Stowell to the New England Hospital, 9 January 1903, Box 13, Folder 6, NEH Collection; and Aldrin Warthin to Stella Taylor, 16 December 1904, Box 14, Folder 24, NEH Collection.

[19]The following discussion of the ex-interns of the New England Hospital is drawn from "Former Interns of the New England Hospital for Women and Children," n.d., Box 1, NEH Collection.

[20]On Alice Hamilton see Barbara Sickerman, ed., Alice Hamilton: A Life in Letters (Cambridge, Mass.: Harvard University Press, 1984).

[21]"Former Interns of the New England Hospital." On women surgeons see Tracy, "Women graduates in medicine," p. 25.

[22]Tracy, "Women graduates in medicine," pp. 25-26.

[23]Elizabeth Kemper Adams, Women Professional Workers (Chautauqua, NY: Chautauqua Press, 1921), p. 65.

[24]Esther Pohl Lovejoy, Women Doctors of the World (New York: Macmillan, 1957), p. 97.

[25]Van Hoosen, Petticoat Surgeon, p. 201.

2

_____

Women in Medicine:
Three Decades in Retrospect

_____

Lissy Jarvik, M.D., Ph.D.

*Professor, Department of Psychiatry and Biobehavioral Sciences and
Chief, Section on Neuropsychogeriatrics, The Neuropsychiatric Institute,
University of California, Los Angeles; and
Chief, Psychogeriatric Unit, West Los Angeles Veterans Administration
Medical Center, Brentwood Division, Los Angeles, California*

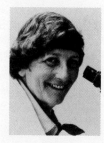

Lissy Jarvik, M.D., Ph.D.

2

——

Women in Medicine:
Three Decades in Retrospect

———

Those of us who have "made it" in academic medicine are accustomed to carefully researched, well-referenced manuscripts--we peruse them, we produce them, they are the *sine qua non* of our professional existence. Rarely are we granted the freedom to use the printed page for personal reminiscences the way I plan to use these pages. I decided to forego the scholarly treatise, and share with you instead recollections of years past and reflections upon years to come.

Viewing the three decades in retrospect, the most obvious change has been in the quantity of women in medicine. Between 1954 and 1984, for example, the proportion of women in American medical schools rose from 4.7 percent[1] to 32.6 percent.[2] Clearly, these national averages hide a great deal of variation. In 1954, some medical school classes contained as many as 10 percent women, others but the single "token" woman necessary to qualify for financial support.

Disregarding for the moment our small numbers, what were the challenges we faced thirty years ago? I think there were three important challenges. The first was: Could we prove that we were as good as any medical man, and therefore, better than most? We had to be better to convince our patients and to convince our colleagues; at least we had to try. Try as hard as we could, however, and succeed beyond our wildest dreams, some of our patients and some of our colleagues would never admit that we were any good at all-- and they still don't. Let me say a word here about financial aid. My school, Western Reserve University, was very generous to me. Without their

aid, I could not have finished medical school even though I worked nights diapering babies in the newborn nursery. I'm glad that the situation has improved substantially since then, and that women currently enrolled in medical schools throughout the country are able to obtain financial aid.

Our second challenge was to answer the question: Is being a woman compatible with being a physician? Or were we really freaks outside the pale of normal womanhood? In my class, one woman dropped out for the very reason that she could not reconcile being a woman, having a family and being a physician. Another married while in medical school, proving that it was entirely possible to be a normal woman, married, and yet be in medicine. And another one went even further and had a baby each year for two years. She had started with an earlier class but ended up in our class and graduated with us. The rest of us just tried to ignore the issue altogether. I found out, as many of my colleagues found out, that denial is really a very good defense.

The third challenge of the 1950's was to prove our right to take a place in medical school away from a man especially since so many men had returned from fighting our war. It was difficult to get into medical school. Those of us who succeeded felt guilty. No matter what we thought, we did feel guilty, and that fueled our intention to be better than anyone else, to work harder, to prove the place had not been given to a woman in vain. But most of the time we tried to ignore the issue. Sometimes that was impossible. Example: In my freshman year the fellow next to me, very shortly after we started biochemistry, turned around and said, "Why don't you get out of here, go back to the kitchen where you belong and give this place to a man?"

In 1977, Mary Walsh published a book entitled, *Doctors Wanted: No Women Need Apply*,[3] pretty late compared to 1950 when I was told quite openly: "We don't want any women here," and later on: "We don't want any women residents here." Mary Walsh wrote: "Any woman who hopes to succeed as a physician must be talented, productive and ambitious; but these qualities which are encouraged in men are perceived in women as aggressive, mannish, and castrating."

In the 1950's women encountered many, many sarcastic responses to their attempts at combining medicine with marriage and pregnancy. But, in general, we tried to ignore them and were awfully glad to have been let into the school in the first place. Consciously, we did not resent the students' or instructors' prejudice. And that was especially true, I think, for those of us who climbed the academic ladder. We were convinced that we were accepted, and that no one paid attention to the fact that we were of the opposite sex.

Even today, many of my women colleagues deny that they experienced any discrimination whatsoever, and they believe it. You could always find a man who was not promoted as rapidly as other men, and occasionally even one who was promoted as slowly as you were. You could always point to a man not having gotten a grant; you could always find a reason why you weren't appointed to one committee or another--and it never occurred to most of us to ask why we hadn't been appointed to *any* of the committees.

I spent fifteen years at Columbia University before I was promoted, and it never occurred to me that my sex had anything to do with that snail's pace. It just never entered my mind, nor was I inclined to wonder why I was not involved in any way in medical education. And it never occurred to me that I should apply for a grant, even though I was in full-time research. How did I finally figure it out? Well, it was my husband who asked me, "Why don't you apply?" And, when I did not succeed, it was he who said, "That's because you are a woman." The first time he told me that, I thought, "That's crazy! Being a woman has nothing to do with it. My application just wasn't good enough." So I kept applying, and eventually received a grant. Even though I had

begun to establish a reputation of my own, I am convinced that for a number of years I was awarded grants only because my husband was part of the "old boys' network," as were nearly all male academicians of some stature. So if I had not been married, had not had my husband's support and help, I doubt that I would ever have made it up the academic ladder.

In retrospect, the greatest challenge to women in medicine in the 1950's was none of the above. It was to become aware that there was such a thing as sexism in our profession and do something about it. Most of us, including myself, remained entirely unaware. We rejected the women's movement as too radical and too alien. We didn't want anything to do with it. And yet, those in the women's movement were actually responsible for awakening the women in medicine. They deserve the credit. For me, the hour of awakening came in 1972, when I moved to UCLA and was invited to join the Association of Academic Women. Suddenly, a new vista opened up to me. Here were faculty women who had thought a great deal about women in academia. And we worked together.

Now, in 1985, I think we have met the challenges facing medical women in the 1950's. What, then, are the challenges remaining for women who enter medicine in the 1980's? They don't have to prove any longer that women can compete with men; they *know* they can, and so do most of their patients and most of their colleagues. They don't have to wonder if being a physician is compatible with being a woman. They *know* it is, and so does everyone else. The logistics of raising a family are still very difficult. It is a challenge on a practical level, but not on a philosophical level. Finally, I don't think many of the women in the class of 1985 worry about the right to take away a place from a man. Instead, they worry about not having proportional representation--32.6 percent is not enough; women constitute over 50 percent of the population, so they would like to have 50 percent of the places in the entering and graduating classes.

But women in medicine in 1985 have other challenges. As I see them, there are three important ones. The *first challenge* is the subtle discrimination which is alive and well and rampant. It is illustrated by an article which appeared in the *Journal of the American Medical Association* under the title, "Hi, Lucille, This Is Dr.

Gold!"[4] There is a tendency to withhold the doctor's title from women. Even I, with two doctorates and clearly a senior appearance, have to remind people that I studied and worked for nearly ten years to earn these titles and have become partial to their use. An article from *The New Physician*[2] tells the following story. In a small New England town, the 65-year-old attending physician--by the way, it could easily have been a 35-year-old attending--introduced the students by saying: "This is student Dr. Jones, and this is student Dr. Goldberg, and this is student Dr. Halloway, and this is Jane." Jane happened to be a medical student, just like the rest of them, except she was a woman. And it happens to me-- all the time. At prestigious meetings--and, the more prestigious they are, the more likely that I am the only woman at the meeting--men will refer to each other as Dr. Green and Dr. Boyd and to me as Lissy. I suspect they are not even aware of it. I wasn't aware of it until somebody pointed out to me what was going on. So, now I call them John and Jim when they call me Lissy.

The *second challenge* is the slow promotion of women in academia. As of June 1983, women constituted 21 percent of assistant professors, 14 percent of associate professors and 6 percent of full professors.[5] The hope expressed in the article from which I got these numbers was that more women will be promoted to the top as more women enter at the bottom. Don't bet on it. It is not going to happen unless women fight for it.

Let's look at the National Institute of Mental Health. According to some figures I happened to see, 30 physicians in total were employed there as of October, 1983, 28 men and two women. Going back to 1977, there was only one other year in which there were any women at all. That was in 1978, and then, too, it was two women. But, that was two out of 16. If the figures are correct, then there was actually a drop from 12.5 percent to 6.7 percent women physicians employed by NIMH. The Third Regional Conference on Women in Medicine, held in New York City in April, 1983, petitioned the National Institutes of Health to increase the representation of women on study sections and advisory councils as well as to set aside contract and grant monies for projects related to women's health. So, that is the second challenge I see for women in 1985: promotion and more rapid advancement for women in academia with representation on prestigious national committees and appointment to positions of influence.

As the *third challenge,* I see something which one would not ordinarily regard as a challenge, i.e., the increased attention being given to women's health issues. We need to watch out for a double-sided sword here. Let us take depression, one issue that has concerned people very much, and legitimately so. Depression is much more frequent in women than it is in men at all ages except the highest ages, i.e., above 75.[6,7,8] Depression is more common in women medical students than it is in men medical students.[9] Similarly, the suicide rate is slightly higher among women medical students and women physicians than it is among their male colleagues,[10,11] even though the suicide rate among men is high, and in general, is nearly always higher in men than in women.[12] In one article published in the *Journal of the American Medical Women's Association* by a couple at Yale University,[13] there are numerous quotes from women physicians interviewed about the high frequency of depression, and some of their comments vividly portray the price paid by a woman in medical school. Here is just one example: "If things go wrong at work, that's your fault, if things go wrong at home, that's your fault, and somehow if you weren't doing both, it wouldn't happen. But then you look around and see people who aren't doing both, and they are really not doing a much better job than you are. But you feel guilty. You pay a large emotional price."

Nowadays, we are no longer dealing with men who openly question the intellectual ability of women (at least not very often!). But male doctors still suggest that women are constitutionally incapable of handling medicine as a career. The bias resurfaces under different guises. Few would now agree with the earlier idea that the menstrual cycle regularly renders women incapable of functioning so that they cannot be trusted with the great questions of life and death.[14] Instead they ask: "Who can trust the great questions of life and death (or perhaps, the even greater responsibilities of full professorship, deanship, or NIH Committee membership) to one who is so prone to melancholy and suicide?" In one guise or another, sexism is still well entrenched.

A report entitled "Depression and Anxiety Among Medical Students"[9] gives the following information. A survey to two medical school classes provided self-ratings of depression and anxiety upon entry into medical school, and again at the end of the second year. At the time they entered medical school, there were no sex differences in depression scores; the students' mean depression scores were within the normal range, although higher than that of a control group of normal non-medical students. At the end of two years, the mean was virtually identical to that at orientation. However, the proportion of students falling into the pathological category had increased from 13 percent to nearly 25 percent, and now, 32 percent of women students fell into the clinically depressed category compared to 16 percent of the male students. After two years, women had become significantly more depressed than men. So for women, the cost of staying in medicine is a significant one.

Having said that, and having said all that I said before about the three major challenges women in medicine face today, I will close with what I consider to be the greatest of all challenges to women in medicine today. It is not one of the three I spoke of before. We who entered medicine in the 1950's entered into a profession dedicated to serve the sick, the poor and the downtrodden, as well as the affluent. There were few third-party payors, no Medicare, no Medicaid. By contrast, those who enter medicine in the 1980's are entering a business, not a profession, a business which is rapidly being usurped by large corporations whose guiding light is not optimum patient care but cost effectiveness which translates into corporate profits. Yes, there are some idealists, but they are so rare that they become the subjects of TV documentaries.

The medical vocabulary has begun to revolve around marketing the product (or services) and "trim points" for DRGs. Where we would have been hard put in the 1950's to find even a single article on medical economics in most of our prestigious journals, in the 1980's we can hardly pick up a copy of the *New England Journal of Medicine* without seeing headings related to money and medicine,[15] corporate for-profit medicine,[16] or DRGs,[17] and *Psychiatric Annals* devoted a whole issue to "The Business of Psychiatry."[18] Stories abound of persons such as the uninsured Savannah house painter with severe burns over 92 percent of his body being refused admission to ten burn centers.[19] To most of us women, this is anathema. I think to most men it is anathema, too, if they think about it. Take the anonymous student: "The

Power of Doctors: As a member of the medical profession I find that what I fear most about the increase of medical commercialism is not that it will cause a loss of control by doctors but that it will erode the ethical foundations upon which our profession rests. The moral commitment of physicians to put their patients' interests first has given the medical profession its 'authority'--that, and its technical competence."[20]

We must do more than note the observations and deplore the state of affairs. We, as women, can exert a major influence. Why? Because for us women there is less stigma attached to being open, sensitive and caring than there is for men. We can use this stereotype to our advantage. We need not be ashamed of our caring attitudes, of being people oriented. What were considered liabilities may become our greatest assets. Perhaps even more important, we are not really part of, have not really been accepted into the medical establishment as full-fledged members. This separation permits us to see the picture of medical education as a process which by-and-large, turns the idealistic, sensitive student into a callous, greedy technocrat who chases after the almighty buck and his own pleasures, forgetting the pain, misery and suffering that lie at the base of his earnings. The roots of this lack of humanity in medical education reach far back. In 1927, for example, Francis W. Peabody wrote:

> *The most common criticism made at present by older practitioners is that young graduates have been taught a great deal about the mechanism of disease, but very little about the practice of medicine--or, to put it more bluntly, they are too "scientific" and do not know how to take care of patients. . . . Where there is so much smoke, there is undoubtedly a good deal of fire, and the problem for teachers and for students is to consider what they can do to extinguish whatever is left of this smoldering distrust.*[21]

Instead of extinguishing the smoldering distrust, the intervening years witnessed how medical education has revived its embers.

To sum up, in the 1950's our challenge as women in medicine was to fight for our professional rights and pave the way for future generations of women as *bona fide* members of the medical profession. In the 1980's, our challenge is not to fight for the survival of women in the medical profession, but to lead the fight for the survival of the profession itself. To lead the fight for the survival of medicine as an honorable, humanitarian profession dedicated to serving the sick, the needy and the helpless is a formidable challenge. Medical women of today have the necessary sensitivities, creativity and guts to meet that challenge--to take up the Gray Panthers' slogan: Health care for people, not for profits.[19] Will they? We will know the answer before the end of this century.

Notes

[1] Rosenthal PA, Eaton J: Women MDs in America: 100 years of progress and backlash. J Am Med Wom Assoc 37:129-133, 1982.

[2] Schapiro R: Women in medicine: The choices and challenges. The New Physician, March 1984, 10-14, 30, 42.

[3] Walsh MR: "Doctors Wanted: No Women Need Apply." New Haven: Yale University Press, 1977.

[4] Natkins LG: "Hi, Lucille, this is Dr. Gold!" JAMA 247:2415, 1982.

[5] In the S'wim 5(2):1, 1983 (published by UCLA Status of Women in Medicine Committee).

[6] Boyd, JH, Weissman MM: Epidemiology of affective disorders. Arch Gen Psychiatry 38:1039-1046, 1981.

[7] Frerichs RR, Aneshensel CS, Clark VA: Prevalence of depression in Los Angeles County. Am J Epidemiol 113:691-699, 1981.

[8] Weissman M, Klerman G: Sex differences and the epidemiology of depression. Arch Gen Psychiatry 34:98-111, 1977.

[9] Salt P, Nadelson CC, Notman MT: Depression and anxiety among medical students. (Presented at the annual meeting of the American Medical Association, May 8, 1984)

[10] Pepitone-Arreola-Rockwell F, Rockwell D, Core MS: Fifty-two medical student suicides. Am J Psychiatry 138:198-201, 1981.

[11] Steppacher RC, Mausner JS: Suicide in male and female physicians. JAMA 228:323-328, 1984.

[12] Fox JE: Revolution in treatment yielding improvements in recovery rate. US Medicine, February 15, 1984, 2, 17.

[13] Brown S, Klein RH: Woman-power in the medical hierarchy. J Am Med Wom Assoc 37:155-164, 1982.

[14] Storer H: Boston Medical and Surgical Journal 75:191-192, 1866, cited in Walsh 1977.

[15] Klein MV, Small GW: Money and medicine. N Engl J Med 311:542, 1984.

[16] Nutter DO: Access to care and the evolution of corporate, for-profit medicine. N Engl J Med 311:917-919, 1984.

[17] Omenn GS, Conrad DA: Implications of DRGs for clinicians. N Engl J Med 311:1314-1317, 1984.

[18] Roeske, NCA (guest editor): The business of psychiatry. Psychiatric Annals 14(5):316-409, 1984.

[19] Kuhn M: Gray Panthers' Project Fund Newsletter, Fall 1984.

[20] Relman AS: The power of doctors (book review). New York Review of Books, March 29, 1984.

[21] Peabody FW: The care of the patient. JAMA 88:877-882, 1927 (reprinted JAMA 252:813-818, 1984).

3

_____

A History of Women
Physician Leaders in Kentucky

_____

Leah J. Dickstein, M.D.

*Associate Dean for Student Affairs and Associate Professor,
Department of Psychiatry and Behavioral Sciences,
University of Louisville School of Medicine,
Louisville, Kentucky*

_____

The author wishes to thank Mrs. Edith Bloch, psychologist at the Bingham Child Guidance Clinic, for sharing information about Lotte Bernstein, M.D., and also wishes to thank other family members of the women described in this chapter.

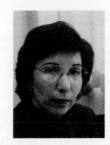

Leah J. Dickstein, M.D.

3

A History of Women
Physician Leaders in Kentucky

The early history of Kentucky medicine does not generally include recognition of women physicians and especially not those who were leaders. Yet in a forthcoming history of women physicians of Kentucky, many unrecognized leaders including teachers, public health workers, and administrators have been discovered. These physicians are interesting because they created positions of influence for themselves in spite of sexist opposition and at a time when there were very few women physicians at all. The very first woman physician in Kentucky, Frances Coomes, is an example, as is Sarah Fitzbutler, the first woman to graduate from a Kentucky medical school. Among the outstanding teachers of medicine in Kentucky are Alice Pickett and Katherine Dodd. Notable early public health physicians are Annie Veech, Lillian South, and Juanita Jennings. Lotte Bernstein led child psychiatry in Louisville for many years. These women made important contributions to health in Kentucky and are valuable as examples of women physicians in leadership roles.

Frances Coomes

Frances Coomes came to Kentucky from Maryland by way of Virginia in 1775 seeking religious freedom with a party which included her husband, William, and another physician, Dr. George Hart. Although always referred to as Mrs. Coomes, she learned her medical skills, which she did not hesitate to use, as an apprentice in the

usual way. Two of her cases are remembered: her successful treatment of her grandson for a rare form of clubfoot and her treatment of a man's chronic leg ulcer with boiling lard. More is known of Dr. Coomes as a leader in education because she started the first school for children in Fort Harrod in 1776.

Sarah Fitzbutler

Sarah Fitzbutler grew up in southern Ontario and married Henry Fitzbutler in 1866. They eventually came to Louisville, where Henry Fitzbutler, with two other black physicians, opened the Louisville National Medical College in 1888. Sarah Fitzbutler entered medical school there when her children were grown and graduated in 1892, the first woman and first black woman to graduate from any Kentucky medical school. She worked with her husband and continued on her own after he died, teaching medicine, supervising nurses' training, serving as director of Louisville National Medical College and on the board of directors of the hospital connected with the school. Three of her children also graduated from this medical school, including two daughters, Prima Washington and Mary Waring.

Alice Pickett

Alice Pickett is known as an outstanding teacher. Born in 1878 on a farm in Finchville, Kentucky, the seventh of ten children, she taught school for a time and then attended Woman's Medical College of Pennsylvania, graduating in 1909. By 1913, she was licensed to practice in Kentucky and was living in Louisville, where she stayed for the rest of her life. She began working at the University of Louisville soon after her arrival as assistant in the out-patient obstetrics clinic, progressing very slowly from this position to professor of obstetrics and gynecology. In 1921, however, with the rank of assistant professor she was made executive of the division of obstetrics and she continued as head until 1946. The titles are confusing here, for in every medical school bulletin in which Dr. Pickett appears as "head," a man is listed as chairman. Investigation did not reveal what the distinction means. From 1946 through 1952, when she retired, Dr. Pickett continued as professor only and was made professor emeritus at her retirement.

In 1952, in an interview for the *Courier-Journal*, Dr. Pickett expressed some reservations about the usual practice of medicine, arguing that physicians ought not to sacrifice everything to their careers and that women are even more likely to sacrifice everything or else quit medicine. She objected that physicians "neglect family, outside interests, recreation and continued study which is necessary to keep abreast of the fast-moving medical world," remarking that "as citizens they're nil." She continued: "The average woman doctor is an even greater victim of professional pressure than the man because she isn't willing to limit her life to her work and the financial obligations to her family. No, she takes on all the responsibilities as wife, mother and citizen." She noted discrimination against women in surgery: "It is quite difficult for women to get adequate surgical training, this in spite of the fact that no one can deny they have cool heads in the operating room and use their hands skillfully."[1]

Dr. Pickett wrote an obstetrical column for the *Kentucky Medical Journal* and contributed many articles demonstrating her no-nonsense views on obstetrics. In an article on postpartum care, she pointed out that the "doctor is apt to fall into what might be called a postpartum slump," and to neglect basic care for the mother once the thrill of delivery is past.[2] She argued against those who believe that finding syphilis will ruin family lives and for routine testing of all pregnant women, saying, "Our nurses and social workers have never been able to discover a single home broken from this cause or a home rendered apparently less happy."[3] In another article, she explained why cesarean section was so popular: "In America, everybody is speed crazy, even the obstetricians. Cesarean section relieves the tedium of long labor for the patient, the family and the attendant."[4] Dr. Pickett was quite proud of her work in the prenatal clinic and presented the results of a survey of mothers from 1923 to 1927: maternal deaths were eight times higher among mothers who never attended the clinic among the 3,217 mothers counted. In fact there were no deaths in 1927 at all among the women who attended the clinic.

Katherine Dodd

Katherine Dodd (1892-1965), who graduated from the Johns Hopkins School of Medicine in 1921-- "admitted to Hopkins because of vacancies in class due to World War I," she joked[5]--is remembered chiefly as a fine teacher. She worked briefly in private practice--"That was during the Depression, so I didn't practice very hard"[6]--and then went to Russia with a Quaker group to help during a famine and malaria epidemic in 1924.

Katherine Dodd began her teaching career at Vanderbilt in 1925 and moved on to the University of Cincinnati in 1943. She is believed to be the first woman chair of pediatrics in the United States at a school other than the Woman's Medical College of Pennsylvania. From 1952 to 1957 she chaired the department of pediatrics at the University of Arkansas Medical Center. In 1957, she came to the University of Louisville as distinguished professor of pediatrics, the first teacher at the School of Medicine to hold this title. When she left, after three years, a colleague said, "She brought us the gift of a brilliant mind and rich experience. She was a gifted teacher. We will miss her."[7] For her work in Kentucky, Dr. Dodd was named Kentucky Woman Physician of the Year in 1957, and in 1959 received the Elizabeth Blackwell Award for teaching. In 1962 the *Journal of Pediatrics* dedicated an issue to her, written entirely by her students, in honor of her seventieth birthday. Her bibliography numbers in all some 58 items. Dr. Dodd went to Emory University after leaving the University of Louisville, but not before she was elected an honorary member of the Alpha Chapter of Phi Chi, an all-male medical fraternity.

Annie Veech

Annie Veech, born into a well-to-do family in Kentucky in 1871, won national fame for her work in maternal and child health. In the 1880's, she and other young women wished to do something worthwhile for the people of Louisville, so they organized a King's Daughters Circle and visited the sick. They were responsible for bringing Louisville its first visiting nurse.[8]

A story is told that Annie Veech at about thirty, single and living at home, and without other work responsibility, withdrew from all activity for several years until Dr. Julia Ingram (Woman's Medical College of Pennsylvania, 1882) came to see her. Annie Veech complained that she couldn't sleep, so Dr. Ingram advised her to keep a paper at her bedside and, every time she awakened, to light a candle, write down the time and go back to sleep. Annie Veech followed these instructions, decided she was sleeping enough, got out of bed and went to the Woman's Medical College of Pennsylvania at 34. There she met Alice Pickett, and they both graduated in 1909. Annie Veech later said, "I decided that happiness lay in thinking of others."

Like Alice Pickett, Dr. Veech went to France with the Red Cross during World War I; they lived together in Louisville and were jointly honored in 1956 by the alumnae association of the Woman's Medical College of Pennsylvania for outstanding medical and scientific achievement.

In 1921, Congress passed the Sheppard-Towner Act, providing matching funds to states for bureaus of maternal and child health. Kentucky's Bureau was formed in 1922, and Dr. Veech became its first director. She was invited to be medical director of the U.S Children's Bureau in 1925, but refused, wanting to devote her medical and leadership skills to Kentucky.

In 1926, Dr. Veech reported on the progress of the Kentucky Bureau of Maternal and Child Health. These were among the many accomplishments:

- 35,152 infants weighed, measured, and examined and their mothers individually advised.
- 866 midwives instructed.
- 182 permanent child health centers established.[9]

In 1929, the appropriation for the Kentucky Bureau was vetoed, but the clubwomen of Kentucky raised $21,000 to keep it going.

One of Dr. Veech's notable projects was an experimental kindergarten in Kentucky's capital, Frankfort, where children learned good health habits by eating nutritious foods and sunbathing as well as by playing. Also under her direction were the annual May Day festivities honoring children and awarding blue ribbons to every child whose health was good enough.

In 1937, Dr. Veech accepted the directorship of the Division of Child Health at the Louisville Health Department. Her goal was a steady decline in maternal and infant morbidity, and this she accomplished for many years through developing innovative and vigorous public health programs. She worked for the Louisville Health Department until her retirement in 1949.

An article Dr. Veech wrote in 1922 offered this philosophy of health:

> *The home is the most important unit in any civilization. The child is the most important reason for a home. Health is attained and maintained by carrying out daily sane health habits, and not by taking medicine. The mother, she who is the director of such a unit and of the destinies of those who compose it, usually goes into this undertaking entirely unprepared to bear her part of the responsibility. The fathers are also unprepared. The results are appalling.*[10]

Lillian South

Lillian South was Kentucky's foremost public health physician for many years. Her father was a physician, and she grew up in Warren County, Kentucky, earning a B.A. in 1897 from Potter College, Bowling Green, Kentucky. She then went to nursing school in New Jersey, and, after receiving her R.N. in 1899, she went on to the Woman's Medical College in Pennsylvania, graduating in 1904.

Dr. South worked with J.N. and A.T. McCormack in Bowling Green from 1906 to 1910. Together they established a 42-bed hospital there, with the headquarters of the State Department of Health in the same building. In 1910 or 1911, the State Department of Health established a Bureau of Bacteriology, and Dr. South was its director from then until 1950 through its move to Louisville.

Her projects at the Department of Health

included a survey in 1912 of hookworm infestation in Kentucky, which merited a $20,000 grant from the Rockefeller Foundation for its eradication. Dr. South also surveyed for malaria and leprosy and worked for rabies prevention.

She organized the first state school for laboratory technicians in the United States and directed it from 1922 until 1952, when it closed and the University of Louisville took it over. So well renowned was Dr. South's school that during World War II General Joseph Stillwell, while in command of Allied Forces in Asia, sent two young Burmese students to Dr. South for training as laboratory technologists. The University of Louisville opened a school of public health in about 1920, and Dr. South taught there as well for several years. Its purpose was to train competent welfare workers rather than researchers or specialists.

Dr. South extended her leadership skills to serve as business manager of the *Kentucky Medical Journal* from 1906 until 1943, then book review editor until 1951. She was the first woman to be elected a vice president of the American Medical Association: she was third vice president in 1913. For many years Dr. South's Kentucky ham breakfasts at the annual AMA meetings were enthusiastically attended.

Juanita Jennings

Juanita Jennings, born in North Carolina in 1899, attended Lincoln Memorial University, Knoxville, graduating with one other woman medical student in a class of 24 in 1911. In her diaries she noted that for two years after graduation she struggled to obtain a hospital position. One male administrator admitted to her that he could not hire her because she was a woman. She worked in Tennessee and West Virginia until 1917, when she came to Kentucky.

In Kentucky, Dr. Jennings worked as a coal company physician in Harlan County, as local health officer and school physician, improving sanitation standards and increasing public welfare. In 1923, she joined the State Department of Health in Louisville as assistant director of the Bureau of Maternal and Child Health and there was responsible for setting up a uniform record-keeping system. In 1935, she was loaned for a year to the U.S. Children's Bureau and helped to organize maternal and child health programs in

several other states. She, as did Annie Veech, refused the offer of directorship of the Federal Children's Bureau. She was also consultant to the county health officers and the public health nurses. She died in 1940.

Lotte Bernstein

Lotte Bernstein grew up in Berlin and studied medicine at Friedrich-Wilhelms University there, graduating in 1924. She trained in psychoanalysis at the Berlin Psychiatric University Hospital of Charity from 1924 to 1928, practicing as an analyst and as a training analyst in Berlin from 1927 to 1935. She emigrated to Norway in 1935 to escape Nazi Germany and there worked as a training analyst until 1942, when she was evacuated as a refugee to Sweden. In Sweden, she worked first as a volunteer consultant in camps where concentration camp survivors were recuperating. Here she began to work with other therapists with art and music and realized their importance as part of mental health care. She gradually focused more of her energies on preventive psychiatry as an analyst to child therapists, social workers, teachers, nurses, and others who worked with children.

In 1951, Dr. Bernstein came to the United States as a lecturer and the University of Louisville Mental Hygiene Clinic among other U.S. institutions offered her a teaching position as clinical director of the Child Guidance Clinic. She established programs for teachers, supervised residents and was consultant to other local agencies. She was very much interested in providing the kind of education for school children that would immunize them against totalitarian ideologies, for she believed that the same education that would fit children for democratic government would also foster mental health. Dr. Bernstein retired from the Child Guidance Clinic in 1964.

It is interesting to note that of these eight early women physicians, five--Frances Coomes, Sarah Fitzbutler, Lillian South, Juanita Jennings, and Lotte Bernstein--were married; three--Frances Coomes, Sarah Fitzbutler, and Juanita Jennings-- bore children; and one, Lotte Bernstein, was very close to and a role model for her stepdaughter. Furthermore, all chose to continue their dual career roles.

What must be highlighted from these individual women's lives and careers are the following factors: they were determined to pursue medical careers despite personal sacrifices and evident societal and personal obstacles. They evidenced creativity and independence from their young adult years onward in gaining and using their medical skills along with their leadership abilities in serving the medical needs of others. Furthermore, they had the ability to function in trail blazer fashion rather than as part of an established group, saw this independence as natural and acceptable, and accepted support from others as it was offered, from men as well as from women, without obvious bitterness and enmity. They also recognized the need for personal sacrifice and, for the most part, bore this weight stoically.

What is most notable about these early Kentucky women physicians is that their successes were not their primary goals; their early pursuits were solo struggles and until recently they have been unrecognized.

References

[1] Are doctors slaves to the public? Louisville Courier-Journal, November 25, 1952.

[2] Pickett A: Routine postpartum care. Kentucky Medical Journal 29:672-674, 1931.

[3] Pickett A: Obstetrical column. Kentucky Medical Journal 21:446-447, 1923.

[4] Pickett A: Indications for cesarean section. Kentucky Medical Journal 28:385-388, 1930.

[5] Thanks, Dr. Katie. Louisville Times, June 11, 1962.

[6] Professor starting 4th medical-school job. Louisville Courier-Journal, September, 10, 1957.

[7] Dr. Katherine Dodd Leaving U.L. post. Louisville Times, July, 12, 1960.

[8] Davidson RC: Analysis of the development of the Visiting Nursing Association of Louisville. (unpublished, University of Louisville Archives and Records), 1942.

[9] Veech AS: Bureau of Maternal and Child Health. Kentucky Medical Journal 24:617-619, 1926.

[10] Veech AS: Public Health Service. Louisville Civic Opinion, December 9, 1922 (WPA Medical Historical Research Project, University of Louisville Archives and Records).

4

Notes on the History
of Women in Psychiatry

Jeanne Spurlock, M.D.

Deputy Medical Director,
American Psychiatric Association,
Washington, D.C.

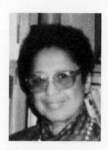

Jeanne Spurlock, M.D.

4

Notes on the History of
Women in Psychiatry

The following notes provide only glimpses of the contributions that women psychiatrists have made/are making to the history of American psychiatry. The sketches do not allow one to look in depth at the contributions of those who have been identified, nor even to glance at the scores of women who have not been named. The author is aware that much has been missed and emphasizes the need for a comprehensive account of the history of women in psychiatry.

Early Sources of Information

Publications about the early history of American psychiatry shed little light on the role of women in the field, perhaps because women psychiatrists were too few in number or because their roles were overlooked or viewed as insignificant. However, in 1908 Ballintine[1] noted that there were available data regarding the number of women physicians providing services in institutions for the insane, in contrast to the unavailability of statistics pertaining to women physicians practicing in other public facilities. At that time 71 women physicians had been appointed to the staff of 61 of the 131 hospitals for the insane. By 1908 eight states had enacted legislation requiring the appointment of a woman physician to the medical staff of mental institutions. Ballintine noted that eight other states had made such appointments in the absence of pertinent legislation. The nature of the specific assignments varied, and to some extent depended on the special needs of each insti-

tution. As Ballintine described them, the typical medical services that these women physicians provided parallel those rendered by today's general practitioner. She, herself, had been appointed to the Rochester (New York) State Hospital, and wrote as a recruiter, as well as a historian.

I wish to especially call your attention to the position of clinical assistant. The appointment is made by the Superintendent, no examination is necessary. This position is not salaried; the incumbent merely has her maintenance. The hospitals afford a vast clinical material for utilization in the study of physical diagnosis; also, experience in general medicines, pathology and psychiatry. The clinical assistant and intern obtains a practical training from her large clientele and from her relations with the friends of her patients, and in addition the discipline that comes from working with a large medical staff.

Those outside the ranks can hardly appreciate the great awakening that has come about during the last few years in the study of psychiatry, and there is every opportunity for women to excel in this work for which she is eminently fitted.

The membership directories of the American Psychiatric Association were thought to be a source of information about our sister pioneers, at least in terms of numbers. However, many members were identified by the initial of their given name(s) and their surname. Thus, it may be that some women members were not identified in this survey. In 1895 four of the 300 members listed were women. The number swelled to 18 in the 1912 listing, but fewer women were listed in the intervening years.

Detailed information about only one (Alice Bennett) of the four first identified women psychiatrists (Alice Bennett, Anne Burnet, Julia Casey, Susan Tabor) has been located. An account of Bennett's contributions is found in a 1933 publication, *Medical Women of America: A Short History of the Pioneer Medical Women of America and of a Few of Their Colleagues in England*.[2] Bennett was appointed to a staff position at the Pennsylvania State Asylum for the Insane (Norristown) in 1880. Her practice patterns clearly identify her as a pioneer and an advocate for patients. She ordered patients to be released from chains and cells to which they had been confined. The success of these measures led other hospitals to follow suit. McGovern[3] provides additional information about Bennett's work in a later publication which noted Bennett's practice of scheduling patients for appropriate leaves during their hospital stay and following them after discharge as well as her campaign against unnecessary sedation. However, there was a "down side," at least from our current perspective. Bennett is said to have advanced the theory that insanity was a symptom of general ill health. Yet, an account of the chronology of events pertaining to unethical charges that were lodged against her suggests that she may have been scapegoated. The State Commission on Lunacy charged her with performing illegal ovariotomies on a large number of mentally ill women without their consent. McGovern notes that Bennett did spend a considerable amount of time in gynecological work, in keeping with the common practice during that period in history. However, six of the surgical procedures which she was charged with performing had been performed by two other physicians, although Bennett had secured permission from the patients' next of kin, and furthermore, each of the surgical procedures had been determined to be necessary because of obvious gynecological pathology. Of particular significance is the fact that during that historical period the majority of the membership of organized psychiatry endorsed the removal of ovarian tumors in psychiatric patients to improve their mental health. Bennett is said to have been

dismayed by the attacks, and moved away from direct clinical practice, redirecting her energies toward combating tuberculosis and campaigning to improve services for the chronically mentally ill.

Of the 18 women psychiatrists listed in the 1912 APA Membership Directory, Mary O'Malley has become more well-known than the others. Ballintine[1] noted that O'Malley was the first woman physician appointed to the Government Hospital for the Insane (now St. Elizabeths Hospital). Her name appears in the transcript of the oral history of Francis Gerty, APA president in 1958-59, who recalls that his brother, also a psychiatrist, spoke of O'Malley as one of his best teachers. O'Malley, for whom the O'Malley Building at St. Elizabeths Hospital was named, was appointed to the post of Woman Assistant Physician there in 1905. An entry in a report from a hospital administrator to the Secretary of the Interior reads:

> It had been thought desirable for some time to have a woman physician connected with the hospital. We have now upward of 600 female patients and in the neighborhood of 300 female employees, many of whom prefer to consult a woman physician. She could, also, as an officer of the institution, inspect the bathing of female patients and look after the sick employees when they are off duty for minor ailments. The Commission was asked to hold an examination for this position, which they did, and made certification of eligibles from their register. Dr. Mary O'Malley, who had already six years of experience in the Binghamton State Hospital, was appointed to begin her duties September 1.

O'Malley had worked with William Alanson White at Binghamton prior to his appointment as Superintendent of St. Elizabeths Hospital. Twelve years after her appointment to the St. Elizabeths staff, O'Malley was promoted to the position of Clinical Director of the Female Service and retained this position until her retirement in 1935.

There are four entries on women in the indexes of the volume, *One Hundred Years of American Psychiatry*:[4] 1) feeble-minded, of child-bearing age; 2) female nurses on male wards; 3) first physician appointed; and 4) physicians. The first woman physician appointed to a psychiatric treatment facility is not identified by name. In a brief statement in the chapter "The History of American Mental Hospitals," it is noted that "assistants came fresh from school or internships, or from private practice. They were all men until 1892 when a woman physician was appointed at Augusta, Maine." The other reference about women physicians is equally brief, and appears in the context of Daniel Hale Tuke's visits to a number of American mental institutions. He is quoted as stating his approval of "staff appointments for women physicians and of the training schools for nurses at McLean Hospital." However, the exact words of Tuke's statement, as they appear in his book, *The Insane in the United States and Canada*,[5] do not reflect blanket endorsement of employment of women as service providers. Tuke refers to Cowles' (Superintendent of McLean Hospital) policy of employing female nurses on the male wards, and notes that Cowles' reasoning for the practice was that "it is unnatural for patients to be placed in asylums under entirely different conditions, in regard to female society, from what they have been accustomed to at home. They [male patients] degenerate in speech and conduct, and the male attendants are also injuriously affected. The presence of female nurses restrains and softens the insane, and enforces self-control." Tuke cautions that

> *the practical carrying out of the system must add greatly to the anxiety of the Superintendent, and that it should be introduced only by one who is confident that he can carry it out successfully. Nor should it be introduced into all asylums. (p. 114)*

However, Tuke adds that the practice was "a valuable feature of this asylum [in] that it forms a training school of nurses."

The "In Memoriam" sections of several early volumes of the *Journal of the American Psychiatric Association* (AJP) highlight the achievements and contributions of a few women psychiatrists. Tribute was paid to Alma Evelyn Fowler in a 1924 volume.[6] Fowler, a 1914 graduate of Tufts Medical School, had been appointed Assistant Physician at Taunton State Hospital, Taunton, Massachusetts, in 1917. She was described as an "enthusiastic student of psychiatry, a faithful and conscientious hospital physician . . . [who] won the respect of all with whom she came in contact."

Anne T. Bingham was memorialized in a 1932

issue of the AJP.[7] Prior to her last administrative post with the Metropolitan Life Insurance Company, she served as Inspector of State Hospitals (New York) in 1912 and 1913. The timing of her death (in 1932) was suggested to be of psychological significance. Bingham, who had been on sick leave because of a cardiac disorder, died less than eight hours after her mother's death and three weeks after the death of her father.

Esther Loving Richards was also eulogized in an AJP issue.[8] A 1915 graduate of the Johns Hopkins Medical School, she was long associated with the Henry Phipps Psychiatric Clinic, where she headed the outpatient services from 1920 until her retirement in 1951.

The reader may have wondered, as has the author, why these women were eulogized in the pages of the AJP and others were not. Efforts to find the answer have been unsuccessful. Currently, the few "In Memoriam" columns are limited to past presidents of the American Psychiatric Association.

The name of Agnes Purcell McGavin is familiar to contemporary psychiatrists since an American Psychiatric Association (APA) award in her name is presented annually to a psychiatrist who has done outstanding work on the preventive aspects of childhood emotional disorders. McGavin, a native of Scotland, came to the United States by way of Canada, where she earned her medical degree at the University of Toronto in 1920. For close to twenty years, beginning in 1931, she served as the Director of the Child Guidance Clinic at Buffalo's Children's Hospital. Her interest in teaching is reflected in her biographical sketch, which lists lectures to nurses and supervision of clinical work of medical students. Obviously, her commitment to children is reflected in her bequest that allows for the annual McGavin Award. The contributions of eleven women have been recognized in the presentations of this award since its inception in 1964: Edith B. Jackson (1964); Lauretta Bender and Margaret Mahler (1969); Marion Kenworthy (1971); Irene Josselyn (1972); Othilda Krug (1975); Eveoleen Rexford and Eleanor Pavenstedt (1976); Viola Bernard (1977); Hilda Bruch (1981); and Stella Chess (1983). These recipients represent academe, administration, and clinical practice as well as research, and most have training in pediatrics and/or psychoanalysis. All have published extensively in topics ranging from rooming-in studies

(Jackson), to childhood psychosis (Bender and Mahler), to community psychiatry (Bernard), to developmental theories (Josselyn and Chess). Josselyn and Rexford ably served as editors of the *Journal of the American Academy of Child Psychiatry;* currently, Chess is the associate editor.

Other women psychiatrists who have been recipients of APA awards include Raquel Cohen, who received the Seymour Vestermark Award in 1976 for her outstanding contributions to education and career development in psychiatry. Stella Chess and her collaborator and spouse, Alexander Thomas, were the 1980 recipients of the Blanche F. Ittleson Prize for research in child psychiatry. Other women psychiatrist-researchers were the recipients of this award in four successive years, from 1982-1985; they were Dorothy Otnow Lewis, Judith Rapoport, Lenore Terr, and Janina Galler.

To date, Nancy Andreasen is the only woman psychiatrist to receive the Samuel G. Hibbs Award, given for the best unpublished paper on a clinical subject. As the 1984 award recipient, Andreasen's presentation was "The Clinical Significance of Thought Disorder." The Founders Award was established in 1977 to honor the APA member "who has made outstanding contributions as author, spokesperson and publicist in the service of the mentally ill and disabled and to the art of the science of helping." Hilde Bruch was selected as that member in 1981. It took a while for the APA to publicly recognize the contributions of women through the Distinguished Service Award which was established in 1965. Anna Freud was so recognized in 1976, then Margaret Mahler in 1981 and Viola Bernard in 1983.

In 1984, Alice Wright received the Warren Williams Award (for the New England Area) for her innovative and effective program as medical director of a community mental health center.

Influences from Europe

The decided influences of European-trained psychoanalysts on American psychiatry became sharpened in the 1930's. In that era more than a few of those who immigrated to the United States were women. Not unlike today, different theoretical concepts and practices were represented in the group. The differences are vividly illustrated in the publications of Helene Deutsch[9] and Karen Horney.[10] Deutsch emphasized a biological factor

as the root of female masochism in contrast to Horney's emphasis on the cultural influences. Margaret Mahler's[11-13] conception of development in relation to the phases of separation-individuation is well known, as is Therese Benedek's[14,15] work which focuses on the psychoanalytic investigation of the sexual cycle of women, and Frieda Fromm-Reichmann's[16] psychoanalytic work with schizophrenic patients. Others of note who immigrated to the United States in the 1930's and 1940's included Berta Bornstein, Ruth Eissler, Dora Hartmann, Edith Jacobson, Marianne Kris, Annie Reich, Melitta Schmideberg, Melitta Sperling, Edith Sterba, and Edith Weigert. Some of their specific contributions to American psychiatry are listed in the bibliography at the end of this chapter.

Some female graduates of European medical schools immigrated to the United States prior to extensive post-graduate training, and pursued psychiatry and psychoanalytic training in this country. Hilde Bruch followed this pattern. Her work on eating disorders is familiar to medical communities throughout the world. It should be noted that some graduates of American medical schools sought psychoanalytic training in Europe and returned to make important contributions to American psychiatry. Margaret Gerard (who returned to Chicago), Flanders Dunbar (New York City), Lucille Dooley (Washington, D.C.), Margaret Ribble (New York City), and Clara Thompson (Washington, D.C., and New York City) are included in this group.

Child Psychiatry

Women have been well represented in what has come to be the sub-specialty of child psychiatry. The names of Lauretta Bender, Margaret Gerard, Margaret Fries, and Margaret Ribble can be found in any list of early pioneers who worked with children. Each made significant contributions as clinicians, researchers, and teachers. Bender's work with schizophrenic children at New York University-Bellevue Hospital is well-known, and other work has supported her theory of the biological foundation of schizophrenia. In their extensive work with infants, Fries and Ribble stressed the importance of mothers' handling of their children as a basis for the development of hyperactivity or inactivity. Ribble emphasized the protection against physiological disorder that is provided by a warm mother-child relationship in a child's first year of life. Gerard was also interested in the damaging influences of the early mother-child relationship, and particularly as they relate to the development of psychosomatic disorders in children.[17] Papers of Berta Bornstein,[18] Edith Buxbaum,[19] Phyllis Greenacre,[20] Eleanor Pavenstedt,[21] and Emmy Sylvester[22] were published in early volumes of *The Psychoanalytic Study of the Child*. The list of women who made significant contributions to the field early in its history also includes Anne Benjamin, Viola Bernard, Stella Chess, Irene Josselyn, Marion Kenworthy, Othilda Krug, and Eveoleen Rexford. In their respective academic positions each left or is leaving a legacy of rich professional literature and well-trained child psychiatrists. Specific references to their broad achievements are to be found in other sections of this chapter.

In relation to the discipline of child psychiatry, an account of Bernard's activities within the American Psychiatric Association (APA) warrants mention in this section. Bernard chaired the APA Commission on Childhood and Adolescence, which was established in 1973 and was to operate for a period of three years. The Commission was charged to assume responsibilities with regard to APA's positions on all matters pertaining to children and youth, for liaison with the professional organizations in allied fields, and for coordination and liaison with the APA's organizational components with regard to child/adolescent aspects of their work. Early in the life of the Commission it was recognized that there was a need for ongoing activity directed toward meeting the stated charges. Primarily because of Bernard's vigorous efforts, determination, and persistence, the APA governing body voted to establish the Council on Children, Adolescents, and Their Families in 1976, whose primary focus is the psychological well-being of children and youth. The identification of families was to connote the constellation of children, youth, and their parents (or surrogate parents). Bernard served as chairperson for the first of her five-year appointments (1976-81) to the Council.

The author is but one of many who developed professionally under the tutelage of Anne Benjamin, Margaret Gerard, and Irene Josselyn, who were training analysts at the Chicago Institute of Psychoanalysis, and with the guidance of Helen Beiser, currently the president of the American Academy of Child Psychiatry and a training analyst at the Chicago Institute. Chess, Krug, and Rexford have trained scores of able child psychiatrists at their respective programs at New York University, the University of Cincinnati, and Boston University.

The list of contemporary child psychiatrists is voluminous and space does not permit identification of all those women who have made and are making significant contributions to the field. Women child psychiatrists have earned leadership roles in research, as illustrated by Stella Chess (longitudinal studies of temperament), by Barbara Fish (longitudinal studies of schizophrenic children), Magda Campbell and Judith Rapoport (psychopharmacological research), Gloria Powell (psychological sequelae of school desegregation), and Elva Poznanski (childhood depression).

Women in child psychiatry have been successful in developing programs and directing activities toward national visibility. Vignettes from the careers of three colleagues are illustrative. Nancy Roeske chaired the APA Task Force on Women, which was established in 1972. It was under her leadership that the members of the Task Force successfully gained the APA Board of Trustees' approval for the formation in 1975 of a Committee on Women, now a critical component of the APA's organizational structure. [The leadership baton was picked up by Elissa Benedek, Elaine (Hilberman) Carmen, Brenda Solomon, Nanette Gartrell, Judith Herman, and Theresa Bernardez, successive chairpersons of the Committee on Women; also by Jean Shinoda Bolen, who chaired the APA Council on National Affairs in 1982-83, and Carol Nadelson, who succeeded Bolen as chairperson in 1983-84.] The work of C. Janet Newman on the survivors of the Buffalo Creek disaster and of Lenore Terr on victims of the Chowchilla kidnaping has provoked interest in the study and care of children subjected to the stress of disasters, both natural and man-made.

Administrators and clinicians who work in public settings are perhaps the most unrecognized and unrewarded. At the risk of reinforcing this pattern, several psychiatrists are listed to illustrate successes in these two areas. It should be noted that more often than not the responsibilities of an administrator and service provider are intermingled, and often they are coupled with a teaching assignment. Ruth Fuller's directorship (1969-78) of the James Weldon Johnson Family and

Child Counseling Center (New York City) is illustrative, as is Virginia Wilking's tenure (1963-82) as Director of the Division of Child Psychiatry at Harlem Hospital Medical Center. Other examples are Elissa Benedek's directorship since 1974 of Research and Training at Ann Arbor's Center for Forensic Psychiatry and Nancy Haslett's directorship of Clinical Services at Louisiana State University's Developmental Disabilities Center (1972-81).

Administration and Academe

In a 1968 publication the late Daniel Blaine, APA Medical Director from 1948-58, noted:

Fewer women psychiatrists are in an administrative capacity, although one can point with pride to the Commissioner of Mental Health for the State of West Virginia, Dr. Mildred Bateman [commissioner from 1962-77], and the ex-Commissioner of Indiana, Dr. Margaret Morgan [commissioner from 1953-58], as well as the superintendent of a number of state hospitals. Dr. Valerya Raulinaitis has been Chief of Staff at the Veterans Administration Hospital, Downey, Illinois for a number of years.

Audrey Worrell was added to the list of women psychiatrists appointed as State Commissioners of Mental Health when she accepted the position in Connecticut in 1981. June Jackson Christmas fulfilled the responsibilities of the Commissioner of Mental Health and Mental Retardation of New York City for six years, beginning in 1972.

Since the 1960's the number of women psychiatrists holding administrative posts has increased considerably. Eight women psychiatrists (Drs. Nellie Anosa, Marla Erball, Ruth Huggins, Carol Hunter, Rena Nora, Danielle Turns, Fay Whita) are currently identified as chiefs of staff at VA hospitals across the nation. Carolyn Robinowitz and Jeanne Spurlock are two of the four deputy medical directors of the APA. Only a few women psychiatrists have held administrative posts in the military but the few are significant. Clotilde Bowen (Retired Colonel) was Chief of the Department of Psychiatry at Fitzsimmons Army Medical Center (1971-74) and Chief of the Department of Psychiatry and Neurology at Tripler Army Medical Center (1979-85). Bowen

was also appointed as a neuropsychiatric consultant to the U.S. Army, Vietnam, and as Assistant Chief of Professional Services to the Medical Command in Vietnam (1970-71). Inquiries directed to several military psychiatrists yielded information that as of August, 1985, three women psychiatrists were serving as service chiefs in army medical centers and one other woman was serving in an acting capacity.

As a beginning of a comparison of the roles of recent appointees to administrative posts and their predecessors, the author made direct inquiries of three colleagues in the Washington, D.C. area. Mildred Mitchell-Bateman has probably had the longest tenure of any other woman psychiatrist who has served as a commissioner (national or regional) of mental health. Prior to her appointment as commissioner she was clinical director of the state mental institution at Lakin, West Virginia, from 1951 to 1952 and superintendent there from 1958 to 1960. Immediately after leaving the commission post she accepted the appointment as Head of the Department of Psychiatry of Marshall University, a newly established medical school in Huntington, West Virginia. Mitchell-Bateman called attention to the significant differences in administration in a governmental post and one in an academic setting. Even with the limitations imposed by the state legislature, she found she was empowered to make more day-to-day decisions as commissioner than she was as a medical school department head. In another context she, noted potential problems that are likely to face a woman administrator:

When things go wrong in an institution administered by a woman, the administrator is confronted with the question: Has this happened because I am a woman, or would it happen to any administrator in this position? . . . When things go wrong with the program, questions will be raised about the woman administrator. This will be true even though she herself may be able to ferret out the solution to the problem; others, she realizes, will still draw their own conclusions about whether or not the problem would have happened had a man been in charge.[23]

Minority people (by gender or race) who are in "in charge" positions are likely to hear references made to their minority status when things are perceived to be going wrong. Mitchell-Bateman recalled relevant statements of associates: "Had you been a man, you would have been fired long ago," "If you had not been a black woman, you would have been replaced long ago." Other informants reported similar experiences, especially since the implementation (alleged or real) of affirmative action programs.

Another woman psychiatrist spoke of her experiences related to being asked to take a top administrative post (in an acting capacity) in a large psychiatric hospital. Presumably, she was asked to take the position because of her earlier record of sound administration in one of the divisions of the facility. Her associates viewed her as competent and deserving of the position, and she was interested in being considered as a serious candidate. Events that followed indicated that she wasn't even in the running for the position. Like Mitchell-Bateman, this administrative psychiatrist had fleeting thoughts about the possibility that she had been passed over because of her gender. But, she was also aware that she had been a victim of the fall-out of a political battle at higher administrative levels. For the most part, her gender has been an asset to her. She remains committed to the idea that early experiences in dealing with controversial issues can serve to foster the development of good administrative skills.

Lucy Ozarin, now formally retired, has held several important administrative posts at the National Institute of Mental Health (NIMH) and the Veterans Administration. At the time of her formal retirement in 1981, she was completing 23 years of service as Assistant Director of Program Development at NIMH. Ozarin sees her greatest administrative skill to be her ability to bring people together and lists three major achievements which stemmed from such efforts: 1) start-up of a family care program "after it was said that it couldn't be done," 2) initiation of the NIMH community support program, and 3) assistance provided in the implementation of community mental health systems. At the time of this writing, this tireless advocate for the mentally ill is a consultant to the World Health Organization (WHO) and NIMH and volunteers as a surveyor of Medicare programs.

To date, three women have been appointed to head medical school departments of psychiatry: Jeanne Spurlock at Meharry Medical College (Nashville), 1966-1973; Mildred Mitchell-Bateman

at Marshall University (Huntington, West Virginia), 1977-83; and Paula Clayton at the University of Minnesota, 1981-present. Four women head large psychiatry residency training programs: Clare Assue (Indiana University), Jean Goodwin (University of New Mexico until 1985), Carol Nadelson (Tufts University), and Patti Tighe (University of Chicago). According to data collected by the Association of American Medical Colleges (AAMC), all full deans of medical schools are currently men. The data do not identify the discipline of the approximately 120 women who are associate or assistant deans. The author knows of two women psychiatrists who currently hold such posts: Leah Dickstein, Associate Dean for Student Affairs at the University of Louisville, and Carola Eisenberg, Dean of Student Affairs at Harvard University. Veva Zimmerman, in the Dean's Office, serves as special advisor on Minority Affairs at New York University. Women psychoanalysts have held important administrative posts at psychoanalytic institutes. The following are illustrative: Joan Fleming, Dean of Education at the Chicago Institute for Psychoanalysis, 1956-59; Doris Hunter, Director of the Pittsburgh Psychoanalytic Institute, 1977-79; Ethel Person, Director of the Columbia University Center for Psychoanalytic Training and Research, since 1981; and Edith Sabshin, Assistant Dean, Chicago Institute of Psychoanalysis, 1974-76.

Some Challengers of Traditional Theories and Practices

We are particularly indebted to Karen Horney[10] and Clara Thompson[24] for their pioneer efforts in challenging the biologically rooted theories of female development and psychopathology. A significant number of other women psychoanalysts have contributed to the data disproving gender-biased concepts and practices. For example, Lucille Dooley[25] and Phyllis Greenacre[20] demonstrated that early in development a girl is aware of her vagina and refuted the then widespread assumptions that this anatomic discovery occurs much later and that a girl's immediate response is that she has been castrated. Mary Jane Sherfey[26] used findings from embryologic research to demonstrate women's biological strengths, in contrast to assumptions that weaknesses predominated. The more recent contributions of Jean Baker Miller[27] must also be noted, particularly her sensitive and succinct volume, *Toward a New Psychology of Women.* The reader gains a fuller understanding of the sociocultural and psychological forces acting on and in women. A detailed account of the contributions of women psychiatrists in this area would fill a volume. The reader is referred to the reference list and selected bibliography. The role of women psychoanalysts as journal editors is also noted. For example, the contributions of Karen Horney as founding editor and Helen DeRosis as the current editor of the *American Journal of Psychoanalysis* are well known, as are those of Mabel Blake Cohen as editor (1949-61) of *Psychiatry.*

Of course, changes do not take place in a vacuum. Influences from the broader society have impacted on the personal and professional development of our predecessors, both female and male, as it has with us and will with our students and our students' students. Spinoffs from the civil rights movements of the 1960's and early 1970's, and the women's movement provide vivid illustrations. Nevertheless, some of our predecessors were "ahead of their times." For instance, Marion Kenworthy, Helen Vincent McLean, Charlotte Babcock, Viola Bernard, and Stella Chess addressed issues of mental health services for the poor and racial minorities long before it was "fashionable." McLean[28-29] contributed to the psychodynamic understanding of the emotional health and impairment of Afro-Americans, a subject later addressed by both Babcock[30] and Bernard.[31-32] Babcock[33] will also be remembered for her work with the Nisei. Bernard, Chess, and Kenworthy, all child psychiatrists, were early activists in the establishment of psychiatric services for black children in New York City. Chess was probably the first psychiatrist to join with the efforts of psychologists Mamie and Kenneth Clark at the Northside Center for Child Development in Harlem. Both Bernard and Kenworthy were very involved in the early days of the operation of Wiltwyck School for Boys and the Bureau of Children's Guidance. Through publications and practices all have contributed significantly to efforts to eradicate the concept that cultural differences are deviances. In this context the contributions of the "first trained" black psychiatrists and psychoanalysts warrant attention: Frances Bonner, training analyst at the Boston Psychoanalytic Institute (1970-75) and the Psychoanalytic Institute of New England (since 1975);

Elizabeth Davis,[34-35] the first Director of Harlem Hospital's Department of Psychiatry (1962-78); child psychiatrist Margaret Morgan Lawrence;[36] and administrators June Jackson Christmas[37-38] and Mildred Mitchell-Bateman. The author lists with modesty her publications that address the aforementioned topic.[39-41]

Elections to Offices of Medical and Health-Related Associations

Women psychiatrists have been elected to the highest office in several national psychiatric and other health-related organizations. As might be expected, the first significant response came from the membership of the American Medical Women's Association (AMWA). Elizabeth Bass (Louisiana) was the first psychiatrist elected in 1921 to the presidency of AMWA as its fifth president. She was followed by Mary O'Malley (1934), Mable Akin (1937), Katherine Wright (1958), Bernice Sacks (1965), and Laura Morrow (1969). Some other presidents of national organizations are listed in Appendix 1 at the end of this chapter.

The career of Marion Kenworthy, who was elected president of three national organizations, warrants additional historical comments. Her administrative abilities have been identified as one of her most significant leadership skills. Early in her career she served as the director of the Mental Hygiene Clinic of the Central School of Hygiene and Physical Education, Central Branch of the YWCA in New York City (1919-21). She later was associate director (1921-1924) and medical director (1924-1927) of the Bureau of Children's Guidance, New York School of Social Work. She was a lecturer at Union Theological Seminary (1925-32) and the Mental Hygiene Institute, Connecticut College (1930-31), and held academic posts at Columbia University's School of Social Work. Her colleagues and students knew her to be a skilled clinician and able teacher. She was awarded two honorary degrees, DMS from the Medical College of Pennsylvania in 1968 and BS from Columbia University in 1973, and received the 1971 Agnes Purcell McGavin Award as noted above. The Marion E. Kenworthy endowed chair of psychiatry was established at Columbia University's School of Social Work in 1957. Dr. Kenworthy will also be remembered as a pioneer in setting up clinical service programs for children and training programs for probation officers. At the time of this writing, plans are underway for developing a study center within the APA library as a living tribute to Marion Kenworthy.

The representation of women elected to serve on the APA Board of Trustees is also of significance, although later in the history of the organization. As noted in Appendix 2 at the end of this chapter, twelve women have been elected to fifteen positions.

Women psychiatrists have been elected to high office in regional medical organizations more often than in national ones. In addition to the district branches of the American Psychiatric Association and state affiliates of the American Academy of Child Psychiatry, women have held offices in general medical societies. Several examples are listed: Barbara Buchanan served as vice-speaker of the House of Delegates of the Missouri State Medical Society for a three-year term, beginning in 1983, and has also been elected to the American Medical Association's Council on Long Range Planning. In 1980 Dorothy Starr was the first woman and first psychiatrist to be elected president of the Medical Society of the District of Columbia.

Discussion

The foregoing notes provide only a brief digest of the contributions of women psychiatrists to American psychiatry. Attention was directed to several sub-specialties; others were not addressed as distinct areas of practice. However, the areas of overlapping warrant emphasis. For example, it was noted that many of the challengers of theory were/are psychoanalysts--as were/are many who also identify as child psychiatrists. It must also be emphasized that scores of male colleagues have supported the efforts of women psychiatrists, and more than a few have been close collaborators.

Indeed, the status of women psychiatrists has been elevated since the early years of American psychiatry, even though there has been relatively little, if any, transfer of power. Nevertheless, there appears to be a definite stability to many of the changes that have been generated by women in the various arenas of psychiatry.

References

[1]Ballintine EP: Women physicians in public institutions. The Woman's Medical Journal. 28(4):79-80, 1980.
[2]Hurd-Mead KC: Medical Women of America: A Short History of the Pioneer Medical Women of America and a Few of Their Colleagues in England. NY: Froben Press, 1933.
[3]McGovern CM: Doctors or ladies: Women physicians in psychiatric institutions 1872-1900. Bulletin History of Medicine. 55:88-107, 1981.
[4]Hall JK, Zilboorg G, Bunker, H, et al: One Hundred Years of American Psychiatry. NY: Columbia U. Press, 1944.
[5]Tuke DH: The Insane in the United States and Canada. NY: Arno Press, 1973.
[6]In Memoriam: Dr. Alma Evelyn Fowler. Amer Jnl Psych 81:784-785, 1925.
[7]In Memoriam: Anne T. Bingham. Amer Jnl Psych. 89(1):652, 1932.
[8]In Memoriam: Ester Loving Richards, M.D. Amer Jnl Psych. 113(1):576, 1956.
[9]Deutsch H: The Psychology of Women: A Psychoanalytic Interpretation. NY: Grune & Stratton, 1944 (Vol. I) & 1945 (Vol. II).
[10]Horney K: Flight from womanhood. Internat'l Jnl Psychoanal. 7:324-339, 1926.
[11]Mahler MS, Pine F, and Bergman A: The Psychological Birth of the Human Infant. NY: Basic Books, 1975.
[12]Mahler MS: On child psychosis and schizophrenia: autistic and symbiotic infantile psychoses. The Psychoanal Study of the Child, 7:286-305, 1952.
[13]Mahler MS: On human symbiosis and the vicissitudes of individuation. Jnl of Amer Psychoanal Assn 15:740-763, 1967.
[14]Benedek T, Rubenstein BB: The correlations between ovarian activity and psychodynamic process: I. The ovulation phase. Psychosomatic Med 1:245-270, 1939.
[15]Benedek T, Rubenstein, BB: The correlations between ovarian activity and psychodynamic process: II. The menstrual phase. Psychosomat Med. 1:461-485, 1939.
[16]Fromm-Reichmann F: Principles of Intensive Psychotherapy. Chicago: University of Chicago

Press, 1950.

[17]Gerard MW: Genesis of psychosomatic symptoms in infancy: the influence of infantile traumata upon symptom choice. In The Psychosomatic Concept in Psychoanalysis, edited by Felix Deutsch. NY: Internat'l. U. Press, 1953, pp. 82-85.

[18]Bornstein B: Clinical notes on child analysis. The Psychoanal Study of the Child. 1:151-66. NY: Internat'l U. Press, 1945.

[19]Buxbaum E: Transference and group formation in children and adolescents. The Psychoanal Study of the Child. 1:351-65. NY: Internat'l U. Press, 1945

[20]Greenacre P: Special problems of early female sexual development. The Psychoanal Study of the Child. 5:122-138, NY: Internat'l U. Press, 1950.

[21]Pavenstedt E, Anderson I: The uncompromising demand of a three-year-old for a real mother. The Psychoanal Study of the Child. 1:211-231. NY: Internat'l U. Press, 1945.

[22]Sylvester E: Analysis of psychogenetic anorexia and vomiting in a four-year-old child. The Psychoanal Study of the Child 1:167-87, 1945.

[23]Mitchell-Bateman M: Women psychiatrists as administrators. Psychiatric Annals 7(4):102-106, 1977.

[24]Thompson C: Penis envy in women. Psychiatry. 6:123-125, 1943.

[25]Dooley L: The genesis of psychological sex differences. Psychiatry. 1:181-185, 1938.

[26]Sherfey MJ: The Nature and Evolution of Female Sexuality. NY: Random House, 1972.

[27]Miller JB: Toward a New Psychology of Women. Boston: Beacon Press, 1976.

[28]McLean HV: Psychodynamic factors in racial relations. Annal Amer Acad Polit & Soc Sci., 244:159-166, 1946.

[29]McLean HV: Racial prejudice. Amer Jnl. Orthopsych. XIV:706-714, 1944.

[30]Hunter DM, Babcock CG: Some aspects of the intrapsychic structure of certain American Negroes as viewed in the intercultural dynamic. The Psychoanal Study of Society. NY: Internat'l U. Press, 1967, p. 124-169.

[31]Bernard VW: Psychoanalysis and members of minority groups. Jnl Amer Psychoanal Assn. 1:256-267, 1953.

[32]Bernard VW: Interracial practice in the midst of change. Amer J Psychiat. 128(8):978-983, 1972.

[33]Babcock CG: Personal and cultural factors in treating a Nisei man. In Clinical Studies in Cultural Conflict, edited by Seward G. NY: Ronald Press, 1958, pp. 409-448.

[34]Davis EB: The American Negro: family membership to personal and social identity. Jnl Nat'l Med Assn. 60:92-99, 1968.

[35]Davis EB, Coleman JV: Interaction between community psychiatry and psychoanalysis in the understanding of ego development. In Psychoanalysis in community psychiatry: Reflections on some theoretical implications. Reported by Ralph Wadeson. Jnl Am Psychoanal Assn. 23(1):177-189, 1975.

[36]Lawrence MM: Young Inner City Families: Development of Ego Strengths Under Stress. NY: Behavioral Publications, 1975.

[37]Christmas JJ: Trying to make it real: issues and concerns in the provision of services for minorities. Presented at the National Conference on Minority Group Alcohol, Drug Abuse, and Mental Health Issues, Denver, Colorado, May 1978.

[38]Christmas JJ: Rehabilitation--general and special considerations. Psychiatric Annals 4(4):49-59, 1974.

[39]Spurlock J, Cohen RS: Should the poor get none? Jnl Amer Acad Child Psychiat. 8(1):16-35, 1969.

[40]Spurlock J, Cohen RS: A reappraisal of the role of black women. Strecker Award Lecture (Inst. of the Penn. Hospital), 1971. Reprinted in Jnl Nat'l Assn of Priv Psychiatric Hospitals. 3(3), Fall, 1971.

[41]Spurlock J, Cohen RS: Black Americans. In Cross-Cultural Psychiatry, edited by Albert Gaw. Littleton, MA: PSG Publishing Co., 1982, pp. 163-178.

A Selected Bibliography

Alpert, Augusta. Reversibility of pathological fixations associated with maternal deprivation in infancy. The Psychoanalytic Study of the Child. 14:169-185, 1959.

Alpert, Augusta. Sublimation and sexualization. The Psychoanalytic Study of the Child. 3(4): 271-278, 1949.

Andreasen, Nancy C. Creativity and psychiatric illness. Psychiatric Annals 8(3):23-45, 1978.

Andreasen, Nancy C. The Broken Brain: the Biological Revolution in Psychiatry. NY: Harper

& Row, 1984.

Andreasen, Nancy C., and Winokur, George, Secondary depression: familial, clinical and research perspectives. American Journal of Psychiatry, 136(1):62-66, 1979.

Beiser, Helen R., Formal games in diagnosis and therapy. Jnl of Amer Academy of Child Psychiat. 18(3)480-491, 1979.

Bender, Lauretta. A Visual Motor Gestalt Test and Its Clinical Use. NY: Amer Orthopsychiatr Assn., 1938.

Bender, Lauretta. Childhood schizophrenia. Nerv Child, 1:138-149, 1942.

Benedek, Elissa P., Barton, Gail, and Bieniek, Christine. Problems for women in psychiatry residency. Amer Jnl Psychiat. 134 (11):1244-1248, 1977.

Benedek, Elissa P., Benedek, Richard S. Joint custody: solution or illusion? Amer Jnl Psychiat. 136(12):1540-1544, 1979.

Benedek, Elissa P. Children of divorce: can we meet their needs? Jnl of Social Issues. 35(4):155-69, 1979.

Bibring, Grete L. Some considerations of the psychological processes in pregnancy. The Psychoanalytic Study of the Child. 14:113-121, 1959.

Bornstein, Berta. On latency. The Psychoanalytic Study of the Child. 6:279-285, 1951.

Bruch, Hilde. Eating Disorders: Obesity, Anorexia Nervosa and the Person Within. NY: Basic Books, 1973.

Bruch, Hilde. Psychiatric aspects of obesity in children. Amer J Psychiat. 99:752, 1943.

Campbell, Magda; Hardesty, Anne S., et. al. Childhood psychosis in perspective: a follow-up of ten children. Jnl of Amer Acad of Child Psych. 17(1):14-28, 1978.

Carmen (Hilberman), Elaine. Rape: A crisis in silence. Psychiatric Opinion. 14(5):32-35, 1977.

Carmen (Hilberman), Elaine; Russo, Nancy Felipe; and Miller, Jean Baker. Inequality and women's mental health: an overview. Am J Psychiat. 138(10):1319-1330, 1981.

Carmen (Hilberman), Elaine; Russo, Nancy Felipe; and Miller, Jean Baker. Mental health and equal rights: the ethical challenge for psychiatry. Psychiatric Opinion. 15(8):11-19, 1978.

Chess, Stella. The plasticity of human development: alternative pathways Jnl of Amer Academy of Child Psychiat. 17(1):80-91, 1978.

Chess, Stella, Hassibi, Mahin. Principles and Practice of Child Psychiatry. NY: Plenum Press,

1978.

Dunbar, Flanders. Psychosomatic Diagnosis. NY: Harper and Row, 1948.

Eissler, Ruth S. Riots: observations in a home for delinquent girls. The Psychoanalytic Study of the Child. 3(4):449-460, 1949.

Fish, Barbara, Shapiro, Theodore, et al. A ten-year follow-up report of neurological and psychological development. Am J Psychiat. 121:768-775, 1965.

Fries, Margaret E. Some factors in the development and significance of early object relationships. Jnl of the Amer Psychoanal Assn. 9:669-683, 1961.

Geleerd, Elizabeth R. A contribution to the problem of psychosis in childhood. The Psychoanalytic Study of the Child. 2:271-291, 1946.

Geleerd, Elizabeth R. Some aspects of ego vicissitudes in adolescence. Jnl of the Amer Psychoanal Assn. 9:394-405, 1961.

Greenacre, Phyllis. Perversions: General considerations regarding their genetic and dynamic background. The Psychoanalytic Study of the Child. 23:47-62, 1968.

Greenacre, Phyllis. Special problems of early female development. The Psychoanalytic Study of the Child. 5:122-138, 1950.

Greenacre, Phyllis. Trauma, Growth, and Personality. NY: Internat'l U. Press, 1952.

Jacobson, Edith. Adolescent moods and the remodeling of psychic structures in adolescence. The Psychoanalytic Study of the Child. 16:164-183, 1961.

Jacobson, Edith. Contribution to the metapsychology of psychotic identifications. Jnl of the Amer Psychoanalytic Assn. 2:239-262, 1954.

Jacobson, Edith. Development of the wish for a child in boys. The Psychoanalytic Study of the Child. 139-152, 1950.

Jacobson, Edith. The Self and the Object World. NY: Internat'l U. Press, 1964.

Johnson, Adelaide M. Juvenile Deliquency. In Amer Handbook of Psychiat., S. Arieti, ed. NY: Basic Books, 1959, pp. 840-56.

Johnson, Adelaide M. Sanction for superego lacunae of adolescents. In Searchlights on Delinquency. K. Eissler, ed. NY: Internat'l U. Press, 1949.

Johnson, Adelaide M., Szurek, Stanislaus A. The genesis of antisocial acting out in children and adults. Psychoanal Quart. 21:323, 1952.

Josselyn, Irene M. The Happy Child: A Psychoanalytic Guide to Emotional and Social Growth. NY: Random House, 1955.

Kaplan, Helen S. Hypoactive sexual desire. Jnl Sex and Marital Therapy. 30(1):3-9, 1977.

Kaplan, Helen S. The New Sex Therapy: Active Treatment of Sexual Dysfunctions. NY: Brunner/Mazel, 1974.

Katan, Anny. The nursery school as a diagnostic help to the child guidance clinic. The Psychoanal Study of the Child. 14:250-264, 1959.

Kestenberg, Judith S. On the development of maternal feelings in early childhood: observations and reflections. The Psychoanal Study of the Child. 11:257-291, 1956.

Kestenberg, Judith S. Vicissitudes of female sexuality. Jnl of Amer Psychoanal Assn. 4:453-476, 1956.

Kirkpatrick, Martha. Equality and genitality, Amer Jnl Psychoanal., 42(2):99-107, 1982.

Kirkpatrick, Martha; Smith, Catherine; and Roy, Ron. Lesbian mothers and their children: a comparative survey. Amer Jnl Orthopsych. 51(3):545-551, 1981.

Kirkpatrick, Martha (ed.). Women's Sexual Development: Explorations of Inner Space. NY: Plenum Press, 1980.

Kirkpatrick, Martha (ed.). Women's Sexual Experience: Explorations of the Dark Continent. NY: Plenum Press, 1982.

Krug, Othilda. The application of principles of child psychotherapy in residential treatment. Am J Psychiat. 108:695-700, 1952.

Lewis, Dorothy Otnow, Shanok, Shelley S. Delinquency and the schizophrenic spectrum of disorders. Jnl of Amer Academy of Child Psychiat. 17(2):263-276, 1978.

Nadelson, Carol C., Notman, Malkah T. Psychotherapy supervision: the problem of conflicting values. American Jnl. Psychotherapy. 32(2):275-283, 1977.

Nadelson, Carol C. The Woman Patient, Vol. II. NY: Plenum Press, 1982.

Notman, Malkah T, Nadelson, Carol C. (eds.) The Woman Patient. Vol. I. NY: Plenum Press, 1978.

Ozarin, Lucy D. Community alternatives to institutional care. Amer Journal of Psychiatry. 133(1):69-72, 1976.

Ozarin, Lucy D. Community mental health center activity in rehabilitation. International Journal of Mental Health. 3(2-3):147-152, 1974.

Ozarin, Lucy D., Sharfstein, Steven. The aftermath of deinstitutionalization: problems and

solutions. Psychiatric Quarterly. 50(2):128-132, 1979.

Person, Ethel S. The influence of values in psychoanalysis: the case of female psychology. In Psychiatric Update/II. Lester Grinspoon, ed. Washington, D.C.: American Psychiatric Press, 1983, pp. 36-50.

Riech, Annie. Early identifications as archaic elements in the superego. Jnl of Amer Psychoanal Assn. 2:218-238, 1954.

Reich, Annie. Narcissistic object choice in women. Jnl of Amer Psychoanal Assn. 1:22-44, 1953.

Robinowitz, Carolyn B; Nadelson, Carol C.; and Notman, Malkah T. Women in academic psychiatry: politics and progress. Am Jnl Psychiat. 138(10):1357-1361, 1981.

Roeske, Nancy C.A., Lake, Karen. Role models for women medical students. Journal of Medical Education. 52(6):459-466, 1977.

Roeske, Nancy C.A. Women in psychiatry: A review. American Journal of Psychiatry, 133(4):365-372, 1976.

Roeske, Nancy C.A. (guest ed.). Women in psychiatry. Psych Annals. 7(4), 1977.

Roeske, Nancy C.A., Sadock, Virginia A. The treatment of psycho-sexual dysfunctions: an overview. In Psychiatry 1982 Annual Review. Lester Grinspoon, ed. Washington, D.C.: Amer Psychiatric Press, 1982, pp. 20-35.

Schachter, Judith S., Butts, Hugh F. Transference and counter-transference in interracial analyses. Jnl of Amer Psychoanal Assn. 16:792-808, 1968.

Seiden, Anne M. Overview: research on the psychology of women. I: Gender differences and sexual reproductive life. Amer Jnl Psychiatry. 133(9):995-1007, 1976.

Seiden, Anne M. Overview: Research on the psychology of women. II: Women in families, work and psychotherapy. Amer Jnl Psychiatry. 133(10):1111-1123, 1976.

Sperling, Melitta. Conversion hysteria and conversion symptoms: A revision of classification and concepts. Jnl of Amer Psychoanal Assn. 21:745-771, 1973.

Sperling, Melitta. School phobias: classification, dynamics, and treatment. The Psychoanalytic Study of the Child. 22:375-401, 1967.

Sperling, Melitta. The analysis of a boy with transvestite tendencies: a contribution to the genesis and dynamics of transvestitism, The Psychoanalytic Study of the Child. 19:470-493,

1964.

Sterba, Edith. Interpretation and education. The Psychoanalytic Study of the Child. 1:309-317, 1945.

Symonds, Alexandra. The psychodynamics of expansiveness in the success-oriented woman. Amer Jnl Psychoanal. 38(3):55-63, 1978.

Symonds, Alexandra. Violence against women: the myth of masochism. Amer Jnl Psychotherapy. 33(2):161-173, 1979.

Appendix 1. Women Psychiatrists Elected to Presidential Positions

American Academy of Child Psychiatry	Anne Benjamin, M.D., 1966-69
	Helen Beiser, M.D., 1983-85
American Academy of Psychoanalysis	Janet Bard, M.D., 1956-57
	Francis Arkin, M.D., 1960-61
	Marianne Eckardt, M.D., 1972-73
	Lillian Robinson, M.D., 1983-84
American Board of Psychiatry and Neurology	Carolyn B. Robinowitz, M.D., 1986-87
American College of Psychiatrists	Evelyn Ivey-Davis, M.D., 1967-68
American Orthopsychiatric Association	Exie Welsch, M.D., 1955-56
American Psychiatric Association	Carol Nadelson, M.D., 1985-86
American Psychoanalytic Association	Marion Kenworthy, M.D., 1958
	Grete Bibring, M.D., 1962
	Rebecca Solomon, M.D., 1979
American Public Health Association	June Jackson Christmas, M.D., 1980
American Society for Adolescent Psychiatry	Ghislaine Godenne, M.D., 1981-82
Association of American Indian Physicians	Johanna Clevenger, M.D., 1982-83
	Catherine Kincaid, M.D., 1984-85
Council of Medical Specialty Societies	Carolyn Robinowitz, M.D., 1981-82
Group for the Advancement of Psychiatry	Marion Kenworthy, M.D., 1959-61
Black Psychiatrists of America	Phyllis Harrison-Ross, M.D., 1978-79
	Andrea Delgado, M.D., 1983-84
Philippine Psychiatrists of America	Rena Nora, M.D., 1979-80
	Norma Panahone, M.D., 1984-85

Appendix 2. Women Elected to the APA Board of Trustees

Year of Election	Elected Position	Person Elected
1965	Vice President	Marion E. Kenworthy, M.D.
1971	Vice President	Viola W. Bernard, M.D.
1973	Vice President	Mildred Mitchell-Bateman, M.D.
1974	Vice President	June Jackson Christmas, M.D
	Trustee, Area II	Henrietta R. Klein, M.D.
1976	Trustee-At-Large	Nancy C. A. Roeske, M.D.
1977	Trustee-At-Large	Mary Ann Bartusis, M.D.
1979	Trustee-At-Large	Rita R. Rogers, M.D.
1980	Trustee-At-Large	Elissa P. Benedek, M.D.
1981	Vice President	Carol C. Nadelson, M.D
	Trustee-At-Large	Martha J. Kirkpatrick, M.D.
1982	Trustee-At-Large	Naomi Goldstein, M.D.
1983	Vice President	Elissa P. Benedek, M.D.
1984	President-Elect	Carol C. Nadelson, M.D.
1985	Secretary	Elissa P. Benedek, M.D.

5

_____

Varieties of Leadership Among
Early Women Psychoanalysts

_____

Nancy Julia Chodorow, Ph.D.

Associate Professor, Board of Studies in Sociology,
University of California, Santa Cruz;
Associate Research Sociologist,
Institute of Personality Assessment and Research,
University of California; and
Berkeley Candidate, San Francisco Psychoanalytic Institute

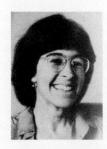

Nancy Julia Chodorow, Ph.D.

5

——

Varieties of Leadership Among
Early Women Psychoanalysts

———————

Among the professions and intellectual disciplines, psychoanalysis remains exceptional in having had, early on, a substantial number of women participants.[1] Many of these women--Melanie Klein, Anna Freud, Karen Horney, Helene Deutsch, Phyllis Greenacre, Edith Jacobson, Margaret Mahler, to name only a few--rank unquestionably among the field's most eminent members. Most research on women in the professions has rightly focused on problems of lack of visibility, tokenism, discrimination, and women's strategies for coping in arenas where "masculine" work styles and forms of colleagueship predominate. In a study of psychoanalysis and its early women practitioners, I have been trying to understand how psychoanalysis came to depart from this "male" professional model, how and why women psychoanalysts were able to participate and be leaders-- to achieve a kind of importance that has been denied to women in most fields--and what the effects of their numbers and prominence have been on the history and nature of the field.[2]

In this chapter, I address a subset of these general questions, those concerning women in leadership roles. I suggest first that a central organizational feature of psychoanalysis, the existence of a variety of routes to leadership, seems to have facilitated women's prominence and recognition. I then examine the patterns in this prominence and recognition. I suggest that women's particular routes to leadership, based both on their own choices and on ideological controls and material constraints upon them, reflected and sus-

tained cultural and psychoanalytic beliefs about women's power, femininity, and women's spheres. Women's prominence thereby remained compatible with expectations of gender difference and gender hierarchy.

I note, to begin with, that psychoanalysts of the early generations themselves agree that their field was unusually open to participation by women, and they are also aware of numbers of women whom they consider important.[3] How did this happen? One of the most striking findings of my research concerns the variety of careers, or what I call "hats," possible within the profession of psychoanalysis. Psychoanalysts became known for and ground their identities in their clinical work, their abilities as training analysts and supervisors, their teaching, writing, and speaking, and their not directly analytic work in psychiatry, child psychiatry, social work, guidance, early child development, and so forth.

In particular, the passing on of the profession has always been of especial importance in the field, so that anyone involved in training is accorded recognition as a leader on an explicit professional basis, and, implicitly, is elevated in importance (whether positive or negative importance is irrelevant for our considerations here) in the psyches of those psychoanalysts-in-training he or she analyzes, and in many cases whom he or she supervises as well.

We can see through ethnographic example that much of the recognition of women psychoanalysts comes from their centrality in teaching and

training. About one Viennese woman who was internationally known but wrote only a few articles,
an English interviewee said, "Every analyst in
New York passed through her hands." Another
interviewee, an American who had been on the
faculty of a university-based institute and who
claimed she "really never fulfilled [her] professional destiny" (she only wrote one book about
training and one other book, and was president of
her society), said of herself:

> I had a husband, I had two houses and I had
> two children. And was teaching and practicing,
> so that I did a little, but mostly my real contri-
> bution has been my personal impact on students,
> and that I think has been considerable. And I
> think people who have known me professionally,
> like my ex-students, would give positive reports
> in terms of what I have been able to give them
> and share with them. But that's been my chief
> contribution.

The impact of many local figures, even if they
are also known for writing and have participated
organizationally in the field, is likewise often
based on their teaching and training. I think for
instance of Frieda Fromm-Reichmann, Edith
Weigert, Lucie Jessner, and Jenny Waelder-Hall in
Washington-Baltimore, Grete Bibring and
Elizabeth Zetzel in Boston, Anna Maenchen in
San Francisco, Sara Bonnett and Lillian Malcove
in New York, Therese Benedek and Joan Fleming
in Chicago.[4]
Statistically, we can also see the role of women
in training. When we compare the percentage of
women in the field as a whole with the number
who have been training analysts, until very
recently women seem to be significantly overrepresented as training analysts in the United States
and either overrepresented or proportionally represented in Europe.[5] But there remains a gender
distinction between reputed clinical skills and
recognition as a training analyst on the one hand
and being formally an official leader of training
on the other: relatively few women, in the data I
have collected so far, have been elected or appointed chairs of training or education committees. That teaching and training are highly valued
in psychoanalysis, then, is an institutional fact
which perhaps helps to account for the relative
prominence of women in this particular profession.

The prominence accorded teaching and training
fits into another feature of the organization of
psychoanalysis which seems to have facilitated
women's prominence and leadership. Unlike many
professions, which are either primarily clinical or
practicing professions, on the one hand, or scien-
tific/research professions on the other, psychoanalysis seems to have maintained both aspects as
centrally important. In the former case, national
and international organization tends to be less important to most practitioners; those for whom it is
important are more likely to be men. In the latter
case, recognition is reserved for writers and
researchers; women, however, concentrate their
energies more locally (as teachers in academia, as
practicing rather than research-oriented doctors).
In the psychoanalytic case, much of its national
and international organization concerns not just
scientific issues, which would single out researchers and writers above others, but also issues of
clinical practice and teaching and training. These
latter practices must originally be local, but
because they are so important, successful local
practitioners often come to have cosmopolitan
recognition. Women have been considered to be
good at teaching and training, and women's
strengths as psychoanalysts are also said, in the
interviews I have collected, to lie particularly in
their clinical acumen, which itself forms the basis
for appointment as a teacher and trainer.[6]
Besides teaching and training, oral presentation
was another avenue of recognition for early
women psychoanalysts. For much of its history,
psychoanalysis has been a face-to-face professional culture; it has stressed the oral transmission
and exchange of knowledge. Women were frequent and active participants in panels at national
meetings, as well as paper presenters and com-
mentators at local meetings. This finding emerged
when I would push and push in the interviews to
find out how some particular woman under discussion, who had never held a national office and
had never published anything, had become so
extremely well thought of and well known. I suspect that as the field of psychoanalysis has gotten
much larger and more formalized and bureaucratized, this avenue of leadership and recognition
is less likely to be open. In so far as women are
less likely to be writers (I discuss this below),
such a formalization represents a real loss in opportunity for expressing in a public forum either
clinical insight or theoretical contribution.

Finally, of course, leadership and recognition come through writing, through written contributions to psychoanalytic theory and practice. I have left this "hat" for last, because it seems to be the one that least distinguishes psychoanalysis from many other fields. That is, the prestige accorded someone by becoming a training analyst and the possibility for achieving universal recognition through oral communication seem to be relatively unusual forms of recognition among modern professions, whereas writing and research are more generally routes to recognition especially in the research-related professions like science, medicine, and the predominantly academic fields. Writing, for psychoanalysts as for these other practitioners, is a major avenue to being seen as a leader, and many people when asked about eminent or prominent women psychoanalysts think of the theoretical giants like Anna Freud, Melanie Klein, Phyllis Greenacre, Edith Jacobson, Margaret Mahler, Frieda Fromm-Reichmann, Karen Horney. Of course some of these writers also had an enormous *personal* as well as theoretical presence, as, for instance, Melanie Klein and Anna Freud in England, or Karen Horney, as she was bursting out of the American Psychoanalytic Association, or Frieda Fromm-Reichmann, whose presence pervaded and invigorated the Washington scene.

But the avenue of writing was not so well trodden by women as were the routes to leadership though training and oral culture, according to my interviewees. Some women were extremely prolific and important, but many found it hard to write, a difficulty attributed to inner inhibitions or to the force of other callings. Several claimed that the great writers had to be either unmarried or "undomestic," because for simply practical reasons, if you had a family to manage and did your clinical work *and* perhaps did training *and* perhaps served on a committee or so, you never had time to write.

Thus, unlike women in other fields, where there was only one route to prominence or where the major routes to prominence did not seem to lie in arenas where women either worked or were seen as particularly gifted, women psychoanalysts benefitted from a variety of possible careers within the field and from the fact that women were seen as especially skilled in the demands of several of these careers.

In one respect, however, women psychoanalysts were very much like women in other fields, and, indeed, like women in the world at large. Women psychoanalysts did not hold official leadership positions proportional to their numbers. For most of the period since 1920, with the exception of the World War II years, women psychoanalysts have been significantly *underrepresented* in both the United States and Europe as officers of psychoanalytic societies, institutes, and associations. Their representation has tended to follow the same curve, with a lower percentage, as their membership. When they have held officerships, these have tended to be treasurer, secretary, or perhaps even vice president of an association or local society. Women are less likely to be president.[7]

Why, in spite of their relatively large presence in the field, and in spite of their clear recognition and eminence as trainers, as models of clinical skill, as face-to-face transmitters of oral knowledge and insight, to some extent as writers, were women not formally recognized through positions of organizational or official leadership? In what follows, I suggest that a variety of attitudes and practices led women, in spite of their significance and recognition, to be less likely to be sought after or perhaps to want formal political leadership. These attitudes and practices turn on an apparent paradox in the relation between psychoanalysis and its early women practitioners: in spite of its unusual openness to women practitioners and its liberating effect on many women patients, psychoanalysis and psychoanalysts have maintained in some respects a quite traditional view of men and women.[8] We can see this in aspects of the theory, and I certainly found it among my interviewees, who almost all professed a belief in profound innate differences between women and men, maintained a traditional division of labor in their home, and, more than feeling that they were challenging women's traditional roles by becoming professional, felt that psychoanalysis was a feminine, or mothering, profession that drew upon women's traditional skills.

My interviewees, both male and female, were able to maintain this traditional gender ideology in the face of what we might see as the serious challenge to it posed by women's extraordinary recognition and prominence. They could do this, it seems, because they were not talking about actual formal organizational and political leadership. As we know from feminist anthropology and political theory, if there is one sphere that might be universally masculine, it is the formally defined, separately institutionalized political sphere; in western society, at least since the Greeks, this sphere is certainly masculine. As other social and cultural gender differences fluctuate and vary historically and cross-culturally, political participation remains the core of masculine control and power in society. Women psychoanalysts seem themselves to have accepted this dichotomy, and men have certainly helped them along.

One American interviewee was quite articulate on the subject. She opened her interview by pointing out that it was true that "women have had a great deal of acceptance in the field of psychoanalysis," partly because of the number of outstanding pioneer women in Vienna. But she goes on, "I must say this, I think that politically, in the inner politics, they aren't accorded the same offices for instance that men are." There has never been a woman president of the local society of which she is a member, in spite of a notable number of prominent women members. She herself was secretary of the society twice, but when she was nominated for president she was defeated, although she had already been president of the local psychiatric society. She claims that she has been asked a half dozen times to run again, but she does not want to. In the first instance, she does not want to deal with all the tensions, which she had enough of when she was in training and the society split. And she thinks that women in general don't want to spend time on "all kinds of internecine fighting," which is all too prevalent in psychoanalysis, in her view. They just aren't so interested:

I think that in general, in the past, women have not been as interested in politics. The time that men put in on politics--and it's very demanding--they would rather be spending with their kids. You know at the time it seems terribly important but a few years afterwards everybody's forgotten that you were president....But your kids are still there, and it's a matter of values in deciding what's more important.

But also, the men don't want them:

So I think that for one thing women have not been as interested. But when they are--look, if

we were to speak in psychoanalytic terms man's castration anxiety still is pervasive. And they don't want to give up to a woman.

So both men's and women's attitudes keep women out of the arena of psychoanalytic politics:

So it's interesting, they had several woman secretaries, because men still think in terms of women as secretaries and it's very hard to eradicate these old impressions. [I asked, "Have the women also been less interested because of the splits, fights, etc.?"] I think if they're smart they'd have been less interested for that reason! I think that's one of the reasons, I really do. And you know there's male chauvinism but there's also a kind of female chauvinism. I find myself saying well, so let them kill each other over it. I'm going to stay out of it, you know, let them get involved in it.

Another woman, who became very active organizationally in the International Psychoanalytic Association after her husband, a prominent leader of the American and International, had died, expressed a similar reticence when I asked her if she had been active along with her husband:

No. As long as he was alive, I stayed out of much of it, except, you know, be a wife and take over whatever things belonged to that. No, that was his bailiwick, his baby. And it wasn't until he died [that I became active].

Or another woman, again specifying a kind of necessity rather than choice, pointed out that after society meetings, when the informal politicking happened, all the men walked home together while each woman grabbed a cab to get home to her family as quickly as possible. Thus, the women, in balancing the demands of home with those of work, often tended themselves not to try to participate in the world of psychoanalytic politics (though several pointed out that becoming a training analyst is itself often a political effort, involving, as one put it, "dickering and bickering").

In interesting ways, cultural ideology about gender also served further to neutralize the power and presence of the women. One mechanism was negative stereotyping. An English man referred to Melanie Klein and her co-workers as "four women who formed a phalanx [and] they all seemed to wear black." A Kleinian woman pointed out that "the Kleinians were treated as a sort of awful regiment of women" and allowed that she herself felt uneasy about such unusual female dominance:

> One did feel uneasy, you see, whereas one didn't feel in the past uneasy if there was the predominance of men. There was this uneasy feeling particularly Mrs. Klein's work centering on the early relation to the mother, this sort of anxiety in others--this regiment of women--and in us, will we be seen as those aggressive, dominating women. [We felt] great relief when bright young men started coming in.

An American visitor described the "little patriarchy" that constituted the Hampstead Clinic under Anna Freud's powerful control, in which everyone sat along a table according to rank, with Miss Freud at the head initiating and controlling the discussion.

A younger Bostonian man referred to the terrifying "Boston matriarchy," who sat together in the back of meetings making collective decisions about everyone's future.[9] Alternately, he claimed to think of them as a "group of Bubbies," thus neutralizing their power not by overstating it but by assimilating them to his Jewish grandmother. In all these cases, we see a kind of ambivalence about female power which must certainly have been transmitted and helped to shape active politics, a seeming exemplification of Horney's claim that the dread of women, bred by fear of the mother, can lead to an exaggeration of female power or to disparagement that denies power (Horney, 1967).

But another aspect to Horney's claim was that, instead of fearing or disparaging women explicitly, men could cope with the dread by idealizing women and putting them on a pedestal: "The attitude of love and adoration signifies: 'There is no need for me to dread a being so wonderful, so beautiful, nay, so saintly' " (Horney, 1967). And this view was also present. One male analyst, a former national officer of the American, talked of every woman he had worked with and known as a "lovely" woman, and claimed that "they were and are lovely and exceptional women, exceptional human beings." Upon noticing his repeated use of the phrase, he claimed, "I find I use the word

lovely about so many of these women. But they were." We also had a confusing interchange about whether any of these women were political, or involved in politics, that gives some flavor of the delicate cultural tightrope walked by powerful women. About one woman:

> R: *I think her sensitivity and her delicacy of perception, her extraordinary intuitions, her awareness of people. So she was a training analyst.*
> NC: *Was she involved in Institute politics?*
> R: *Not overtly...not manifestly. She was interested, but she didn't--she was friends with everyone.*
> NC: *So she was powerful without being officially...*
> R: *She was training chairman for quite a number of years, chair of the education committee.*
> NC: *That's pretty active, isn't it?*
> R: *I didn't mean to give the impression that she was passive.*
> NC: *But you said not manifestly.*
> R: *I thought you said political. One can be a chairman of the education committee without being a politician.*

About another woman, one of the few who held a major national officership:

> I have the greatest respect and admiration, a woman of wonderful integrity, absolutely dedicated to analysis, absolutely dedicated to education, to learning, clearly interested in teaching and supervision, and very clear, very firm, not an ounce of politics in her body.

In this man's view, then the "lovely women" were not political. They had been very active, but *organizationally,* not *politically.* The former involves responsible commitment to the organization and practice of psychoanalysis, the latter participation in partisan battles and maneuvers to obtain power.

Similarly, the other side of the awful regiment of obviously aggressive and unfeminine women is a tradition of super-feminizing of important women. This begins early in psychoanalytic history. Although there were only a few women in the early period, people do not tend to remember most of them, including those who were actually participants in the Viennese or other societies.

The one woman who stands for all really early women analysts is Lou-Andreas Salome, a woman known generally for her femininity and male-directed intellect--the "poet of psychoanalysis," according to Freud. Other mythologized women include Marie Bonaparte, "the Princess," who could hold meetings of the International Psychoanalytic in her living room, and Beata Rank, about whom accounts always describe the marvelous parties she gave and the gaggle of adoring young students who fetched her car, took her coat, and so forth.

But it was not just the men who cast women into feminine, or mothering roles (nor do I mean to say that the women I am discussing were not recognized for their professional acumen and expertise; they were). One woman I interviewed took on the responsibility of overseeing the decoration of the local institute when it moved. A younger man told of sitting down, with trepidation but with great curiosity, with the female powerhouses of the institute where he was in training, wondering what they would talk about, to find them talking about the different kinds of cookies each would bake for the next week's fund raiser. Conflation of analytic and feminine roles was, then, another "hat" that women donned to help soften the cultural contradiction in their being strong leaders.

I have discussed a number of aspects of the question of leadership among early women psychoanalysts. I start from the perception, shared by most of the people I have talked with, that women were indeed leaders in the field. Compared to many other fields, women's leadership was much more widely accepted in psychoanalysis. This seems to be a result of the variety of careers that psychoanalysts could follow. But that leadership was not reflected in the holding of official political positions, seemingly because some of the women themselves, as well as some men psychoanalysts, accepted our culture's traditional separation of spheres in which women retain more particularistic roles that seem to grow out of their domestic, or feminine, capacities, as teachers, trainers, good at face-to-face communication while men locate themselves more universalistically in the public, political sphere and the sphere of written, non-face-to-face communication. Ambivalence toward women's leadership was reflected not only structurally, in their disproportionate exclusion from official leadership positions, but also ideologically, in some of the language used to characterize important women and in women's own choice of "appropriate" spheres of activity and leadership. As women of a later generation strive to overcome the gender division of spheres, it seems clear that women psychoanalysts, like other women, have both a structural and ideological battle to fight in their attempt to gain power and attain positions of formal, official leadership in their field.

However, feminists have argued that we must revalue and redefine what our culture considers important, and psychoanalysis enables us to do just that, because it values a number of kinds of leadership, some of which were more likely to be avenues of recognition for women, and which were also more easily assimilated to cultural expectations of femininity, or appropriate female roles and activities. I suggest that the psychoanalytic case should lead us not only to be wary of arenas where women are excluded. It should also lead us to valorize and work to maintain face-to-face aspects of our increasingly depersonalized, rationalized, and bureaucratized professions, and to honor training and teaching as a personal passing-on of a craft--as an important form of professional generativity.

Reference

Horney K: The dread of women, in Feminine Psychology, Harold Kelman, ed., New York, W.W. Norton, 1967, pp. 133-146.

Notes

[1]From 1920 to 1970, women averaged 20 percent of psychoanalysts in the United States and 30 percent in Europe. In the United States, their numbers began to increase in the twenties, rose to a peak of around 30 percent in the late forties and early fifties, and have gradually decreased since that time. In Europe, there has been, after the initial rise in the twenties and thirties, fairly consistent fluctuation at around 37 percent. In the United States during this same period, doctors averaged around 4-7 percent, lawyers around 1-5 percent, and Ph.D's around 10-15 percent, decreasing from the twenties through the sixties (these figures can be found in a wide variety of secondary sources on women and the professions). In Europe, where there were many more

women professionals in most countries than in the United States, and where the percentage of women in medicine was often considerably higher than the percentage of women in other fields, it is still the case that, in general, the percentage of women psychoanalysts was higher still than in medicine. (I cannot support such a sweeping statement in the context of this short article, since it would require participation rates for a variety of countries over a multi-decade period. The data I do have are spottier than those for the United States, but they do include information on France since 1930, England since 1940, the Netherlands and West Germany since 1950, and some isolated figures for different countries from before 1930. I have had to extrapolate backwards from these, and from impressions about women in the professions provided by interviewees. More systematic data would have been an entire study in itself. For the purposes of my claims in this chapter, I believe the general assertion I make above is sufficient; I will reproduce the back-up data more extensively in later writing.)

[2]The research upon which this chapter is based has been supported by the Russell Sage Foundation and the National Endowment for the Humanities. A Fellowship at the Center for the Advanced Study in the Behavioral Sciences, where I was also supported by grants from the National Institute of Mental Health, 5-T32-MH14581, and The Spencer Foundation, and a Faculty Research Grant from the University of California, Santa Cruz, also helped at an early stage. The Institute of Personality Assessment and Research provided me with space and facilities. Andrea Press and Avril Thorne performed the remarkably difficult task of gathering the numerical data I refer to in this paper. I also thank them and Barrie Thorne for comments and suggestions.

[3]My study is based on over 75 interviews, about 50 with women trained in the twenties through mid-forties and another 25 with men of their generation and with some of their offspring who are themselves therapists or analysts. These interviews have all been with the "orthodox": I have interviewed only members of the American and International Psychoanalytic Associations.

[4]Several of these--Fleming and Benedek, Bibring, Fromm-Reichmann--wrote books explicitly concerned with teaching. There is also the massive study of psychoanalytic education conducted by

Helen Ross and Bertram Lewin. I learned of the importance of local leadership in training and teaching partly through experience: I never interviewed Lillian Malcove, though she was alive when I began my study, because, in setting priorities among a master list of older women psychoanalysts, I was choosing to interview women whom I had heard of, which usually meant that they had written something or that they were part of the early mythic Viennese period of psychoanalysis. Lillian Malcove was neither, but I later heard from several interviewees that she was considered to have been a major power in the New York Institute, through her committee work and role in the training of candidates. As an outsider who knew psychoanalysis through its literature, then, I had a very different knowledge and conception of importance than practitioners, a situation that would not be the case in my own field and other academic fields, where recognition is almost entirely through writing.

[5]In recent years these numbers are coming together, so that women on both continents are training analysts in rough proportion to their numbers. My data on membership, officerships, and training analysts comes from the *International Journal of Psycho-Analysis, The Journal of the American Psychoanalytic Association*, visits to and correspondence with individual institutes and societies, and especially for the early periods, from secondary sources on the history of psychoanalysis. The membership data seem quite reliable, as does the data on officerships. It has been hard to collect reliable data on training analyst status, particularly from the European societies that I have not been able to visit, since these data are not usually kept in easily accessible form, and pre-World War II data have sometimes been lost or destroyed.

[6]There were also men whose reputations and prominence were earned by the same route. My point here is that men were as likely or more likely to gain recognition through the originally universalistic route of science whereas women's recognition was much more likely to be through the more particularistic local route. As I also discuss below, men's recognition was also more likely to be reflected in formal organizational terms in officerships.

[7]There have been no women presidents of the International Psychoanalytic Association, although

there does seem to be a pattern in which men presidents choose women as their secretaries, and there are currently several women vice-presidents. There have been only three women presidents of the American Psychoanalytic (Marion Kenworthy, Grete Bibring, and Rebecca Solomon) and few of other national societies. Sara Bonnett and Joan Fleming are the only women who have been chairs of the American Psychoanalytic Association's Board of Professional Standards. Within the United States, different locales seem to have differed in their acceptance of or tolerance for formal recognition of women leaders. For my research as a whole, I have been drawing upon a sample of six of the larger and more important societies (Baltimore-Washington, later Baltimore-D.C. and Washington; Boston; Chicago; Los Angeles, later Los Angeles and Southern California; New York; and San Francisco) to construct membership and other data. Of all the women presidents of these societies, 30 percent are from Chicago, and 30 percent from Baltimore-Washington, and these mainly before 1960; all but one are members of the cohort of early women psychoanalysts trained in the twenties and thirties. Within Europe (my sample here

consists of the British, German, Hungarian, Paris/French, Swiss, and Viennese societies before World War II, with the addition of the Dutch and Swedish societies after), the British society is likewise exceptional, and provides a large proportion of the European totals. In both Europe and America, Sylvia Payne, in Great Britain, is something of an exception: she was the first president of the British society after Ernest Jones' lengthy twenty-year tenure, and she served as president two other times. Payne is also credited with the notable accomplishment of preventing a split in the society between the Melanie Klein and Anna Freud factions.

[8] I discuss psychoanalysts' views of women further in " '70's Questions for '30's Women: Gender Consciousness and Gender Blindness in Early Women Psychoanalysts and in One Feminist Sociologist," unpublished paper.

[9] In fact, there were major tensions between some of the most dominant women in the Boston society, and I did not otherwise hear that all the Boston women of the early generation functioned as this kind of unit. But this was the impression created upon a young analyst by the notable existence of a number of very powerful women.

6

Helene Deutsch, M.D.: Biographical Hindsight

Paul Roazen, Ph.D.

*Professor of Political and Social Science,
York University,
Toronto, Ontario, Canada*

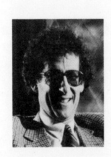 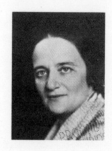

Paul Roazen, Ph.D.   **Helene Deutsch, M.D.**

6

Helene Deutsch, M.D.:
Biographical Hindsight

Biographical reconstruction does not stop when a biography gets published, and it is a tribute to the importance of my subject that there is an opportunity now for me to reflect on how I chose to approach Helene Deutsch's life.[1-6] When one reviewer called her "arguably the most important woman in the history of psychoanalysis,"[7] for a moment I felt that I had let Helene down. For, although my book examined both her writings and her leadership, I had made no such claim for Helene. The other obvious candidate for the title accorded Helene Deutsch by that reviewer was, of course, Anna Freud. Yet, despite Anna Freud's immense public standing, especially in America, I do think her contribution has been exaggerated out of loyalty to her father's memory. There is no doubt that Anna Freud and her school of child analysis had a notable impact. But it is striking that virtually no critiques of her have appeared in spite of the fact that--especially her work on jurisprudence--her ideas have enshrined middle class values of an exceptionally conformist nature. (Some French analysts have been savagely unblinkered in their view of Anna Freud as a calamity.)[8]

Whatever standing future historians may in the end assign to Helene Deutsch, certain features to her career are not in dispute. She was the first psychoanalyst to write a book on female psychology. When she was completing her manuscript in 1923, she wrote to her husband Felix, "It brings something new to this *terra incognita* in analysis-- I believe, the first ray of light on the unappreci-

ated female libido."[1] For her to refer to female libido in that period was implicitly to challenge Freud's own outlook. At the same time, Helene Deutsch was pioneering in her emphasis on the role of motherhood. Other analysts around that time, such as Otto Rank, Sandor Ferenczi and Georg Groddeck, were also intrigued by the neglected role of mothering, but Helene Deutsch was the only one to insist on its significance for female psychology.

Almost simultaneously with the completion of her first book, Helene became the first head of the Vienna Psychoanalytic Society's Training Institute. For over ten years she was the foremost leader, aside from Freud himself, in training future psychoanalysts in Vienna. When she left for Boston in 1935, Anna Freud and Edward Bibring shared the teaching roles Helene had left behind. In America, she became a prominent analyst, helping to make the Boston Psychoanalytic Society a flourishing center for training. But Helene was not interested in founding any kind of personal school among her following. She remained tolerant of divergent outlooks and participated in no doctrinal splits. In a field as controversial as psychoanalysis, Helene Deutsch stands out for her catholicity and lack of dogma.

At the same time Helene was not a mere mouthpiece for Freud's own views. Right from the first, when she came to Freud for a personal analysis in 1918, she did so with the self-respect which accompanied her success in academic psychiatry. All her work was distinctively her own, although she expresses herself within the framework of ideas that Freud laid down. Helene's mind was subtle and well-educated, and she felt no need to challenge Freud intellectually or organizationally. It is especially striking how her two-volume book, *The Psychology of Women,* which is loyal to psychoanalysis as a tradition of thought, at the same time succeeded in expressing Helene's own outlook on women, which was directly derived from her own experience. Before becoming an analyst, she had led a full and complicated emotional life, and despite her capacity for entering the lives of her patients vicariously, Helene kept on making new friends and acquaintances right up to her death in 1982 at the age of ninety-seven.

Her old age was as remarkable as any other feature of her life that one could talk about. In her nineties she could spontaneously burst out singing with her Armenian housekeeper. At the time I was writing my book about her, I wondered if I were not making a mistake by not interviewing even more people who had known her in America. But here I had to make a decision which really hinged on the kind of documentary evidence that I had available. Curiously enough, for her earlier years there was more material than for the last forty-seven years of her life. This is because, after she came to America in 1935, she fit more or less into the culture of the New World, as a result of which, there are fewer and less poignant letters from the period of her life in Boston. One of a biographer's central objectives is the recreation of his subject, and I thought that the letters from her early Polish lover, Herman Lieberman, and the correspondence between herself and her husband Felix did the best possible job of presenting her personality.

The publication of my book was in itself an occasion for second-guessing, since in reading the reviews, I naturally wondered whether my book had succeeded in the job as I had seen it. One old-line feminist critic of Helene's really proceeded as if my book had never been written. She ignored her life and its struggles, passed over my re-examination of her writings and proceeded to denounce her as a traitor to her sex. What seems progressive in the history of women, as opposed to reactionary, depends very much on the cultural and historical sophistication in the eyes of the beholder. On the whole, I think the reviewers were generous both to my book and Helene. By

coincidence, the same spring my book appeared, there was an article in a feminist journal re-examining Helene's *The Psychology of Women* along the lines I myself had followed.[9]

New evidence is, from a historical point of view, especially precious, and Helene's physician--whom I had interviewed earlier with her permission and that of her son--recently gave me a copy of a letter Helene had sent him two weeks before she died. It seems to me remarkable that this articulate woman was still capable of writing such a letter, communicating her inmost thoughts and feelings. I would have thought she had lost that capacity by then. She wrote it mostly in German; the envelope is addressed "to Dr. Zetzel with love." As I interpret her leaving him this bequest, she was trying to thank him for having been her doctor for almost fifty years. He had been a physician for many Boston analysts, his second wife had also been a psychoanalyst and his step-son had been a schoolboy rival of one of Helene's grandsons.

Dear Lou, my warmest greetings for you--
so far things in our families haven't gone so
well--
miserably, in fact--.
A few days ago I saw and spoke with "the
Professor"--
he also hasn't gotten any younger--
Rather a somewhat foolish old gentleman.
I have a huge correspondence to get rid of--
so greetings and love from an old, worried
woman.

  Yours,
  Helene

Helene was being frank about what she considered the failure of her private life that I wondered whether I had unnecessarily failed to be more explicit in my biography. I had, however, used a quotation from George Orwell: "Any life when viewed from the inside is simply a series of defeats." When she commented about how she thought things had gone miserably in her family, she had in mind how she felt she had failed with her only son Martin as well as her two grandsons' inability to establish themselves in accord with a heterosexual pattern. Like Freud, she could not reconcile herself to things in her family that she could accept clinically.

Yet no sooner had she admitted to Zetzel what

she knew he would readily understand, than she turned to the triumph of her life, her relationship with Freud. As a psychoanalyst, she had been fulfilled. In the act of professionally living with others, she had succeeded in unfolding all her talents. As a writer, she found Freud's world expansive enough to permit her to express her own thoughts and ideas. One of the books from her library which she loaned me was entitled, *How to Travel Incognito*, by Ludwig Bemelmans, and I consider it a peculiarly suitable title for the story of Helene's career as a psychoanalyst.

Helene had a remarkable sense of humor. One of the physicians who happened to see her in a hospital near the end was appalled at the shrunken size of her body but impressed enough by her name to bring her a copy of *The Psychology of Women* for autographing. She so startled him by a bit of her wit that he exclaimed, "Dr. Deutsch, you still have a sense of humor!" She quietly contradicted him by remarking, "I have a sense of humor." The doctor said he never again had treated a dying patient as if death had already taken place.

For those who knew Helene, it will come as no surprise that although she remained loyal and devoted to Freud, she still could be irreverent about him. Whether she had dreamt of a conversation with Freud or had a waking vision is less important than the significance he retained in her life. She was more distant from him than many others who had surrounded him, and certainly his own daughter Anna could not be expected to appreciate any jokes about "the Professor."

The "huge correspondence" that she refers to in the letter to Zetzel means the letters from Lieberman that she had asked to be returned to her. Initially she told me, when I was interviewing her in 1964 about Freud and the history of psychoanalysis, that she intended to destroy this correspondence out of deference to her late husband. But when I was working on my biography of her, I found that she had in fact been unable to do away with the letters. They were all saved, outside of their envelopes, in a separately catalogued folder which also contained photographs. Had she known she still had them she could have at least used a photograph of Lieberman for her *Confrontations With Myself*, an autobiography which appeared in 1973. Helene had obviously reread the letters over the years, and when I went over them all with her, checking them for dating

as well as examining their substance and translations from the Polish, she knew some of the expressions by heart.

After her death her son and daughter-in-law could not find the Lieberman letters in her house. I had, in fact, when her daughter-in-law Suzanne told me Helene wanted the originals back, returned them to Helene's house; Helene knew that I had made Xerox copies, but nonetheless she proceeded to destroy the originals. (Incidentally, since Helene saved hundreds of Suzanne's letters from Los Alamos, presumably there are many letters to her from Helene which Suzanne will someday add to Helene's papers at the Schlesinger Library for the History of Women in America at Radcliffe College.)

Helene's letter to Zetzel makes me think of life imitating art. For she had not read, as far as I know, D. M. Thomas's *The White Hotel* and his fictional use of Freud as an old man. And she could not have known about Thomas' poem about my *Brother Animal: The Story of Freud and Tausk*, which Thomas called "Fathers, Sons and Lovers," since it did not appear until after her death.[10] Thomas in his poem was giving his version of the Tausk "problem," and Helene's own part in the struggle between Tausk and Freud.

Helene died having long since accepted the inevitability of death, and yet she was still searching for understanding. Perhaps she was unnecessarily harsh on herself, "masochistic" in evaluating her own human frailties. But her early psychoanalytic essay, "A Two-Year-Old Boy's First Love Comes to Grief,"[11] was an autobiographical account of how her involvement as a psychoanalytic psychiatrist interfered with her mothering her son Martin. However much Martin gained from her, his own mature antagonism toward his mother (matched only by Helene's own hostility to her own mother) serves as evidence for the extraordinary strain in their relationship. If she had neglected Martin, she overdid things with her eldest grandson; and to the end of her life she was as unforgiving of herself as of her own mother, whose dire warnings about her as a young woman seemed to have been fulfilled. In extreme old age Helene consciously regretted not having had more children, which would have suited what her husband desired as well; and she brooded over the miscarriages she had had, which were attributed to psychogenic causes. The absence of any great-grand children spoke for itself.

Yet of all the men in Helene's life perhaps Freud was the most important. In my biography I discussed how her tie to Freud was patterned on her idealized relationship to her father; and Helene consciously saw her second analysis with Karl Abraham in 1923-24 as a renewal of a father involvement. (Although she interpreted her affair at that time with Sandor Rado as a sign of her "masochism," she did not see, nor did I when I wrote my book, that for her to have a sexual relationship with another patient of Abraham's might reflect an "acting out" of her feelings for Abraham.)

Helene was so mature a woman when she came to Freud at the age of thirty-four that she could hardly blame him for any of the twisted courses her own life had taken. On the contrary, she found in his system of ideas an explanation of why things had gone the way they had. If she allowed her career to replace her life as a mother and a wife, then she need not recommend her example to others. She identified with Tolstoy's Anna Karenina's guilt feelings as a mother; and had she left her husband, Felix, she might have lost her son Martin. Her writings on the conflicts in a woman between parenting and professional life remain enduring insights into human psychology. And as fathers nowadays take over more of the parenting functions, they too will experience more regularly the tensions between success in the outside world and competency at home.

Although Helene has been misinterpreted as a naive defender of old-fashioned family life, her biography shows how daring she was in defying traditional sexual roles and stereotypes. The early Freudians, like the English Bloomsbury circle, were apt to ignore everything that had been thought conventional about femininity and masculinity. In terms of her own intimate family, it was her husband Felix who provided basic early mothering for their son Martin. And Helene felt she had had to wear the pants in the family professionally. My biography, and her letter to Zetzel, were in a sense posthumous expressions of her power. Helene was convinced that her choices had been humanly costly for her. If she had been more accepting of herself, it might have led her to ideas about human development and normality that would match the unconventionality of her own experience, and entitle others to feel more at ease in defying conformist pressures. Within the profession she chose for herself she became one

of the best mothers in the history of psychoanalysis.

Much of my research on Helene hinged on my interviewing her. I first met her in 1964 for the sake of my research on Freud and the history of psychoanalysis. It was only in 1977-78 that the idea of a biography of her began to take shape. Perhaps she had had me in mind as a biographer long before I formally put the question to her. My interviewing demand on Helene had always been the same: that she be brilliant and original. (Sometime late in my work on Freud she jokingly volunteered that the evening before I used to see her weekly, she would worry about what she had to offer me the next morning.) My work on Helene's life proceeded on the conviction that behind all the letters she had saved, and out of the implicit autobiography of her professional writings, there had to be a story of her life as interesting as the woman I knew.

It was only after I finished my book that I fully realized how different were her own ideas from those of Freud; in my "Epilogue" I went through her *The Psychology of Women* to show how it departed from classical psychoanalytic thinking. But I had all along sensed that recent feminists had given Helene a raw deal and that they were even capable of ignoring how respectfully a pioneering feminist like Simone de Beauvoir had treated Helene's work.

My research on Helene was a part of my long-standing interest in historical underdogs. I first became interested in Freud as a neglected figure in my own profession, political science.[12-14] I then wrote, with Helene's cooperation, a book on Victor Tausk's tortured relationship to Freud, on the grounds that Tausk had been neglected historigraphically.[15-18] My book on Freud and his circle was in large part an attempt to correct preceding distortions.[19] And when I wrote a study of Erik H. Erikson, it was because I thought his ideas and their relationship to psychoanalysis needed clarifying.[20,21]

Feminism often seems as much a political movement as an intellectual approach, and therefore we have grown accustomed to feminist writings which color reality to suit ideological purposes. When it comes to psychoanalysis feminists have already succeeded in achieving a major social impact. Starting in the late 1960's and extending throughout the 1970's, feminists established once and for all the sexist biases implicit in

Freud's framework. Although women had all along held high positions as analysts throughout this century (and perhaps more so in Freud's lifetime than now), Freud's ideas were long ago challenged by a few so-called dissident analysts discontented with his approach to feminine psychology. Feminism has so fundamentally altered the way Freud's work is now perceived that Freud's stature has unnecessarily suffered a relative decline.

In recent years, however, feminist writers on psychoanalysis have tended to shift. Now that their battle against Freud's sexism has been won, feminism is allowing itself to see other aspects to analysis than those it had been assaulting. Psychoanalysis has come to be seen not just as a defense of patriarchal culture, but as a critical source of insight into traditionalist injustices.

Despite how easy it can be to pass judgment by today's standards on a woman born over a century ago, Helene Deutsch's writings were the authentic outgrowth of her most intense personal experiences. In social context she herself was a leading feminist. In 1924, when Helene had just made a presentation on "The Menopause,"[22] her old lover Herman Lieberman wrote her:

> *I was very happy and proud about your success at the conference of psychoanalysis, just like in the old times and just as if you still belonged to me. Do you remember, Halusia, your speech at that meeting in Vienna, about allowing women to study law? I was very proud of your success at that meeting then, and now I had the same feeling when reading the report of the conference.*[1]

Helene had, even as a medical student (1907-13), spoken in behalf of her sex. No doubt she would have delighted to see Alix Strachey's comment in a letter to her husband James about Helene's Menopause paper, "a great success, only capped by her evening gown (from Paris they all said) . . . . She's a remarkable woman."[23]

As a pre-World War I psychiatrist Helene had proposed founding a special institution for young girls; as she wrote to her husband:

> *Young girls suffering from neuroses and psychoses are the unhappiest creatures in the world. They are sent to unsuitable places, places which make their illness worse. If they have a neuro-*

> *sis, they are in real trouble. They are sent to sanatoria where instead of psychiatric treatment they are given hydro-electric therapy. Flirtations with doctors and affairs with other patients spoil these girls for life. Where real medical care could bring about a miracle in dealing with the complaints, unscientific approaches cause havoc.*

> *And psychoses: all these schizophrenics, these split personalities who could live peacefully until they succumb entirely in their insanity! And all those in an observation period when we don't know if we are dealing with a hysteria or a dementia praecox? The many who are at the borderline and who are crying for help while they can still feel their individuality and their being. I know already: only a woman can understand and help them. That is the most wonderful aspect of my profession--I can feel my power and know what I can do.*[1]

Even before World War I, Helene had grown disappointed with feminism as a movement; it was not sufficiently idealistic for her, and too bread-and-butterish. She grew up in an ideology that saw the emancipation of women as part of a general human awakening. A trade-union mentality embarrassed her. It seemed to her that her freedom as a woman had followed rather than preceded her liberation as a proud individual; as she wrote Felix in 1914, "now I am a *free woman*--in order to become that, I had to be a *free human being.*"[1]

In terms of her life and career, Helene became a powerful leader and an inspiration to many younger women and colleagues. In 1928 she presented a public lecture in Vienna, "George Sand: A Woman's Destiny."[24] This paper about a great French writer filled out some of Helene's purposes as a thinker; in the course of making the subject of women her specialty, she had to come to terms with the life of the woman she credited with being "the first systematic feminist." Ironically enough George Sand herself, like Helene after her, has been attacked in our time for not being a feminist. I think that Gustave Flaubert's memorable words about George Sand are worth repeating: "One had to know her as I knew her to realize how much of the feminine there was in this great woman, the immensity of tenderness to be found in this genius." Helene did herself espouse certain conventions of her time about the nature of maleness and femaleness. But she was working from the premise of the universality of bisexual trends. And in trying to account for the sources of the formation of George Sand's conflicted personality, Helene was at the same time reflecting self-critically on the underside to her own immensely successful career.

Helene's gentleness in expressing herself meant that only in the course of a footnote did she defend herself against Karen Horney's gloss on Helene's ideas:

I should like to defend my previous work against a misinterpretation. K. Horney contends that I regard feminine masochism as an 'elemental power in feminine mental life' and that, according to my view, 'what woman ultimately wants in intercourse is to be raped and violated; what she wants in mental life is to be humiliated.' It is true that I consider masochism 'an elemental power in feminine life,' but in my previous studies and also in this one I have tried to show that one of woman's tasks is to govern this masochism, to steer it into the right paths, and thus to protect herself against those dangers that Horney thinks I consider woman's normal lot.[1]

For Helene it went almost without saying that "all those to whom the ideals of freedom and equality are not empty works sincerely desire that woman should be socially equal to man." None of her idealism, however, meant that she did not have the courage to elaborate on what she considered some of the essential differences between men and women. The kind of masochism that afflicted her own life, for instance, would in principle be different from male masochism. (By "masochism" she was writing with a technical psychoanalytic concept in mind.) Although she has been attacked for her views on female "narcissism," Helene thought of it as a counter-weight to masochism; and "passivity" was, Helene held, a special source of insight for women which led them to a kind of intuition unknown in men. But isolated terms like "masochism," "narcissism," and "passivity" are apt to be as misleading about Helene Deutsch's ideas as Freud's concepts of id, ego, and superego are a superficial approach to the import of psychoanalysis.

Helene was in reality as surprisingly unorthodox in practice as she was in theory. She wrote about

anorexia nervosa,[25] argued against rigidities in training,[26] and grew distrustful of long-term analyses as therapy.[1] Only a conscientious examination of all her life and work shows how unlike a stereotyped Freudian she was. She moved beyond accepting penis envy as a biological entity or a useful theoretical construct. When she talked about a "masculinity complex" it was largely out of dissatisfaction with her own life. Feminine psychology remained her special field until the end of her life.

Helene Deutsch was an original figure in the history of psychoanalysis, and she exerted a special influence on modern psychiatry. The example of her life makes an enduringly valuable object of admiration and identification. She will be remembered as one of Freud's unusually independent followers who, without the need for rebellion, heroically coped with the idiosyncracies of her private life as she carved out of Freud's teachings a special niche for herself in the history of ideas.

References

[1] Roazen P: Helene Deutsch: A Psychoanalyst's Life, N.Y., Doubleday, 1985, N.Y., New American Library, 1986.

[2] Roazen P: "Helene Deutsch's 'Two Cases of Induced Insanity,' " International Journal of Psychoanalysis, Spring 1981, pp. 139-150.

[3] Roazen P: "Helene Deutsch's 'On the Pathological Lie,' " Journal of the American Academy of Psychoanalysis, July 1982, pp. 369-386.

[4] Roazen P: "Obituary of Helene Deutsch," International Journal of Psychoanalysis, Fall 1982, pp. 491-492.

[5] Roazen P: "In Memoriam: Helene Deutsch," American Journal of Psychiatry, April 1983, pp. 497-499.

[6] Roazen P: "Helene Deutsch's 'A Case That Throws Light on the Mechanism of Regression in Schizophrenia,' " Psychoanalytic Review, Spring 1985, pp. 1-8.

[7] Kimmel M: "The Loyal Analyst," Psychology Today, August 1985, pp. 73-74.

[8] Roustang F: Dire Mastery: Discipleship from Freud to Lacan, Baltimore, Johns Hopkins Univ. Press, 1982, pp. 11-12.

[9] Webster BS: "Helene Deutsch: A New Look," Signs, Spring 1985, pp. 553-571.

[10] Thomas DM: "Fathers, Sons and Lovers," in

Selected Poems, N.Y., Viking, 1983, pp. 14-17.

[11]Deutsch H: "A Two-Year-Old Boy's First Love Comes to Grief," in Neuroses and Character Types: Clinical Psychoanalytic Studies, N.Y., International Universities Press, 1965, pp. 159-164.

[12]Roazen P: Freud: Political and Social Thought, N.Y., Knopf, 1968, reprinted with a new Preface, N.Y., Da Capo Books, 1986.

[13]Roazen P: "Psychology and Politics," Contemporary Psychoanalysis, pp. 144-57.

[14]Roazen P: " 'As if' and Politics," Political Psychology, Oct. 1983, pp. 685-692.

[15]Roazen P: Brother Animal: The Story of Freud and Tausk, N.Y., Knopf, 1969; N.Y., New York University Press, 1986.

[16]Roazen P: "Reflections on Ethos and Authenticity in Psychoanalysis," The Human Context, Autumn 1972, pp. 577-587.

[17]Roazen P: "Orthodoxy on Freud: The Case of Tausk," Contemporary Psychoanalysis, Jan. 1977, pp. 102-115.

[18]Roazen P: "Reading, Writing, and Memory: Dr. K. R. Eissler's Thinking," Contemporary Psychoanalysis, April 1978, pp. 345-353.

[19]Roazen P: Freud and His Followers, N.Y., Knopf, 1975; N.Y., New York University Press, 1985.

[20]Roazen P: Erik H. Erikson: The Power and Limits of a Vision, N.Y., The Free Press, 1976; The Free Press, 1986.

[21]Roazen P: "Erik H. Erikson's America: The Political Implications of Ego Psychology," Journal of the History of the Behavioral Sciences, Fall 1980, pp. 333-341.

[22]Roazen P: "Helene Deutsch's 'The Menopause,' " International Journal of Psychoanalysis, 1984, pp. 55-62.

[23]Meisel P and Kendrick W (editors): Bloomsbury/ Freud: The Letters of James and Alix Strachey, 1924-25, N.Y., Basic Books, 1985, p. 87.

[24]Roazen P: "Helene Deutsch's 'George Sand: A Woman's Destiny,' " International Review of Psychoanalysis, Fall 1982, pp. 445-460.

[25]Roazen P: "Helene Deutsch's 'Anorexia Nervosa,' " Bulletin of the Menninger Clinic, Nov. 1981, pp. 499-511.

[26]Roazen P: "Helene Deutsch's 'On Supervised Psychoanalysis,' " Contemporary Psychoanalysis, Jan. 1983, pp. 53-67.

7

Karen Horney, M.D.:
An Early Leader

Edward R. Clemmens, M.D.

*Fellow of the American Academy of Psychoanalysis; and
Training and Supervising Analyst,
The American Institute for Psychoanalysis
and the Karen Horney Clinic,
New York, New York*

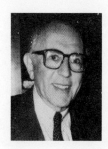 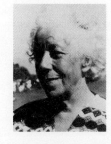

Edward R. Clemmens, M.D.   **Karen Horney, M.D.**

7

Karen Horney, M.D.:
An Early Leader

How can we do justice to Karen Horney, as we try to account for her greatness? For great she was, creative, full of an indomitable spirit, original, self-reliant and enormously sure of the rightness of her ideas. Much is known of her professional career, of the admiration and loyalty that she inspired in those colleagues who saw her as an innovator and a leader, and in the masses of lay people to whom she gave hope and who adored her. And much is known also about the enemies she made, the powerful opposition she met in the psychoanalytic establishment which endures to this day and which continues to deny her the recognition she deserves as a pioneer.

A fair amount is also known about her beginnings, her family, her genealogy, her childhood and adolescence,[1] and finally we are fortunate to still have access to the recollections of those people who were close to her. Her daughter, Marianne Horney Eckardt, M.D., a past president of the American Academy of Psychoanalysis, has repeatedly shared with us impressions and memories of her mother and she has done so again in preparation for this essay.

However, a troubling question remains unanswered: Does all this knowledge offer us a better understanding of how Karen Horney became the person she was? I submit that such knowledge does not further our understanding very much, because we have only a dim awareness of the complex interplay of nature and nurture. We know next to nothing of the genetic underpinnings which are as chancy as a lottery and which

may lead to luck or misfortune. We are only a bit better informed about the positive value of parental care and support versus the character building school of hard knocks with its concurrent need to overcome adversity. It would seem that Karen Horney had a goodly share of most of these factors. We have no record of how she herself perceived their interplay, nor whether such considerations mattered to her. We do have, however, her own candid description of her inner experiences, an intensely private communication, about which I have written elsewhere.[2] If Horney were alive today and we were to ask her what it was that shaped her, she might not know. Even if she answered, would her subjective perception be any more valid than are the suppositions of hagiographers and novelists? Those readers who wish to learn more about the facts of Karen Horney's life will find abundant material in Jack Rubins' and Harold Kelman's books.[3,4] This essay will contain no more than a brief summary. It will use particularly Marianne H. Eckardt's recollections and thoughts, as she expressed them in a recent interview with Leah J. Dickstein, M.D., co-editor of the present volume.

Karen Horney was born in Hamburg, Germany, in 1885. Her father was a sea captain, a native of Norway, who had four children by an earlier marriage. He was 50 years old, when Karen was born. Intensely religious and authoritarian, he was resented by his young wife and his daughter. During his long absences at sea he was never missed. The parents' marriage was unhappy in the extreme. Karen's mother was 17 years younger than her husband. She was of Dutch stock, came from an educated and fairly affluent background that included well-known professionals. She chafed for years under her husband's oppressive influence and eventually left him. The older branch of the family never accepted her, nor her children. Karen's father was opposed to his daughter's seeking an education and he actively stood in her way. Her mother was too preoccupied with her own unhappiness to become a positive influence in Karen's educational pursuits. She was, at best, accepting of her daughter's plans.

Karen, however, was intensely self-motivated from an early age. At age 15 she wrote in her diary, "I have a wish that I would go to the gymnasium [High School], but my father doesn't want me to, but he can't forbid me to study. I will study to be a teacher, and after I am a teacher for two years I can be on my own. I'll go into my final exam and then study medicine, and then I will become a doctor." She knew that she was gifted and bright. She considered herself lucky to be part of an elite of women, not a feminist striving for feminine rights. She loved her teachers and her school. She was happiest away from home, with her friends and at school, and she engaged early in a vast array of intellectual pursuits. In her teens she developed a love for the theater and hoped for awhile to become an actress. (Her oldest daughter is a famous German actress.) She also read avidly and, as her horizon expanded, quickly surpassed her mother and her older brother in sophistication. In the early years of the 20th century she already believed in sexual freedom. She had intense crushes, wrote lengthy romantic entries into her diary, discussed philosophy and religion and was in a constant ferment of growth and development.

Her bubbly enthusiasm persisted well into her early years of medical studies, but it came to a sad end during her analysis with Karl Abraham. For several years she seems to have been moderately depressed and the entries in her diary end on that note. When she began to publish papers during her early years as an analyst in Berlin, her depression seems to have lifted. There is an air of confidence and solidity in her writings, although the bubbly exuberance of her youth never returned. The intellectual climate of Berlin during the years of the Weimar Republic was stimulating and so was New York in the late Thirties and Forties,

when her fame in the United States grew. As Marianne Eckardt put it:

She was not one to worry about whether her thoughts would be right: she first thought her thoughts. She was always questioning and working and debating and discussing, and that went on throughout her life. She knew the inner satisfaction of thinking and debating. She was a beautiful lecturer: she always had notes, but she never read her lectures, and they always made a circle. She was at home in her own creative concepts.

And further:

I think she very much believed in the system that she developed, which happened to be her last book before she died of cancer. The chances are that she would have written more books. Each book is a sequence and a buildup-- it has a tremendous logic--in the foreword or the postscript she writes exactly how she started, what she first thought, when she changed her mind. I think her totality of ideas was what meant most to her. She was always a little bit depressed if she began to write a book and couldn't progress. She didn't hem and haw any more than anybody else, but she would complain about not having written and feeling lethargic; nevertheless, she produced, so that was purely her own frustration at not being able to write rather than being able to accept that there is a period of gestation before writing.

I thought of one other thing--it has to do with her sense of exceptionality which comes through very often in the diary. She says, 'I believe that a spiritualized great sensuality is a sign of a great personality, or can be. Limited people will show themselves to be limited in sensuality, too. Other great personalities will feel a great desire of the senses and will combat it because they think it is wrong. If they manage that, it is certainly one of the greatest victories within a person.' She believed that what she called spiritualized sensuality is a sign of a great personality, and she opposed the sense of limitedness. In her own home, growing up, she was aware of its limitedness--the prejudice, the middle-class average household. She definitely was above it.

What remains to be discussed is the issue of Karen Horney's leadership qualities. They were, indeed, of a very special kind. What stood out about her was the impact of her personality, the impression that she had something important to say. In my own contacts with her I found her to be enormously convincing, almost spellbinding as a speaker and a discussant, lucid and clarifying, never verbose or nebulous, but simple and direct. In meeting other people she often was reserved, but she could be warm at times. There was an air of cosmopolitanism about her, a friendly, yet slightly ironic worldliness which reminded me of the intellectual style of Berlin in the 1920's. Her sincerity was contagious, so that in her presence people tried to bring out the best they were capable of. These are leadership qualities, to be sure. She also was the undisputed head of the psychoanalytic school she had founded, both in a moral and in a scientific sense. Administrative details, however, bored her. She was not much interested in politics, in implementing and solidifying structures. She was first and foremost an individualist. Her life's work with its emphasis on the REAL SELF is a mirror image of her own strong personality of which she wrote so eloquently in her adolescent diaries.[1]

With the advent of women's liberation in our generation we have come to conceive of women in leadership roles as reclaiming a position in society that is rightfully theirs, as standing up to male prerogatives and fighting for the rights of other women. Karen Horney did not do any of these things. Her fights for acceptance and recognition were intense, but they were individual, they were for her own sake, not collective or for the sake of other women. She had little feeling for what has since come to be known as the "sisterhood," so that she was indifferent to the gender of her associates. This does not mean that she ignored entrenched male prejudices. Her early psychoanalytic work constituted an intense refutation of Freud's ideas about feminine psychology.[5] She did not believe that most women's psyches are shaped by penis envy, or that masochism is a natural condition of women. It was this clarity of her views, the strength of her convictions that accounted for her following. Among her admirers gender made no difference. Her leadership was based solely on the quality of her contributions. We can only speculate, whether she would have participated in efforts such as female conscious-ness-raising had she lived in our current generation. I think it would have been unlikely.

Life in many ways had been good to her. While she had to overcome serious obstacles, she never had to face closed doors. This was sheer luck and it happened repeatedly. She entered into a Gymnasium (high school) for girls, when it hardly had opened, and she was admitted to the Medical School of the University of Freiburg two or three years after they had started to accept women, at a time when the University of Berlin was still closed to them. When she moved to Berlin to begin her psychiatric and psychoanalytic career, there were four senior analysts only. Thus she became part of the movement almost at its inception and she participated in its ferment and rapid growth. Had she gone to Vienna instead, she would have been one of many candidates and might well have been squeezed into oblivion.

She arrived in the United States to help Franz Alexander found the Chicago Psychoanalytic Institute. Upon moving to New York she was still several years ahead of the wave of refugee psychoanalysts who had fled from Europe following Hitler's rise to power. When her disagreement with the New York Psychoanalytic Association (Freudian) made her links with them more precarious, the New School for Social Research offered her an immense opportunity to lecture and to become widely known beyond the circle of her colleagues. The blossoming of the New School, in turn, was due to its having become a University in Exile for many refugee social scientists, whom she had previously known in Europe.

This does not mean that Horney does not deserve credit for what she did and that everything was just a chain of lucky coincidences. Her clear vision enabled her to recognize opportunities and to seize them at a propitious moment, which is the essence of "kairos." To be able to do this requires a measure of inner freedom, a relative absence of neurotic shackles, courage, and a taste for decisive action. Such qualities are not common. They are even less common among thinkers and scientists. Horney combined a talent and a liking for research and pure thought with a practical and pragmatic bent. She was at home in both worlds, just as she was on both sides of the Atlantic. An individualist, a scientist, a thinker and a doer, hers was indeed a rare combination of leadership qualities.

References

[1]Horney K: The Adolescent Diaries of Karen Horney. Basic Books, Inc., New York, 1980.

[2]Clemmens ER: Book Essay, The Adolescent Diaries of Karen Horney. Journal of the American Academy of Psychoanalysis. Vol. 10, No. 1, 1982.

[3]Rubins JL: Karen Horney, Gentle Rebel of Psychoanalysis. The Dial Press, New York, 1978.

[4]Kelman H: Helping People, Karen Horney's Psychoanalytic Approach. Science House, New York, 1971.

[5]Horney K: Feminine Psychology. W.W. Norton & Co. Inc., New York, 1967.

8

Frieda Fromm-Reichmann, M.D.:
Pioneer in Psychiatry and Psychoanalysis

Sylvia G. Hoff, L.C.S.W.

Social Worker,
Chestnut Lodge,
Rockville, Maryland

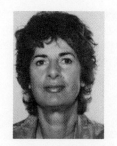 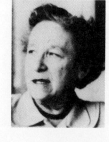

Sylvia G. Hoff, L.C.S.W.   Frieda Fromm-Reichmann, M.D.

8

Frieda Fromm-Reichmann, M.D.:
Pioneer in Psychiatry and Psychoanalysis

When Frieda Fromm-Reichmann appeared on a ward at Chestnut Lodge, the mental hospital to which she devoted the last twenty years of her life, "people moved back as if she were parting the Red Sea."[1] They moved back in awe before this plump, elderly refugee woman who was less than four feet eleven inches tall. It will be the subject of this article to examine the sources of the energy, creativity and confidence which fueled the achievements of this pioneer in the field of psychiatry and psychoanalysis.

The list of her achievements is impressive. Born in Karlsruhe, Germany, in 1889 at a time when the patriarchal edict of contemporary society proclaimed that women's sphere was to be confined to "Kinder, Kirche, Kriche" (children, church, kitchen), she graduated from the Albertus University in Koenigsberg, East Prussia. She specialized in psychiatry and neurology. By 1916, at the age of 27, she had become physician-in-charge of Koenigsberg's new 100-bed hospital and dispensary for brain-damaged soldiers. This laid the groundwork for her later understanding of psychotic panic states.

After the end of World War I, she continued to publish scientific papers with Goldstein at the University of Frankfurt, but a growing commitment to the study and practice of psychoanalysis led her to accept a position as staff psychiatrist and psychoanalyst at the sanatorium Weisser Hirsch, outside Dresden. Her employer was J. H. Schultz, the father of "autogenic training," a form of relaxation therapy. In addition to this full-time

position and the pursuit of her scientific studies, she commuted regularly to Berlin to complete her training analysis under Hanns Sachs. In 1923, she served as a visiting physician at Emil Kraepelin's psychiatric clinic at the University of Munich.

Initially, Frieda Fromm-Reichmann's enthusiasm for psychoanalysis included a belief that this new technique for the exploration of the human soul would not only alleviate individual suffering, but could also be a tool for social change. While working at Weisser Hirsch she analyzed many members of socialist Zionist youth groups and initially continued these efforts in her spare time, while running a small private psychoanalytic sanatorium in Heidelberg from 1924 to 1928.

Perhaps we should take a brief look at the particular nature of these facilities which, although quaint and peculiar to our modern eyes, played an important part in disseminating the new method of psychoanalysis to a wider public. There was and is a long tradition of sanatoria in Europe, usually not places for the severely ill, but instead comfortable and sometimes luxurious hotel-like structures, spas, mountain retreats, and seaside villas. Here the wealthy have traditionally sought relief from the after-effects of over-indulgence of one kind or another, as well as from a variety of nervous afflictions.

Frieda Fromm-Reichmann, with the help of the social philosopher Erich Fromm who became her husband in 1926, established a facility in which several weeks of intensive analysis were offered to the residents. As the sanatorium kitchen was strictly kosher, it became a magnet for wealthy Jewish burghers from all over Germany.

By the late twenties, Frieda Fromm-Reichmann and Erich Fromm had tired of the superficiality of work in the sanatorium. They also abandoned, after much study and reflection, the practice of orthodox Judaism.

Together they had organized, with several colleagues, the Frankfurt chapter of the German Psychoanalytic Society in 1926. Three years later, Frieda Fromm-Reichmann participated in the founding of the Psychoanalytic Institute of South Western Germany. By now, they had become disillusioned with the usefulness of psychoanalysis as a political method.

After Hitler came to power in 1933 and the persecution of the Jews as well as the psychoanalytic movement began to gather momentum, Frieda Fromm-Reichmann escaped with only two small suitcases of belongings to Strasbourg, France, where many of her patients followed her to continue their treatment. Erich Fromm had already left for Switzerland several years earlier because of an exacerbation of his tuberculosis, a condition with which he had waged a long struggle. Although they were to remain life-long friends, their life together had ended at this point and they were to be divorced in 1942.

In 1935, Frieda visited Israel where her mother and sister, Greta, had settled but then decided to depart for the United States. She believed that there she would find a larger arena for her work which would not only benefit the field of psychoanalysis as a whole, but would enable her to earn the means to help friends and family members who were suffering deprivation in many parts of the world as a result of Nazi persecution.

She arrived in New York in 1936. Several months later, with Erich Fromm acting as an intermediary, she was engaged as a staff psychiatrist at Chestnut Lodge in Rockville, Maryland. Her employer was Dexter Bullard, Sr., who was in the process of transforming the traditional sanatorium his father had founded into an up-to-date facility for the treatment of severe mental illness through intensive psychoanalytic treatment.

Chestnut Lodge was to provide the stage for most of her pioneering efforts with schizophrenic and manic-depressive patients, individuals who had formerly been considered hopelessly beyond the reach of individual psychotherapy. Here she was to exchange ideas with Harry Stack Sullivan during weekly seminars which continued for years. Sullivan's emphasis on the interpersonal nature of human development was to have a profound influence on her own work in deciphering the mysterious verbal and non-verbal communication of the mentally ill.

Frieda Fromm-Reichmann was an extraordinarily gifted and emphatic clinician. Joanne Greenberg, her most famous patient, described her vividly as the therapist Dr. Fried in her autobiographical novel, *I Never Promised You A Rose Garden*. As a training analyst and lecturer, she became an inspiring teacher to a whole generation of psychoanalysts and lay students. She gave a memorable lecture series about "the assets of the mentally handicapped" at the William Alanson White Institute in New York and The Washington School of Psychiatry, both institutions she helped to organize.

Although the major part of her energies was spent as a clinician and teacher, two important works containing some of her many papers were published: *Principles of Intensive Psychotherapy* (1950) and *An Intensive Study of Twelve Cases of Manic Depressive Psychosis* (1954).

Frieda Fromm-Reichmann's lifelong passion for music, the visual arts and literature fueled her interest in the relationship between art and mental illness, but she never romanticized this interplay. She was never seduced by colorful and dramatic symptoms, but was a partner to her patients' efforts in the struggle to regain the true source of all creative effort, a sound, cohesive sense of self.

Now let us look at the origins of the particular combination of qualities which shaped her life as a leader and pioneer in the field of psychoanalysis. Freida Fromm-Reichmann was born into a solidly middle class family, almost exactly nine months to the day after her parents, Adolf and Klara Simon Reichmann's marriage. The robust, blond, blue-eyed infant was warmly received into a large extended family of solid, Jewish merchants. On the surface, it was the most conventional setting. Appearances were of the greatest importance. Klara continued to help Adolf as cashier in his iron-ware shop in order to be able to afford the housemaid who was, in white cap and apron, indispensable in a respectable household.

Frieda was to combine the best characteristics of both parents in a particularly fortuitous manner. Adolf Reichmann was a sensitive, gentle man with a passion for literature and music. He always regretted that he had to leave school early to assume the support of his mother and siblings after his father died because he would have preferred to devote his life to his studies. Clearly, he had been influenced by the values of his grandfather, Seligman Feuchtwanger, who had closed his silverware shop as early as possible every day. He turned away further customers after earning a modest subsistence for himself, his wife Fanny, and the eighteen children, in order to devote himself to the study of the Talmud.

Adolf's business acumen was questionable and the family moved from Karlsruhe to Koenigsberg on the Baltic Sea when Frieda was nine years old. Here Adolf was initially a complete failure in the business end of the bank in which his brother-in-law, the director, offered him employment. Only when he became personnel manager did he come into his own. The special sensitivity, warmth and tact, which were to be Frieda's inheritance, earned him the love and respect of his fellow employees.

It was Klara Simon who was to be the driving force of Frieda's life. On the surface, she was a conventional wife and mother, but her ideas were ahead of her time. Klara had been trained as a teacher, but in her middle class milieu, there was no expectation that she would ever use her skills. The only hope for a secure, respectable future was a suitable marriage. She was to tell her daughters often how bitter she had felt about her lack of options. She would say that it was "terrible" that women were forced into marriage. She explained that she still felt this way even though she loved her husband and valued their life together. With the greatest confidence, she expected her daughters, Frieda and the younger Greta and Anna to fulfill the dreams of professional success and independence which had been denied her. "Our children will be musical," Klara announced. "How do you know?" asked Adolf. "They will be, I promise you that," Klara answered.

In addition to self-confidence, Klara enjoyed unflagging energy, a sharp wit and remarkable willpower. She was the dominant figure in the Reichmann household. Adolf worshipped his clever wife and deferred to her judgment. Frieda, like her mother well under five feet tall, perceived the tiny Klara as an all-powerful force. Frieda was almost middle aged by the time she gained enough distance to perceive herself as a

creative, productive person in her own right and could begin to regard her mother as something less than perfect. For many years she felt that the only reason she accomplished anything was because her mother had arranged everything so wonderfully for her.

The expectation of her parents that she was to compensate for the disappointments of their lives, that she owed them a generous return for their investment of love and attention provided a powerful motivating force for Frieda. She responded by becoming a model student as soon as she entered school and remained at the top of her class throughout her academic career. She rarely missed a day of school, because she had inherited her mother's strong constitution. Klara was of sound health until her death in her late eighties; she was a powerful swimmer who supposedly once crossed the Rhine fully clothed. She continued to swim until her eightieth year when she stopped because she felt it was no longer seemly for a woman of her age.

Greta, the Reichmann's second daughter who arrived two and a half years after Frieda was not as fortunate as her older sister. She was a plain child and her delicate nature, so different from Klara's own, was alien to her mother. The same firm molding and prodding to which Frieda responded so well caused her sister to withdraw and to droop. She needed considerable tutoring to keep up in school and she grew up to be a self-deprecating, unworldly spinster who devoted her whole life to an obscure, fruitless research project on the lute. Later Anna, the youngest, who was born eight years after Frieda, even failed to pass a grade in high-school. This provoked such an intense family crisis that Frieda had to return home to intervene because she was concerned that Anna would be psychologically crushed by the weight of her parents' disappointment.

Frieda had been thrust into a leadership position at the age of two-and-a-half when her sister Greta was born. In spite of her modern thinking, Klara enforced an Old Testament adherence to the importance of the position of the first-born. The two younger children were not allowed to contradict Frieda. "Don't argue with her, she is the oldest," Klara would say firmly. The three girls were usually dressed alike, but Frieda's costumes would always receive an extra ornament of some kind, an additional embroidered flower, some extra lace or ruffle. Frieda tried to protest against this special treatment, but Klara remained adamant. Shouldering increasingly heavy responsibilities, being always somewhat set apart as an authority figure became a way of life for Frieda from that early point on.

In addition, Frieda was to say later that she had been a psychiatrist since the age of three. As the oldest child and the one closest to her mother, she had become aware quite early of the subtle emotional currents and counter-currents between her parents. Around the turn of the century, there were few distractions; family members lived constantly in each other's presence. In the evenings, Adolf read aloud from the classics while Klara embroidered.

The girls were constantly observed, admonished and praised. They were never free from the weight of their parents' expectations. On the other hand, the girls also focused their own close attention on their parents. Frieda became a mediator between them early on. Her father was often preoccupied and might overlook a particular surprise which had been prepared for him. Occasionally, he could be short-tempered. Klara would nurse her wounded feelings until Frieda moved back and forth between them, explaining, humoring and finally establishing the usual equilibrium.

Frieda believed that she knew all her parents' secrets. Later she heard them sharing their worries about the hereditary deafness which began to afflict both of them quite early. This kind of handicap in both parents would prejudice the girls' marriageability considerably, particularly as they were already deficient in the matter of a proper dowry.

Klara started to become deaf after Anna's birth. She bore her impediment with her usual aplomb. Riding the train in England in her eighties she would wear a large sign around her neck asking her fellow passengers to, "Please put me out in Birmingham." Adolf, more sensitive and painfully aware that his whole family depended on his capacity to earn a living in an occupation which required the ability to communicate, became increasingly depressed. In the last years of his life his desk was covered with useless, complicated contraptions which were to help him bridge the growing gap between himself and others. In 1924, shortly before his retirement, he was mysteriously killed in a fall down an elevator shaft at the bank. Frieda later said that he had been despondent and

might have contributed, at least unconsciously, to his own death.

The same hereditary deafness which had afflicted her parents also cast its deepening shadow over the last decade of Frieda's life. It was a major, if by no means the only factor causing the increasing sadness and isolation of those years.

Back in Koenigsberg, more than forty years earlier, Klara had to organize a group of progressive Jewish matrons to get a private tutorial group started for their daughters when Frieda reached high school age. The public "gymnasium" was still closed to girls. Frieda passed the "Abitur," the University entrance examination, with flying colors. When it was time to decide what course her future career should take, a family conference was called. The position of language teacher was considered, as Frieda had a natural aptitude for this, but--for once--Adolf prevailed with his opinion that medicine would provide the widest opportunity for a young Jewish woman at a time when there was still considerable discrimination in the public school system.

Frieda entered medical school at the University of Konigsberg daringly attired, with the progressive Klara's approval, in "reform" dresses without the stiff collar and whalebone underpinnings which were customary at that time. There was only a handful of pioneering women among hundreds of male students. She was teased and harassed by many of the elderly male professors and even her fellow students occasionally let a door fly in her face. Yet, along with the struggles, there were dances and flirtations, but Frieda knew what was expected of her. She was well-launched on her course to fulfill her parents' dreams and an early marriage was not part of their plans for her.

Frieda's maternal, nurturing yearnings were already strongly developed. During her obstetrical training, she became entranced with the infants and would irritate the nurses by competing with them for the infants' care. The fact that she was to have no children of her own was particularly tragic for someone who loved them as much as she did. During the early years of her career she would temporarily adopt various waifs and strays, always with the greatest confidence, but occasionally with questionable results.

Because her tiny stature precluded a career in obstetrics, she chose the field of psychiatry for which she felt equal enthusiasm. Early on she had recognized her special gift for communicating with disturbed individuals. When she observed the famous Kraepelin interviewing a patient during her fourth year of medical school, she found him insensitive and thought confidentially to herself, "This I could do better."

She was licensed to practice psychiatry and neurology in 1914, just before the onset of the First World War. As we have seen, she began her career with many assets. Good health, energy, self-confidence, talent, sensitivity, a boundless capacity for hard work and the fervent desire to fulfill her parents' expectations. She was well equipped to assume a position of leadership in a field still dominated by men.

Yet she also carried with her certain liabilities which were to prevent her from having as complete and rich a life as she might have wished. Her mother's message that marriage is "terrible" even under the best of circumstances must have found its mark. Frieda was the close friend, protege and collaborator of several much older married men before she married at 35, when she already looked plump and elderly, the charming, brilliant, 24-year-old Erich Fromm. He had initially been her analysand. It was well known in the Reichmann family that Fromm disliked children. This marriage certainly closed the door to any hope she might still have had for children of her own. Although Frieda remained on friendly terms with Fromm, the end of the marriage, when she was about 40 years old, caused her great pain and as far as we know she never again attempted to establish a life with another man.

She was an endless source of strength and support for her family, friends and patients. During the years of Nazi persecution, when hundreds of friends and relatives were scattered all over the world, she often supported as many as a dozen individuals at a time with regular monthly stipends, in addition to more sporadic help for many others. She was somewhat in the role of the oldest sister,

the authority figure, and she found it difficult to lean on others, to share her own sorrows and disappointments. Her friends would notice a hurt look when a young godchild turned away from her; they worried about the merciless way in which she drove herself even as she got older. The light in her cottage on the grounds of Chestnut Lodge would burn until late at night and they knew she was sitting up working on a paper or a lecture, chain-smoking and drinking strong coffee. The end came unexpectedly at age 68 with a sudden heart attack when she was alone in the cottage.

Frieda had enjoyed her success. She liked being an authority figure before whom "people moved back as if she were parting the Red Sea." Years earlier, she had felt that the walls would part before her mother as Klara approached them. She had fulfilled her mother's as well as her own expectations, but, like many other women pioneers, she had also paid a price. She would have been pleased to hear the 27-year-old Perri Klass, Harvard medical school student, published novelist and mother of a young child say in a recent interview: "Women are not pioneers in medicine any more. The burden that falls on pioneers is not ours. Pioneers have a special kind of heroism which absorbs all their energy. They dare not be the first one to go home at night, or to have a baby . . . ."[2] Perri Klass, aware of the debt she owes to Frieda Fromm-Reichmann and other women pioneers is finally allowed to have it all.

References

[1]Draft of a paper by Laurice McAfee, M.D., reporting on an interview with Joanne Greenberg. Presented at Chestnut Lodge Symposium, October, 1985.
[2]New York Magazine, October 14, 1985, p. 63.

9

Marion E. Kenworthy, M.D.:
Trailblazer for Psychiatric Social Work

Viola W. Bernard, M.D.

Clinical Professor Emerita,
College of Physicians and Surgeons,
Columbia University,
New York, New York

This chapter was originally published in June 1979, shortly before Dr. Kenworthy's death in 1980, as the first in a series of profiles of famous living American psychiatrists, in PSYCHIATRIC ANNALS Vol. 9, No. 6. The profile is reprinted here, with minor revisions, with the kind permission of PSYCHIATRIC ANNALS and of SLACK, Incorporated.

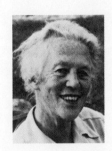 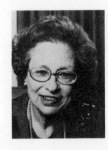

Marion E. Kenworthy, M.D.   Viola W. Bernard, M.D.

9

Marion E. Kenworthy, M.D.:
Trailblazer for Psychiatric Social Work

It seems appropriate indeed that a profile of Dr. Kenworthy, as a pioneer leader in academia as well as president of national organizations, be included in this historical review of medical women's leadership roles. The evolution of psychiatry in America has been achieved by a succession of noted pioneers. Study of their contributions not only is of absorbing interest but also can serve as a crucial corrective to our tendency to repeat mistakes and to rediscover the wheel. To learn about the lives and achievements of these early forebears of our discipline, we have to resort, for the most part, to writings by and about them. Happily, some of us came to know, as older colleagues, those outstanding figures in our field whose long careers represent a significant portion of psychiatric history in this country. They brought that history to life more vividly than could the printed page alone, through their own recollections and through their myriad personal and professional relationships with many of us, in so many ways over so many years.

But younger generations of analysts, psychiatrists, and other mental-health professionals--or those still in training--have lacked the privilege of such relationships; many are unaware of these pioneering leaders and of their influential impact on present-day psychiatry and its allied fields. Through this book, younger colleagues can become better acquainted with these remarkable women, and learn why they deserve a permanent place in the history of American psychiatry.

Looming large among them is Marion E. Kenworthy, M.D., the subject of this chapter. The editors of this volume sought not a eulogy, but a real-life picture that could convey Marion's professional significance and stature in human, personal terms.

Perhaps a good way to begin is to give an example of how, from her youth, Marion was always ahead of her time in recognizing human needs, devising new ways to meet them, and going into vigorous action to do so. Thus, a pressing concern for psychiatry now, in the idiom of today, is to innovate and monitor transitional settings for deinstitutionalized patients to improve their return to community life. Some 70 years ago, young Dr. Kenworthy originated a family-care program for patients who no longer needed hospital care but who were not yet well enough to live independently without an intervening sheltered and supervised environment. Twice a month, she drove her horse and buggy around the country byways, even in the fierce New England winters, making rounds of her family-placed patients.

Marion was born on August 17, 1891. Her parents were of English background, her mother a descendant of early settlers who had come over on the Mayflower, her father a businessman. The family lived not far from Concord, Massachusetts, the home of Ralph Waldo Emerson, whose writings meant much to Marion throughout her life, and to whom she was related on her mother's side. It was here that she first developed talents in taking care of animals and other growing things. Later, as a medical student in 1912 or so, she developed a therapeutic gardening program for mental patients.

Marion later said that her determination to become a physician originated early in her childhood, when her mother died of tuberculosis. If she became a doctor, the little girl decided, she would be able to help people get well. A look back at the childhood decision today, some 85 years later, makes it clear that Marion Kenworthy spent a lifetime doing just that!

It was unusual and hard for women to be doctors in those days, but Marion would not be deterred. She scorned her father's suggestion that she study nursing instead, and she entered medical school. She obtained her medical degree from Tufts Medical School with honors in 1913 and was the first woman physician at the Gardner [Massachusetts] State Colony for Chronic Mental Patients. It was at Gardner that she originated the family-care plan mentioned above.

Marion Kenworthy is most renowned today for her unique, pioneering and sustained contributions to the development of psychiatric social work and its relationships to psychiatry. Often referred to as the Mother or Patron Saint of psychiatric social work, she first introduced psychiatry into the curriculum of a school of social work. This was back in 1929, at the New York School of Social Work, later the Columbia University School of Social Work. She retired from the University 36 years later as Professor Emeritus in Psychiatry, with the Marion E. Kenworthy Professorial Chair established in her honor.

The immense impact of this one person on the whole of social work, and the areas of human welfare with which it entwines, continued on after her retirement and her death in 1980. The ripple effects of what she set in motion can be seen today in the teaching of the leading social work educators who were her students, and in the greater respect for social work and social workers among psychiatrists, which she brought about. This respect can be seen in the attitude held by many psychiatrists today, an attitude she transmitted through personal example that demonstrated the all-out responsiveness to human need that Marion believed was basic to the "helping professions."

Marion Kenworthy was an important part of my own personal and professional life since the early 1930s and so, rather than attempt any systematic chronology of her life and work, I shall draw on my own recollections and those of others close to her, aided by conversations I had with Marion herself in the months before she died. I would also recommend to readers a 1956 booklet written by Albert Deutsch, himself a gifted writer and devoted friend of Marion's.[1] The booklet contains, in addition to Deutsch's warm and discerning biographic sketch, a final section of letters "from the tribunal of her contemporaries." The writers make up a roster of leaders--all her close associates--in American medicine, psychiatry, child psychiatry, social work, mental health, and public life. Among those in the latter category are the late Eugene Meyer, then publisher of the *Washington Post*, a long-time friend and an ally in publicly airing urgent psychiatric problems; David Heyman, president of the New York Foundation, which supported many mental-health projects on Marion's advice; and President Dwight Eisenhower, who wrote in appreciation of Marion's "work and counsel on the role of women in the armed forces" and of her "long and dedicated service to the welfare of our country."

The purpose of the brochure was "to memorialize for public appreciation the highlights of the remarkable career of an outstanding figure." This "remarkable career" by no means stopped with Marion's retirement from Columbia. She continued a busy private practice and a huge amount of organizational and consultative work. Her many honors after her retirement included the honorary degree of Doctor of Medical Science from the Woman's Medical College of Pennsylvania in 1968, the 1971 Agnes Purcell McGavin Award of the American Psychiatric Association for outstanding contributions to child psychiatry and, in 1973, the honorary degree of Doctor of Science from Columbia University.

Deutsch's account not only covers the range of Marion's accomplishments up to 1957 but also catches the flavor of her personality. I cannot refrain from retelling the revealing and endearing anecdote with which he opens his portrait. It concerns a piglet, the runt of a litter, that could not have survived had not Dr. Kenworthy brought it in from the country to her beautifully furnished city home, nursing and feeding it with an eye dropper until it could return to the farm, where it flourished. As Deutsch recognized, "The incident reflects Dr. Kenworthy's love for living things--plant, animal, or human--her instinct for doctoring, her basic optimism, her readiness to accept a challenge in the face of heavy odds." Although some might think it peculiar to rear a pig in a Fifth Avenue apartment, Deutsch goes on to say, "Far from being eccentric, she is an archetype of the down-to-earth, matter-of-fact, pragmatic American."

By the time I came to know Marion, in the late 1920s, she was already a psychoanalyst, living and teaching in New York City, having moved from Massachusetts in 1919. Those earlier professional years engaged her in what Deutsch referred to as "an exuberant cross-fertilizing fellowship in an exciting period of professional ferment." Psychiatry was changing under the impact of psychoanalysis. Ernest Southard, who Marion said influenced her most profoundly, was stressing the significance of the social environment and the value of social workers in the study and care of mental patients (community and social psychiatry were *not* born, full-blown, in the 1960s); Healy and Bronner, pioneers in child psychiatry and delinquency studies, had founded the famous Judge Baker Guidance Center in Boston, where Marion worked during the summer of 1920. Meanwhile, significant changes in social work--its theory and practice, especially casework--were bringing it closer to psychiatry. This convergence was furthered by the Mental Hygiene Movement founded by Clifford Beers in 1909.

In 1921 Marion took an important step that led to her developing the specialized field of psychiatric social work. A Bureau of Children's Guidance was established by the New York School of Social Work, supported by the Commonwealth Fund. Dr. Bernard Glueck was named its director, and Marion was its associate director and later its medical director.

The Bureau conducted a child guidance clinic for the study and treatment of children with behavior problems. The clinic, in turn, provided a fieldwork setting for practical training in psychiatric social work. This project--nearly 600 disturbed children were treated--was the first clinic run by a school of social work. Marion described it, in collaboration with Porter Lee, then head of the social work school, in their book *Mental Hygiene and Social Work*.[2] It includes a formulation by Marion of her psychoanalytically oriented ego-libido method for casework assessment of personality. This became central to her teaching for many years.

In the course of time, generations of social-work educators, many of them her former students, came to challenge the validity of this method, which was hard for Marion to accept. However, as one of the more outstanding scholars among them, Professor Gordon Hamilton, is quoted as saying, "When social workers needed desperately to understand the human personality in structural terms, she gave them that structure in her ego-libido method. I happen to believe this method is now outmoded . . . but none can deny the great value of her original contribution."

As a first year medical student in 1932, my intent was to become a psychiatrist and psychoanalyst, and I was deeply disappointed by the dull and descriptive nature of my first year psychiatry course at medical school. I therefore wangled my way into the evening section of Dr. Kenworthy's dynamic course, "Personality and Behavior," for social work students at the New York School, and audited it throughout the year. Thus began a long association packed with far more in the way of personal and professional experiences than can be conveyed in these pages.

Marion's focus on the interactions of psychodynamics and environmental variables in the development and functioning of personality, her stress on prevention, child development, and family dynamics, and her adherence to a clinical-team approach markedly influenced my own career. From the outset, she gave constant encouragement and opened many opportunities for me. Early in my career she invited me to teach a section of her course at the social work school, and I took over her teaching assignments during World War Two, when she went on a flying mission to military installations in the Pacific for General Eisenhower. General Marshall had become impressed by Marion at a meeting on psychiatric issues of the WAVES and WACS, when she exploded with an undeleted expletive at some foolishness, and had recommended her to Eisenhower. This distinguished and gracious lady could, indeed, swear like a trooper when her sense of righteous indignation was aroused, something that occurred fairly often.

As I review the decades after that, it is striking to note the many and varied ways in which I worked with Marion. This made it possible to see her in action in a wide range of important professional positions: as Professor of Psychiatry at Columbia University School of Social Work, as the first woman vice president of the American Psychiatric Association, as president of the Group for the Advancement of Psychiatry, as president of the American Academy of Child Psychiatry, and as president of the American Psychoanalytic Association. (She was the first woman to serve as president of the last three organizations.)

Readers may wonder how one person could fill so many high offices. The wonder grew for me as I came to see and appreciate--through my own activities in each of these organizations--the quality and commitment of her leadership. For Marion, such posts were not medals to wear but rather opportunities to work harder than ever for progress in psychiatry. She drove herself and her co-workers to efforts that were extraordinary (and sometimes rather taxing for the rest of us mere mortals).

In 1932 I introduced a friend of my childhood, Justine Wise Polier, to Marion. They became fast friends and close associates in many endeavors. As Judge Polier became active in larger areas of work--juvenile justice, child welfare and human rights--both Marion and I worked closely with her. Related efforts in law and psychiatry developed. This was especially true as we tried to integrate mental health concepts and services inside and outside the Juvenile Court, in cooperation with many colleagues and concerned citizens. Some of the committees, agencies, and *ad hoc* groups in which we joined forces were the Wiltwyck School for Boys; the Citizens' Committee for Children of New York; Louise Wise Services, a multi-service children's agency; and the *ad hoc* Non-Sectarian Committee for Refugee Children. This last group sought to rescue children from the Nazis through federal legislation that would permit thousands of them to enter this country. Marion worked indefatigably on this effort, for which she brought together an influential group that included Marshall Field, Rabbi Stephen Wise, Louis S. Weiss, an attorney, Ben Cohen of the Washington "Brain Trust," and Clarence Pickett, director of the American Friends Service Committee.

Many innovative projects were hatched and efforts launched during long evening meetings held in Marion's living room. These included a series of efforts to strengthen mental health services both in the Children's Court and in the public schools. In the Children's Court, for example, a treatment clinic was begun in cooperation with the School of Social Work. A demonstration men-

tal health project was carried out in three Harlem schools. When funds were needed for causes that Marion considered important, one of her frequent expressions was that she would take her "little tin cup and raise the money." The cup seemed bottomless.

Even when she was deep in her eighties and too plagued by illness to continue her practice, Marion still responded to a telephone call from a former patient like a firehorse to the bell, with characteristic concern and helpfulness. Shortly before she died, I asked her what she felt was her most characteristic trait. Without a moment's hesitation she replied, "My stick-to-it-iveness." She was absolutely right. When Marion believed in something or someone, her commitment was profound and enduring. Her staying power on behalf of her goals and convictions was extraordinary. "You don't let yourself be disappointed," she said, "and you stay with it." Stay with it she always did!

The same was true of her personal loyalties and, I should add, of her antipathies. These were unshakable to the point, at times, of diminishing the objectivity of her judgment, for I do not wish to portray Marion as an idealized paragon of perfection. One's faults often stem from one's virtues. Her "stick-to-it-iveness" was a fundamental source of her unique strengths; yet she could also be unduly stubborn, and she had trouble changing her long-cherished convictions, even on occasions when it seemed appropriate. But these minor flaws were insignificant to those of us who saw Marion in her human totality.

By juxtaposing two disparate kinds of tributes that she evoked, I can perhaps convey some sense of that totality. On Marion's living room mantle stood two framed photographs: one of General Marshall, the other of President Eisenhower. Both photos bore autographed messages that conveyed the feelings for her of these two world figures. Another kind of tribute came from Kitty, a girl with little schooling, who worked in Marion's household for many years. Kitty came from a country village and was a devout Catholic. Once, on her return from a trip to Ireland, she told a friend, "The priests say only Catholics go to heaven. But I'm sure they couldn't have meant to leave out Dr. Kenworthy just because she's Protestant."

And so, Marion Kenworthy's childhood goal to study medicine was richly fulfilled by this truly admirable woman and the physician she became.

References

[1]Deutsch, Albert. *Dr. Marion E. Kenworthy: A Commemorative.* New York: New York School of Social Work, 1956. (Two of Deutsch's books, *The Shame of the States* and *The Mentally Ill in America*, were forceful weapons in the fight to reform patient care.)

[2]Lee, P. R. and M. E. Kenworthy. *Mental Hygiene and Social Work.* New York: Commonwealth Fund Division of Publications, 1929.

10

Clara Thompson, M.D.:
Unassuming Leader

Ruth Moulton, M.D.

*Training and Supervising Analyst,
William Alanson White Institute,
New York, New York*

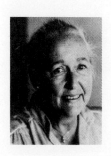 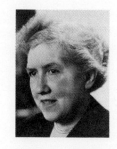

Ruth Moulton, M.D.   Clara Thompson, M.D.

10

Clara Thompson, M.D.:
Unassuming Leader

Clara Thompson was born in the rural outskirts of Providence, Rhode Island, amid the tensions of a large, extended family. They all belonged to the same Baptist church but her mother was the strict religious observer and the disciplinarian of the family, while her father whom she adored was more imaginative, a successful, self-made man who rose to be president of an outstanding drug company. Her paternal grandfather had been a rigger of whaling ships. She identified with her father, loved the sea as he did and enjoyed vacations in Orchard Beach, Maine. However, she had constant conflict with her mother. Her brother, nine years younger, was her mother's favorite and was never close to Clara. Clara was both a serious student who joined the debating team, and also a "tomboy" who enjoyed swimming, boating and basketball. In high school she intended to become a medical missionary and stood at the head of her class in every subject.

In 1912 she began her pre-medical course at Pembroke, the college for women of Brown University, and continued to live at home. During this time she was seen by her friends as warm and quiet, with an undemanding level of friendliness but also as lonely and embittered. She gave up going to church, abandoned the idea of being a missionary and thus precipitated an estrangement from her mother that lasted 20 years. A major in the U.S. Medical Corps fell in love with her and asked her to marry him but only if she would give up her medical career. She was very fond of him, but felt she could not make this sacrifice.

They ended their relationship, but she remained deeply troubled, guilty about rejecting him, not sure that she had done the right thing for herself and uncertain of her future as a woman doctor. She was graduated from college in 1916, a member of Phi Beta Kappa and Sigma Xi, seen as brilliant but unhappy. In the yearbook she said her future plans were to "Murder people in the most refined way possible." This would seem to be an effort to overcome her early role as "the dutiful child" quietly suppressing her rebellion and wishing to be more assertive. (Note paper, "Dutiful Child Resistance" in *Psychoanalytic Review*, 1941.)

When Clara entered the Johns Hopkins Medical School in 1916 she had not decided on a specialty, although she had worked one summer with mental patients at Danvers State Hospital in Massachusetts. In her second year at Hopkins she met Lucille Dooley, who had taken her doctorate in psychology at Clark University under G. Stanley Hall and had participated in the 1910 conference where she heard Freud, Jung, and Adolph Meyer. Dooley was the first person who could discuss psychoanalysis with Clara in a knowledgeable way. This resulted in Clara's working at St. Elizabeths Hospital, Washington, D.C., in the summer of 1918 where she met William Alanson White, superintendent, and Edward Kempf, his associate. White was a fine clinician, an excellent teacher and had a broad interest in the social sciences which appealed to Clara. Harry Stack Sullivan also developed deep respect for White when he came to St. Elizabeths in 1921. White modernized St. Elizabeths, popularized psychoanalysis while criticizing its rigidities, led the mental hygiene movement, initiated a training school for nurses, taught Sullivan and encouraged Clara. Phipps Clinic was fully integrated into the Johns Hopkins Medical School and Dr. Adolph Meyer, as Chief, was able to develop a comprehensive psychiatric curriculum and used his theory of "psychobiology," which also emphasized the importance of environmental factors in patients' lives and emotional illnesses. Clara had her psychiatric residency under him from 1922 to 1925 and was in charge of his private patients in 1924. In 1923, she met Sullivan who became a trusted colleague and life-long friend. They were drawn together by their experiences of loneliness and their interest in therapy with very sick patients. (Her first paper was on "Manic-Depressive Psychosis," 1930.)

Also in 1924 Clara entered psychoanalytic treatment with Dr. Joseph C. Thompson, with whom she had great rapport. Meyer's disapproval of this led him to dismiss her from Phipps in 1925. Sullivan was of great help to her during this crisis and later suggested that she go to Ferenczi who had lectured at the New School for Social Research in New York City in 1927. She went to Budapest, Hungary to work with Ferenczi during the summers of 1928 and 1929 and then left Baltimore to complete her treatment with him in 1931. This ended with his sudden death in 1933 at which point she started private practice in New York City. Ferenczi had espoused the need for a more open, sincere relationship between analyst and patient that was very compatible with Sullivan's concepts on interpersonal relationships. Ferenczi had a much more positive regard for the role of women and mothers as compared to Freud; he believed in a reconstructive emotional experience in analysis and eventually came to a new approach called "relaxation therapy." In 1932, his paper, "Confusion of Tongues between Adult and Child," attacked the professional hypocrisy of psychoanalytic detachment and precipitated his open break with Freud. Thus, Ferenczi, with his emphasis on parents and early family atmosphere, added yet another dimension to Clara's humanistic, pragmatic point of view. None of her significant mentors or colleagues accepted an orthodox stand. A common interest "to put psychoanalysis into a social context" was shared by White, Sul-

livan, Ferenczi, Horney, and Fromm.

In New York City in 1933 Clara renewed her contacts with Sullivan and Silverberg, both there from Washington, and became friends with Karen Horney who had left Chicago and her association with Franz Alexander. They formed a "Zodiac Club"--Sullivan was a horse, Silverberg a gazelle, Horney a water buffalo and Clara a puma, based on her love of cats. Eric Fromm later joined them and taught psychoanalytic psychology at the New York School for Social Research. Clara tried at this time to analyze Sullivan, but found it difficult and short-lived. He was trying to establish a White Foundation in New York City but found it infeasible even after acquiring a brownstone in the East Sixties to house it. He returned to Washington in 1937 when White died and developed the Foundation there.

Clara taught basic readings in psychoanalysis at the New York Psychoanalytic Institute from 1934 to 1941. This was based on Freud and his early followers--Jung, Rank, Adler, and Ferenczi. Careful appraisal of Freud's early libido and instinct theories led to an increasingly critical evaluation, less acceptable to the American Psychoanalytic Association. The end result was Clara's book in 1950, "Psychoanalysis: Evolution and Development," with Patric Mullahy, which became the text for her first year course at the William Alanson White Institute for many years.

Horney published "New Ways in Psychoanalysis" in 1939 and Fromm's book "Escape from Freedom" was translated into English in 1941. Both books provoked the New York Psychoanalytic Institute, then under the sway of the orthodox European analysts, and precipitated the first "split." Training privileges were withdrawn from Horney, who was popular with students but seen by the hierarchy as disruptive. Clara resigned along with Karen Horney (see her letter of spring, 1941), Sarah Kelman, Harmon Ephron and Bernard Robbins who marched down Fifth Avenue after a final meeting, singing "Go Down Moses . . . ." They were joined by other dissidents such as Harold Kelman, Judd Marmor and a group of students of Thompson, Horney and Kardiner who, somehow, had never "graduated" from the New York Psychoanalytic Institute because they did not totally agree with the orthodox concepts. Together they formed the Association for the Advancement of Psychoanalysis with Silverberg of New York Medical College as first president. Horney was dean of this new group and a rivalry developed between her and Fromm, a popular teacher at the New York School for Social Research. Clara soon discovered that no new students were being referred to her or to Fromm. Horney then deprived Fromm of his training status in 1943, presumably because he was not an M.D. and thus was a threat to the liaison with Flower-Fifth Avenue Hospital. Stephen Jewett, then head of their Department of Psychiatry, however, said he had no prejudices against qualified Ph.D.'s. The M.D.-Ph.D. issue was probably a red herring because two years later Horney and Kelman founded their own training school, dropping the medical affiliation.

In the spring of 1943, Thompson, Janet Rioch and Fromm, with the help of David Rioch, Sullivan and Frieda Fromm-Reichmann from Washington, formed the New York Branch of the Washington School of Psychiatry. Ralph Crowley joined the group in 1946 after his service in the navy. He had been a training and supervising analyst in the Washington-Baltimore Psychoanalytic Institute since 1935. The only students to leave Horney were Ruth Foster and Ruth Moulton who followed their analysts. Clara's male students (Gene Eisner, Leon Goldensohn, Ed Kasin, Meyer Maskin, Ed Tauber and Ed Weinstein) were still in the armed forces.

Clara became the executive director of the New York branch which she remained until her death in 1958. This was a period of real fulfillment for her. She worked six days a week, attended many classes, went to Washington to teach every two or three weeks, welcomed veteran candidates back from the war, entertained on Sundays in the City and on New Year's Eve, trying to bring people together in an informal atmosphere. She may have feared that she overdid it, as shown in her paper about "An institute is not a home."[1]

In terms of contributions to the psychology of women, the decade of the forties was one of fruition for Clara. She had many sources of inspiration other than her own struggles as a professional woman in a culture, still patriarchal, which made it hard to combine career with marriage and motherhood. She also had unique sources of inspiration beginning with the influence of Lucille Dooley, who was the first woman in America to write on "The Genesis of Psychological Sex Differences." Dooley had made observations of two three-year-old girls, who instead

of envying the little boy's penis, mistook it for a tag of hanging flesh. She thus joined Horney in saying that penis envy was not the universal cornerstone on which female sexuality rested. Freud had found American women "unfeminine" but Jones had found more "femininity in the little girl than most analysts liked to believe."[2] Ferenczi also had a more positive, admiring attitude toward women, saying that they had a harder role than men because they had to become the *mother* while men could always get a mother by having a wife who could satisfy their dependency needs in a culturally acceptable, hidden fashion.[3]

In 1939 Clara reviewed Ferenczi's paper on "Thalassa, A Theory of Genitality." She was also able to discuss with Horney the latter's papers on female sexuality written in German from 1924 to 1933. With this background, Thompson made her own perceptive observations on women within their cultural milieu and wrote her own papers which were lucid and pragmatic: "The Role of Women in This Culture," (1941) and "Penis Envy in Women" (1943) and others (see bibliography). Among her pithy phrases were "The unconscious of woman lags far behind" (1941), "There is a new restlessness in women, typical when an old role in the culture begins to fail" (influenced by Fromm), "The penis may be a symbol of aggression and penis envy is often the envy women have of the position of men in our society," "Woman's problem is not to become reconciled to the lack of a penis but to accept her unique sexuality in its own right." These concepts now have much more widespread acceptance but were quite exceptional in their clarity and clinical usefulness in the 1940's.

Another important aspect of her decade of greatest happiness were her close friendships in Provincetown. Clara bought an old saltbox cottage on the bay in Provincetown, Massachusetts, which she dearly loved. The interchange between the Portuguese fishermen and the artists, beginning with Hawthorne, made for a zestful, lively community, so different from the tight New England atmosphere of Chatham and Hyannis. One important person for her was Henry Major, a Hungarian painter, who used her garage as a studio. She entertained a mixture of artists and analytic folk on Saturday nights--evenings that were most stimulating. She swam twice daily, following the love of her father's family and scheduled her patients to fit the tides. Another loyal friend was

Philip Malicoat, a painter and student of Hawthorne who loved the use of subtle shades in landscapes and seascapes. He also did carpentry and made her picture window and benches for her cottage, redid her worn-out desk (a painting of the latter, buffeted by waves, hangs in the White Institute, W.A.W.I.). She willed her cottage to him, and his sculpter son, Conrad, made her unusual and controversial tombstone.

These happy days came to an end with the death of a man she cared for in the late 1940's. Clara fought against loneliness and immersed herself in the problems of the new Institute. Then Sullivan died in January 1949, and Fromm moved to Mexico. The American Psychoanalytic Association became increasingly stringent in its standards, allowed only one analytic institute per city and refused the application of the W.A.W.I. (William Alanson White Institute) to be included as a training group. There was debate as to whether it was better to belong and work from within or separate and grow autonomously. Only the latter, without risking loss of identity and integrity was possible. When the American Psychoanalytic Association tried to rescind the training status of the W.A.W.I. senior analysts in 1952, Abe Fortas brought a lawsuit against them for "restriction of trade," for labeling the W.A.W.I. "unethical" when there was no definition of "psychoanalysis" agreed upon (1953-54).

Clara deeply wanted a national organization to accept her graduates, Ph.D's included. This resulted in the formation of the Academy of Psychoanalysis in 1956 with Janet Rioch as first president. Clara found the Academy a disappointment, as a group of rather chauvinistic men managed to arrange that only M.D.'s were acceptable as members. It was founded as a liberal organization, a free forum for scientific interchange, but Ph.D.'s could only be scientific associates. This political division has influenced the peace of mind of the W.A.W.I. ever since and the entrenched power of the medical community grows with current inflation and the disillusionment with psychoanalysis as oversold in recent decades.

Clara died of metastasis of a malignant rectal polyp in December, 1958. Few could call this the result of a "broken heart" but it might almost have been so.

Clara had a multifaceted personality. She dubbed herself "the silent Swede," a reticent, shy girl who felt like an outsider in a tight, religious New England family. She rebelled against authority and the church, only to lose contact with her mother, with bitter feelings and loneliness. She always had a capacity to be a warm, understanding, non-judgmental friend and was very encouraging and supportive to her students and analysands almost to a fault. Some felt she never confronted them sufficiently with their hostility. She was renowned for her integrity and honesty; she said what she meant and never played politics. She refused to pretend she did not train Ph.D.'s in order to appease the American Psychoanalytic Association, who did so only under a discreet, misleading cover. She refused to be tactful and ambiguous in 1951-1952 when negotiating with the American Psychoanalytic Association. She preferred to "go her own way" unfettered by pretensions. Only history will tell whether her preference for independence "paid off" in the long run or caused isolation, separation and inbreeding. It certainly gave the W.A.W.I. its distinction and autonomy. We may have more resilience to face future stress since the institute began with the conviction that psychoanalysis was still in an experimental stage of development, dogmatism in psychoanalytic education was to be avoided, and premature crystallization of theories would restrict growth. (See May 1941 letter of resignation from the American Psychoanalytic Association.) Clara wanted her colleagues not to be misled by an illusion of certainty, but to share her belief in the continuing evolution of ideas.

References

[1]Thompson C: A Study of the Emotional Climate of Psychoanalytic Training Institutes. Psychiatry Vol. 21, 1958, pp. 45-51.
[2]Moulton R: Survey and Re-evaluation of the Concept of Penis Envy. Contemporary Psychoanalysis. Vol. VI, No. 1, Fall, 1970.
[3]Moulton R: Early Papers on Women: Horney to Thompson 1921-1951. Amer Jnl of Psychoanalysis, 35, 1975, pp. 207-223.

Bibliography

Green M, editor: Interpersonal Psychoanalysis: The Selected Papers of Clara Thompson. (Her biography and bibliography are at the end). Basic Books, 1964.

Perry HS: Psychiatrist of America: The Life of Harry Stack Sullivan. Harvard University Press, 1982. (See Chap. 24, "Clara Thompson, Dear Colleague and Friend").

Quen J and Carlson E, editors: American Psychoanalysis: Origins and Development. Brunner-Mazel, 1978. (See esp. pp. 136-138 and pp. 156-158 on the formation of the Academy of Psychoanalysis)

Thompson C: History of W.A.W.I. for Sullivan Society. March, 1955 (Mimeograph copies in Institute).

Thompson C: On Women. Mentor Books, 1971.

William Alanson White Institute Newsletter, Thompson Memorial Issue, Vol. 7, no. 1, March 1959.

William Alanson White Institute Newsletter, on Twenty-Fifth Anniversary. Vol. 3, no. 1, Fall 1968.

William Alanson White Institute Newsletter, Thompson paperback published. Vol. 6, no. 2, Winter 1971-2.

William Alanson White Institute Newsletter, Clara Thompson, Analyst and Friend by Ruth Moulton. Vol. 8, no. 1, Fall 1973.

11

Anna Freud:
Bold Investigator and Model Builder

Albert Solnit, M.D.

*Sterling Professor of Pediatrics and Psychiatry,
School of Medicine and Child Study Center,
Yale University,
New Haven, Connecticut*

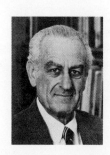

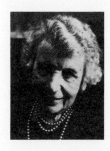

Albert Solnit, M.D.
Photograph by T. Charles Erickson

Anna Freud

11

Anna Freud:
Bold Investigator and Model Builder

Although Anna Freud's leadership in psycho-analysis was well established before she and her family moved to England, her creativity came to full flower in England after the death of her father in 1939. Throughout her long career Anna Freud had a clear preference for privacy. However, she was willing to make a reasonable compromise of this preference if it would help to support and disseminate the works and findings of psychoanalysis, particularly child analysis.

In 1977 she wrote to her long time friend and colleague, Muriel Gardiner:

> *I get letters from strangers from time to time urging me to write my memoirs, almost as if it were my duty to do it. But of course that is the last thing I would be able to do. I cannot share my feelings with the reading public and there is too much feeling bound up with the past, and above all the part of the past in which others would be interested. So, I allow myself the privilege of taking it all with me.*[1]

Thus, a preference for privacy and an insistence that her scientific, clinical and teaching activities be judged by their results, rather than by her personal charisma, were hallmarks of her leadership.

Born in Vienna, Austria, on December 3, 1895, the youngest of 6 children of Sigmund and Martha Freud, Anna Freud was the only one to become a psychoanalyst. She began her professional career as an elementary school teacher, stimulated by the contributions of Maria Montessori. She was educated at the College Lyceum, a Viennese girls' school where she also taught for many years, exercising a strong influence on teacher training and directly on many of the teachers. During this period she also began a training analysis, and in 1922, at 26 years of age, she became a member of the Vienna Psychoanalytic Society. She practiced, taught and took a leading role in that Society until the Nazis forced her and her family to leave in 1938 because the Freuds were Jewish.

Overall, Anna Freud's work can be considered: 1) as guardian, advocate of and enriching contributor to her father as the creator of psychoanalysis--she was his psychoanalytic heir; 2) as pioneer in establishing child psychoanalysis; and 3) as an original, natural scientist and psychoanalyst.

Thus, Anna Freud's contributions, can be viewed in these three overlapping sectors:

1. Anna Freud was the guardian and advocate of her father and his work in creating psychoanalysis. She wrote *The Ego and the Mechanisms of Defense*,[2] first published in 1936 as an 80th birthday gift for her father. It was a brilliant seminal contribution to the enrichment and advancement of psychoanalysis as a general psychology of man. After reading the book, Sigmund Freud wrote to Arnold Zweig on April 2, 1937, "She has become an independent person who has been granted the gift of recognizing that which only confuses others."[3]

2. She was a pioneer in establishing child psychoanalysis, a new method leading to a greater knowledge about children, focusing on their inner emotional and intellectual lives. Her creation of child psychoanalysis has enabled us to know the characteristics of the healthy and the disordered developing child, and to add to and to modify our knowledge about the reconstructed child derived from adult psychoanalysis.

3. Anna Freud was also a strikingly original, natural scientist and psychoanalyst. Her innovative thinking and active collaboration in child care and health, in education and the law, and her extraordinary capacity to be practical in providing care for children caught up in "experiments" of nature and man-made catastrophes were brilliant applications of psychoanalytic theory in the service of children and their parents.

In this context, as her father's psychoanalytic heir, *Normality and Pathology in Childhood*[4] was a vital link in Anna Freud's systematizing original scholarship. She explained that *The Ego and the Mechanisms of Defense* could not be revised to incorporate newer knowledge and questions "without carrying out large-scale revisions and without incidentally destroying the unity and present circumscribed usefulness of the book."[5] In 30 years what had been new, original thinking about the functions of the ego had become accepted as everyday working knowledge in psychoanalysis.

> *If, in 1936, it was sufficient to enumerate and illustrate ego mechanisms, to inquire into their chronology, and to assess the role of the defense organization as a whole for the maintenance of health or illness, this no longer can be done today without relating the ego's defensive achievements to its other aspects, i.e. to its primary deficiencies, its apparatuses and functions, its autonomies, etc.*[5]

Thus, Anna Freud's reflection in 1966 indicated that the 1936 book, *The Ego and the Mechanisms of Defense*, was not only a classic but that it was still useful as an integral part of current psychoanalytic thinking, especially to remind psychoanalysts that "defense" is not only associated with pathology but also with normal aspects of development and coping behavior. Over and over she emphasized the unity of the child's growing personality.

Embracing her father's enlarged view of man and his world and the method that made it possible, Anna Freud elaborated and applied psychoanalysis with her own originality. Her genius encompassed psychoanalytic theory and practice, spanning the gap between them with a concentration, lucidity and scientific productivity that has been evocative and demanding. Her search for truth was intense, sustained and passionate, fortified by her penetrating logic and imagination. At the same time, she was never satisfied. She could concentrate on a motivational state, line of development or theoretical issue, and just as it appeared that she had dealt with the topic comprehensively, she reminded herself and those with whom she worked that now it was time to examine the context and the whole child, not at one age, but at least over, as she once said, "the first dozen years of his growth."[6]

Contributions to Child Analysis

Anna Freud viewed herself primarily as a psychoanalyst, not as a child or adult analyst, not as a specialist in ego psychology or psychoanalytic child development. She was a generalist in the best sense of the word. She acknowledged that psychoanalysis as a science rested on clinical, empirical findings starting as a psychology of the unconscious, of the id. In this historical perspective, she pointed out that such a restricted definition

> *immediately loses all claim to accuracy when we apply it to psychoanalytic therapy. From the beginning, analysis as a therapeutic method was concerned with the ego and its aberrations: the investigation of the id and its mode of operation was always only a means to an end. And the end was invariably the same: the correction of these abnormalities and the restoration of the ego to its integrity.*

She added,

> *We should probably define the [scholarly] tasks of analysis as follows: to acquire the fullest possible knowledge of all the three institutions of which we believe the psychic personality to be constituted and to learn what are their relations to one another and to the outside world. That is to say: in relation to the ego, to explore*

*its contents, its boundaries and its functions,
and to trace the history of its dependence on the
outside world, the id and the superego; and in
relation to the id, to give an account of the
instincts, i.e. of the id contents, and to follow
them through the transformations which they
undergo.*[5]

Even before Anna Freud introduced child psychoanalysis, there had been the effort to apply what had been learned from reconstructions in adult analysis to the upbringing of children. The preoccupation of adult analysts with

*early happenings in life . . . raised hopes in
many quarters that analysts would become experts on childhood, even when they were engaged in the therapy of adults only. Their
knowledge of the processes of mental growth,
and their understanding of the interplay between the external and internal forces which
shape the individual, were expected to qualify
them automatically for being knowledgeable in
all instances where a child's emotional stability
or normal functioning were in doubt.*[4]

These efforts gave one-sided emphasis to

*the detrimental influence of many parental and
environmental attitudes and actions such as dishonesty in sexual matters, unrealistically high
moral standards, over-strictness or over-
indulgence, frustrations, punishments or seduc-
tive behavior.*[4]

Anna Freud corrected such a misuse of psychoanalytic knowledge when she said, "In spite of the many partial advances psychoanalytic education did not succeed in becoming the preventive measure it set out to be." According to psychoanalytic tenets, there is

*no wholesale 'prevention of neurosis.' . . . By
definition, the various psychic agencies are at
cross-purpose with each other, and this gives
rise to the inner discords and clashes which
reach consciousness as mental conflicts. These
latter exist therefore wherever complex structural personality development has come into
being. There are of course instances where an
'analytic upbringing' helps the child toward
finding adequate solutions which safeguard*

*mental health; but there are also many others
where inner disharmony cannot be prevented
and becomes the starting point for one or the
other kind of pathological development.*[4]

Ironically, as Anna Freud pointed out, the analyst of adults should be in no danger of becoming an environmentalist with regard to children:

*The power of mind over matter, i.e. of the in-
ternal over the external world, is presented to
him in an unending series of examples by his
[adult] patients: in changing aspects of the
circumstances of their real life which is brought
about by their mood swings from elation to
depression; in the use made by them of elements in the environment to fit and feed unconscious fantasies; in their projections which
turn harmless, indifferent or benevolent fellow
beings into persecutors; in the distortion of the
analyst's own image which serves an irrational
and at times delusional transference, etc. It is
especially the latter which accounts for the
[adult] analyst's readiness to believe that also
in the patient's childhood similar forces were at
work, and that internal not external factors are
responsible for the causation of his illness....In
short, the analyst of adults is a firm believer in
psychic, as opposed to external, reality. If anything, he is too eager to see during his therapeutic work all current happenings in terms of
resistance and of transference, and thereby to
discount their value in reality.*[4]

With the introduction of child psychoanalysis, Anna Freud indicated there could be the integration of direct and reconstructed data for a fuller understanding of psychoanalytic child psychology, especially in connection with how the past influences present attitudes and how current experience may reshape the influence or perception of the past.

In her pioneer work in child psychoanalysis, Anna Freud viewed its tasks, in principle, to be the same as those outlined above for adults. However, she pointed out "analysis where children are concerned, requires certain modifications and adjustments, or indeed can be undertaken only subject to specific precautions."[7]

Historically, Anna Freud reported,

In Vienna, from 1927 onward, a group of analysts, later joined by colleagues from Budapest and Prague, held regular meetings with me to discuss the child-analytic technique I had suggested, to report on cases treated with this method, to compare results, and to clarify the theoretical background of our clinical findings.[8]

When Anna Freud felt she had made an error or changed her mind, like her father, she set forth clearly the corrections and reasons for them. For example, in 1974 she said,

If I now look back to my first book from the vantage point of almost a half century of psychoanalytic experience, I can only repeat here what I have affirmed on other occasions, namely that a number of statements made in my Four Lectures on Child Analysis *in 1926 have to be modified. It is no longer true that child analysts work in a psychological vacuum and cannot trust either parents or teachers to supplement their analytic efforts with the necessary educational and supporting ones. The latter burden which in earlier years used to fall on the therapist can now be shared with the child's environment in most instances. Similarly, it is much easier than it used to be for the child analysts to gain entrance into the child's hidden internal world. What used to be effected by a prolonged introductory or preparatory phase to the treatment proper is now almost invariably brought about by the scrutiny and analysis of the patient's defensive mechanisms and manuevers.*[8]

In this same introduction she indicated another change of mind when she stated:

I now agree fully that during analytic treatment children regard their analyst not only as a new object for their affectionate or hostile, sexual or aggressive impulses, or as a helping person with whom they can establish a working alliance, but that, with therapy conducted within the correct limits, multitudes of transference phenomena appear--that the child displayed toward his original objects. I cannot say the same of my convictions concerning the full-blown transference neurosis as we expect it to develop in adult neurotics who undergo psychoanalytic treatment in its classic form. I believe

that in child analysis it is extremely rare that we see the original neurotic formations, [i.e. the one] linked with the parents disappear altogether to be replaced by new symptoms centered exclusively around the person of the analyst.[8]

Anna Freud's interests in the child's external world had started in the home and in the school with a concern for child-rearing, child-parent relationships, a safe nurturing environment and the care and education of the child in the nursery, day care center and school. Her dissatisfaction with understanding the child only in terms of manifest behavior was significantly overcome by her use of child psychoanalysis and her contributions to our understanding of the child's internal world. Characteristically, Anna Freud, as a generalist, advanced from the special magnified focus to the overall view of the child and his external and internal world; from the past to the present and future and from the present to the past; from viewing the burdens of childhood as they take their role in adulthood, and from tracing forward and backward the patterned interactions of id and ego-superego in a variety of developmental and historical contexts.

In speaking and writing of child analysis and mental growth, Anna Freud stated,

...normality or pathology of development is seen to depend largely on four factors: (i) on the constitutional and experiential element in the life of an individual not departing too far from what is average and expectable; (ii) on the internal agencies of the individual's personality maturing at approximately the same rate of speed, none of them being either delayed or precocious compared with the others; (iii) on external intervention being well-timed, coming neither too early nor too late; (iv) on the ego's mechanisms used to achieve the necessary compromises being age-adequate, i.e., neither too primitive nor too sophisticated.[9]

It was also characteristic of Anna Freud's scientific thinking that she started with empirical data and then modified theoretical assumptions and questions if they failed to account for her empirical observations. Next she tested them in clinical settings and applied them in practical situations. Thus, her interest in *Normality and Pathology in Childhood* led her to a more coherent view of the continuum and differentiation of healthy and deviant development as a crucial basis for the concept of developmental lines. She said, "For useful answers to the parent's questions concerning developmental issues, the external decisions under consideration [by parents] need thus to be translated into their internal implications."[4]

Anna Freud's search for a more useful and systematic method of assessing health and pathology in adults and children was unending. In adults she had made it abundantly clear that technically and diagnostically "the proper field for our observations [in the psychoanalytic situation] is always the ego."[2]

However, she also repeatedly found that attempts to use the classifications of psychopathology from adult disorders for children were unsatisfactory. She knew that even more in children than in adults the same symptom may have different meanings especially at different developmental levels, e.g. negativism or a sleep disorder, while the same underlying disorder can be expressed in different ways by different children or even at times by the same child. As a forerunner to the developmental lines, she introduced a balanced inventory of functional strengths and weaknesses of a child's personality. This inventory required that each child's psychic structures be described, qualifying these characterizations according to the individual's particular developmental capacities. This Diagnostic or Metapsychological Profile[4] became a practical "instrument which imposes balance, completeness and comparability . . . in assessment of factors within an individual case and between individual cases, and comparability of reliable assessment between analysts, with each other and in time." Its potential uses "include assessment of change over time, compilation of similar cases, comparison of differing conditions and as a training aid."[10]

The Hampstead Psychoanalytic Index, conceived by Dorothy Burlingham and co-sponsored by Anna Freud, established a systematic method of reducing psychoanalytic data in order to make reliable comparisons of children treated psychoanalytically. Of the Index, she said,

What we hope to construct by this laborious method is something of a 'collective analytic memory,' i.e. a storehouse of analytic material which places at the disposal of the single thinker and author an abundance of facts gathered by many, thereby transcending the narrow confines of individual experience and extending the possibilities for insightful study, for constructive comparisons between cases, for deductions and generalizations, and finally for extrapolations of theory from clinical therapeutic work.[11]

As Lustman pointed out, "Coming to grips with issues of categorization in data collection, data storage [data banks] and data reduction--brought Anna Freud to the concept of developmental lines,"[10] which established a basis for more rigorous studies in psychoanalysis by providing for the organization and hierarchical ordering of data collection, reduction and storage.

Thus, developmental lines is a conceptual tool that is derived from clinical observation that permits a substantial integration of knowledge. These lines have become a crucial foundation for improving our capacity to bring improved order into elaborating and refining criteria of healthy and deviant development. With this method for organizing our clinical data into appropriate hierarchies of significance, we are able to improve our nosology of neurotic illness and to use a systematic diagnostic inventory as a means of making more rational recommendations regarding treatment of other interventions. Also, the concept of developmental lines opened up a more useful view of the relationship and the continuum of childhood and adult development.

Consequently, developmental lines provided a theoretical construct from which one could examine psychoanalytic and non-psychoanalytic settings (home, day care centers, schools, etc.) with regard to the child moving from dependency to emotional self-reliance and adult object relationships; from sucking to rational eating; from wetting and soiling to bladder and bowel control; from irresponsibility to responsibility in body management; from ego-centricity to peer companionship; from the body to the toy and from play to work.

Anna Freud formulated further questions in this connection in 1981 when she said,

The child's relationship to his own body might recommend itself as a next topic. Does it not strike all teachers how willing children are to endanger themselves, and that even their six- and seven-year olds need constant watchfulness

from an adult even if this is of a less exhausting kind than the role of ever-present guardian angel which is enforced on the mother of a toddler.

Anna Freud continued,

Is there consensus about the age when the developmental steps toward recognition of danger are finally undertaken? Or, more meaningfully, how long does a child's advance in motoric skill outstrip his appreciation of potential danger?

  Another topic for developmental exploration which I can recommend is the young child's attitude toward the satisfaction of body needs such as sleep and hunger. At which level of development can we expect children simply to go to bed when they are tired or to eat when their body demands nourishment? How well known is it that toddlers have to fight sleep since, at this early date, it threatens them with separation from their objects, and somewhat later, with giving up ego functions which are extremely precious and valued as very recent, still insecurely anchored acquisitions.

Thus, in her contributions to child analysis, reaching a vital nodal point in *Normality and Pathology in Childhood,*[3] Anna Freud extended her findings by "carrying out scientifically valid research in psychoanalysis *in the absence* of laboratory conditions, quantification of results, the setting up of control groups, and other limitations."[8] This accomplishment was clearly documented by Seymour L. Lustman[10] in his paper, "The scientific leadership of Anna Freud." He further stated, "The scaffold and texture of Anna Freud's writings represent the most proficient, knowledgeable and functional grasp of the epistemological structure and function of theory [concerning development]--and may well represent her most influential long-term contribution."[12]

Applied Analysis

In reviewing Anna Freud's contributions to applied psychoanalysis, we become aware that this sector of her accomplishments, more dramatically than any other, provided a biographical/ historical account of her personal responses to children in crisis situations. To these catastrophic "experiments" created by nature and man she brought an extraordinary blend of humanitarian concern guided by her quiet courage, daring imagination and rigorous demands on herself and others that they be guided by their best knowledge in providing needed services and care. As a passionate scientist she insisted that services be critically reviewed, i.e. assessed, in order to improve the care and simultaneously to advance understanding and knowledge--to improve competence through practice and review.

In her work in applied analysis, Anna Freud was a bold investigator and model builder. In a vital sense she also prepared a future agenda for research and teaching in psychoanalysis. The agenda implied a model of psychoanalytic education, training and research. Such a model sets standards that could be used as guidelines to move forward our institutions of psychoanalytic education from part-time to full-time, in spirit if not immediately in form.

With regard to applied psychoanalysis, Anna Freud was clear and autobiographical when she said in 1966:

In this respect, I have been especially fortunate all my life. From the very beginning, I was able to move back and forth between practice and theory. I started out as an elementary school teacher. I changed from that to the field of analysis and child analysis. From then on, I moved constantly back and forth, from the theoretical study of these problems to their practical application. I agree that one has to have special luck to do this, and that most people do not have this. Personally I have to be grateful to a number of persons and institutions for giving me that opportunity. When I was still very young in my psychoanalytic studies but had learned enough to apply at least some of the knowledge, I was asked by the city of Vienna [in 1926] to make that knowledge available to teachers of nursery schools and elementary schools. I was given the opportunity to work with small groups of teachers, to discuss their practical problems with them in easy, theoretical terms. This proved to be useful to them and was immensely useful to me.[13]

  Apart from these . . . developments, Vienna had at that time also become a fertile ground for the analytic study of normal child develop-

ment and for the application of these new findings to education. *Many of us had for years been listening to inspiring lectures for teachers and youth leaders given by Siegfried Bernfeld, and many young and enthusiastic workers had joined in his educational experiment in 'Kinderheim Baumgarten', a camp school for children made homeless by World War I. Thus, the* Four Lectures for Teachers and Parents . . . *were not an independent venture of mine but were commissioned by the Board of Education of the City of Vienna, and were furthermore followed by a regular seminar for nursery school teachers conducted by Dorothy Burlingham and myself . . . . To these ventures were added in 1937 an experimental day nursery for toddlers, founded and maintained by Dr. Edith Jackson, and administered by myself in conjunction with Dorothy Burlingham and the pediatrician Dr. Josephine Stross.*[8]

At another time she extended her comments about the day nursery when she said:

(It was experimental because at that time group care for children of that age [one and two years of age] was unheard of.) The children we worked with were the most underprivileged children that could be found in Vienna. For such children, to begin education and therapy at three is much too late. Our entrance requirement was ability to walk--not necessarily to walk well, but to be able to get from one place to another, to have a certain amount of free movement. This was an excellent opportunity for us to learn and to test out some of our theoretical ideas in an active plan of day care.[5]

Thus, the sequence of her applications of psychoanalysis was significantly determined by the opportunities to respond to children's needs. As Anna Freud said:

Promising as these undertakings seemed at that time, they came to a natural end when Hitler invaded Austria in 1938. This meant not a cessation of the work itself, but rather the emigration and spread of numerous analytically trained workers to other countries and continents, foremost to England and the United States.[7]

In 1938 the Freud family was forced by the threat of the Nazis to leave Vienna. Sigmund Freud, as a Jew and as the most prominent psychoanalyst, was in great danger. After a long argument, Anna Freud succeeded in persuading the Nazi officials to take her instead of her ailing father to the Gestapo office. She returned safely the next morning after many hours of grueling and threatening interrogation.

Of Anna Freud it could be said, as she wrote of her heroic friend and colleague Muriel Gardiner:

It is possible even for lone individuals to pit their strength successfully against the sinister forces of an unjust regime...for every gang of evil-doers who take pleasure in hurting, harming and destroying, there is always at least one 'just' man or woman to help, rescue and sacrifice his or her own good for fellow-beings.[14]

Child Care

Anna Freud commented further:

World War II prompted us in England to create a direct heir to the Jackson Nursery in Vienna, i.e., the much enlarged, residential war nurseries, known under the name of 'Hampstead Nurseries' where more than 80 war babies and young children were housed from 1939-1945.[8]

This opportunity was provided, not by a person or an institution, but by an emergency, the emergency being World War II. This, of course, was a marvelous opportunity, for if anybody wanted to try out a scheme of residential care for children, what better excuse for it was there than war conditions, when the children had to be separated from their parents for reasons of safety. These war conditions, combined with the generosity of an American charity, the Foster Parents' Plan for War Children, made it possible for me and some colleagues to try out a residential scheme for a period of five years. We learned intensively and extensively how to care for 80 resident children from birth to the age of 5.[4]

This provided an unprecedented and unending source of observational material for all of us who shared in the care of [these children]. Records of these observations are laid down in the Monthly Reports to the Foster Parents' Plan for War Children, Inc....These were published in full...with the intention of offering the reader a detailed view of attempts at a psychoanalytically inspired upbringing of infants and young children, so far as this was feasible under the adverse conditions of a worldwide war. The Monthly Reports, filled as they are with accounts of coping with practical difficulties, shortages and threats from enemy action, lay no claim to scientific value. What proved of value nevertheless were the conclusions drawn by us concerning a number of topics that have vital relevance to normal and abnormal child development: the effect of separation of infant and mother at a time when the biological unity between the two partners is at its height; a comparison between developmental progression under family and residential conditions; the reactions of toddlers of community life in which the relationship to peers takes the place of the normal ties to parents or other adults in parental roles; the oedipal development in the absence of oedipal objects, especially fathers.

With the return of peace conditions, and after the Hampstead Child-Therapy Course and Clinic had taken the place of the Hampstead Nurseries, therapeutic child analysis and an intensive form of training for it came into their own once more. Maintaining the balance between clinical and applied psychoanalytic work... [gave] evidence of my spread of interest from pathology to normality in childhood; to careful assessment of the various developmental stages and their dependence on the interaction between the appropriate environmental and internal factors: to diagnostic statements based on meta psychological assessments of the immature personality; to a schema of diagnostic categories that are divorced from adult psychopathology and linked to the degree of deviation from the expected norm in childhood.[8]

This introduced me again to the whole range of problems: of day care in nurseries for normal children and for handicapped (that is, blind) children of well baby clinics and of outpatient treatment of problem children, mostly neurotic. This had two advantages for me personally. It provided an opportunity to maintain a close connection between theory and practice, to check constantly on theoretical ideas by practical application and to widen practical handling and practical measures with the growth of theoretical knowledge. It also had

another advantage. Having worked in day care, in residential care and in outpatient care, I had all the vested interests combined inside myself. If they conflicted with each other, they conflicted in me, and I could argue them out with myself without hurting anybody's feelings when finding that one or the other was better or worse than the rest.[5]

Lottie Newman,[3] in her incisive biography of Anna Freud for an international encyclopedia, described how Anna Freud used her theoretical knowledge to provide group care for children separated from their parents during World War II.

When Anna Freud found that the children's development lagged, that they were slow in overcoming reverses, she attributed these difficulties to the lack of a stable mother relationship and accordingly introduced small 'family groups,' in which about 4 children were assigned to specific workers who, as substitute mothers, were solely responsible for the physical care of these children.

The result of this arrangement was astonishing in its force and immediacy. The need for individual attachment with the feelings which had been lying dormant came out in a rush, and in the course of one week all six families were completely and firmly established. But the reactions in the beginning were far from being exclusively happy ones.

Since all these children have already undergone a painful separation from their own mothers, their mother relationship is naturally burdened with all the effects of this experience. To have a mother means to them equally the possibility of losing a mother; the love for the mother being thus closely accompanied by the hate and resentment produced by her supposed desertion.

The children showed all the signs of possessiveness, anxiety and jealousy that arise when attention has to be shared, and the formerly peaceful nursery reverberated with the weeping of children whose 'mother' had left the room, for instance, to get something from the next room, and whose absence was mourned as if she would never return. Fights among children multiplied in frequency and intensity.[15]

Under these conditions few workers would have

had the courage to persist in their conviction, but Anna Freud did. Gradually the children realized that their new "mothers" really belonged to them and the frenzy subsided. "At the same time children began to develop in leaps and bounds."[3]

Anna Freud summarized her outlook on applied analysis when she said:

After extending my interest from adult to child analysis and from clinical to theoretical problems, I also turned to the various applications of analysis. Beginning in Vienna and continuing in England and the United States, I tried to select from analytic knowledge what can be useful for education, for teaching, for pediatrics and for the law.[16]

As with so much of Anna Freud's life and work, her contributions were useful as model services. They also became the basis for the revision of, or additions to, psychoanalytic theory. Together these contributions constituted a creative mosaic of clinical practice and teaching of original, rigorous research and theory building and of useful applications embedded in model services for children and their parents.

The Child and the Law

Anna Freud's interest and involvement in the child and the law were closely related to her lifelong interest in the interactions of children and their parents and in the psychoanalytic theory of object relations. From her work in Vienna with toddlers of poor working mothers, with children in war-torn London whose safety required them to be separated from their parents and with pediatricians concerned with the child in hospital, she had become expert in understanding and assisting children who needed to cope with such separations and losses. She also had substantial experience with children of divorced parents and with neglected, abused and abandoned children. Thus, child placement conflicts and the law were logical extensions of her long-term interests in the applications of psychoanalysis, especially in a period of history in which the apparent increase in the instability of the family was a daily threatening crisis for the huge number of children experiencing neglect, abuse, abandonment or the divorce of their parents.

In her collaborative work with those concerned

with children and the law,[4,17-19] Anna Freud emphasized the nature of the parent-child interaction, developmental lines and the interdependence of id and ego-superego aspects of the child's developing personality. She worked closely with her colleagues in separating out value preferences, e.g., minimizing the state's intrusion into the privacy of the family and when the child's interests shall be paramount, from those applications of psychoanalytic theory that are formulated as "the child's need for continuity of relationship" and "the child's sense of time."[17,18] In this collaboration, as in all of her work, she insisted on facing facts. Thus she accepted and made good use of Joseph Goldstein's[17] formulation of "least detrimental alternative" as the realistic way of describing the child's best interests when there are conflicts of placement.

She was equally emphatic in asserting the preference that "So long as the child is part of a viable family, his own interests are merged with those of the other members. Only after the family fails in its function should the child's interests become a matter for state intrusion."[18] As implied in this formulation, she also contributed substantially to making explicit the child's need for autonomous parents and the importance of respecting and supporting the integrity of the family in raising children.

At the same time, she brought to this collaboration, as she did in all her applied works, a keen sense of the limits of psychoanalytic knowledge and its applications, especially when it is used by experts to assess the nature of the child-parent relationship, once the privacy of the family is breached. With her collaborators she recognized that such assessments are carried out in coercive settings without the protection of confidentiality. In the last years of her life she worked steadfastly with her collaborators in examining the usefulness and the limitations of experts evaluating and resolving child placement conflicts.[19]

Pediatrics

Anna Freud's work with pediatricians extended over more than three decades as she wove together her knowledge about the child's feelings about his body and the fundamental unity of body and mind--how the psyche is embedded in the body and mind--how the psyche is embedded in the body and how the body is embedded in the child's mind. The Hampstead Clinic's current collaborative studies of children with chronic illness, e.g. diabetes mellitus, is an example of one of the directions of this life-long interest. Recognition of this sustained dialogue with pediatricians was formally acknowledged when she was given the C. Anderson Alderich Award of the American Academy of Pediatrics in 1974. She responded with a summary of the needed collaboration between pediatricians and child analysts, emphasizing the indivisibility of the body and the mind. She concluded by saying, "In fact, the children themselves have never left us in doubt that their bodies and minds, their physical and mental growth were anything except indissoluble unities."[20]

Education

As already indicated, Anna Freud's keen interest and involvement with the child's education began with her own training as a teacher. In her book *Psychoanalysis for Teachers and Parents*,[13] she reflected upon her understanding of what teachers needed to know from psychoanalytic theory about how children develop and learn. On several occasions in New Haven she visited the public primary schools, talking to and with teachers in such a spirited, imaginative way that their dialogue had to be interrupted in order to keep her busy schedule intact.

In each instance where she creatively and humanely responded to the needs of young children in depriving, threatening, disruptive situations, like an artist she designed an appropriate setting into which she intuitively poured her psychoanalytic knowledge and judgment, adapted and applied, e.g. in designing a temporary replacement for children of their parents and home. Characteristically she also set up systematic evaluative observations and procedures that resulted in publications useful to others, with theory-building and refining formulations and with descriptions of practical models of family, school, health and law services for children.

She had that immense capacity to keep theory and applications in a constant interchange of refinement and elaboration. What she learned from analyzing a child she also made useful for teachers in understanding their students and for pediatricians in relating to their patients and in sharpening their diagnostic and therapeutic effec-

tiveness as they worked with children and their parents.

Anna Freud's methods of applying psychoanalytic theory and insights are superbly summarized in the introductions to *War and Children*[21] and *Infants without Families*.[22] Here one can witness her steady commitment to children's needs, her creative boldness in building new models of service and her investigative vigor in pressing forward in theory-building that has heuristic value and consolidative, integrating impact.

In New Haven in the mid-1960's, Heinz Hartmann gently chided Anna Freud for making clear and simple what was complex about early child development. Anna Freud responded by saying that if one could find the clear, simpler description and explanation about a developmental process there would be ample opportunity to complicate it in applying the concept.[23]

Conclusion

A great deal of Anna Freud's work was unique and original, very much her own. She was a pioneer and leader. As a founding editor of *The Psychoanalytic Study of the Child*, she helped both authors and editors with her cogent comments and suggestions. She trained several generations of analysts and exerted a direct influence on the large number of people to whom she lectured. Her personal impact was so immense because she vividly conveyed a unique combination of charm and humor, secure knowledge and great modesty, an unflinching willingness to look at facts, unbounded curiosity and a relentless quest to learn and enormous pleasure in and a total commitment to hard work. She was also an extraordinary collaborator, bringing out the best in her colleagues and students, in her spirited search for, and love of, truth. In her own person she combined life's experiences, dedicated energies, and independent critical mind and a soaring creative imagination. Her leadership and originality as an investigator, teacher, clinician, founder of child psychoanalysis and as builder of models of intervention that advanced humanitarian and scientific aims are acknowledged by the many honorary degrees she was granted as well as by the C.B.E. (Commander of the British Empire) awarded by the Queen of England. Her honorary degrees were received from the following institutions: Clark University, Jefferson Medical

College, University of Sheffield (England), University of Chicago, Yale University, University of Vienna and Harvard University.

Anna Freud insisted on looking at the facts with an unyielding commitment to children. Her passionate interest in every sector of child life and experience enabled her to weave together beautifully and vigorously the clinical and theoretical themes of child and adult development.

As a psychoanalyst Anna Freud had a long, productive life, making vital contributions to psychoanalysis and its allied fields. She pioneered in the development of child analysis and in ushering in psychoanalytic ego psychology. She inspired and trained several generations of psychoanalysts and exerted a direct influence on colleagues in related fields of scientific work and humanitarian service. She made original contributions to psychoanalysis and to putting theory into practice. To the end she loved her work and all that it entailed.

Anna Freud's genius encompassed the study and understanding of children and adults, spanning the gap between theory and practice. Her *Collected Writings*[24] in eight volumes provides us with a rich legacy of her scientific, clinical and educational contributions.

Until her last days, she was able to work effectively, though toward the end with great effort and with the support of loyal friends and collaborators. Having made a significant clarifying suggestion about the revision of a chapter in an ongoing collaborative project, in July, 1982, she conveyed to Professor Joseph Goldstein her immense pleasure in hard work and her insistence on facing facts when she said, "We could have done so much more together. I'd love to be going with you."[25]

References

[1]Personal note to Gardiner M, 1977.
[2]Freud A: The ego and the mechanisms of defense. In The Writings of Anna Freud, Vol. 2. New York: Int. Univ. Press, 1936.
[3]Newman L: Anna Freud. In International Encyclopedia of Psychiatry, Psychology, Psychoanalysis, and Neurology, ed. Wolman BB. New York, Aesculapius, 5:90-94, 1977.
[4]Freud A: Normality and pathology in childhood. In The Writings of Anna Freud, Vol. 6. New York: Int. Univ. Press, 1965.
[5]Freud A: Residential vs. foster care. In On Rearing infants and young children in institutions, ed. Witmer HL. Washington D.C.: HEW Children's Bureau Research Reports #1, 1967, pp. 47-55; and in The Writings of Anna Freud, Vol. 7.
[6]Freud A: The past revisited. Annual Psychoanal 10:259-265, 1982.
[7]Freud A: Four lectures on analysis. In The Writings of Anna Freud, Vol. 1. New York: Int. Univ. Press, 1926 (1927).
[8]Freud A: Introduction. In The Writings of Anna Freud, Vol. 1. New York: Int. Univ. Press, 1974 (1922-1935).
[9]Freud A: Child analysis as the study of mental growth, normal and abnormal. In The Writings of Anna Freud, Vol. 8. New York: Int. Univ. Press, (1970-1980), 1979 (1981).
[10]Freud A: Preface to The Hampstead Psychoanalytic Index. Bolland J & Sandler J, eds. New York: Int. University Press, 1965.
[11]Freud A: Preface to The Hampstead Psychoanalytic Index, Bolland J & Sandler J, eds. New York: Int. Univ. Press, 1965.
[12]Solnit AJ & Newman L: Anna Freud: the child expert. In The Psychoanalytic Study of the Child, ed. Solnit AJ et al., Vol. 39. New Haven, CT: Yale University Press, 1984.
[13]Freud A: Four lectures on psychoanalysis for teachers and parents. In The Writings of Anna Freud, Vol. 1. New York: Int. Univ. Press, 1930.
[14]Freud A: Foreward. Code Name Mary by Gardiner M. New Haven, CT: Yale University Press, 1983.
[15]Freud A: Infants without families. In The Writings of Anna Freud, Vol. 3. New York: Int. Univ. Press, 1973.
[16]Freud A: Doctoral award address on receiving an honorary doctor of science degree. Jefferson Medical College, Philadelphia, PA, June 12, 1964.
[17]Goldstein J, Freud A, & Solnit AJ: Beyond the Best Interests of the Child. New York: Free Press, 1973.
[18]Goldstein J, Freud A, & Solnit AJ: Before the Best Interests of the Child. New York: Free Press, 1979.
[19]Goldstein J, Freud A, & Solnit AJ: In the Best Interests of the Child: Chapter 1, The Problems and our questions. Bull. Hampstead Clinic, 6:129-133, 1983. Also Chapter 1 of In the Best

Interests of the Child, New York: Free Press, 1985.

[20]Freud A: Remarks on receiving the C. Anderson Alderich Award. Pediatrics, Oct. 21, 1974.

[21]Freud A & Burlingham D: War and children. New York: Int. Univ. Press, 1943.

[22]Freud A & Burlingham D: Infants without families. New York: Int. Univ. Press, Vol. 3, 1944.

[23]Personal communication, Provence S, 1983.

[24]Freud A: The Writings of Anna Freud, Vols 1-8. New York: Int. Univ. Press, 1974-1981.

[25]Goldstein J: Anna Freud, 1895-1982. Bull. Hampstead Clinic, 6:34, 1983.

12

Margaret S. Mahler, M.D.: Original Thinker, Exceptional Woman

Judith R. Smith, C.S.W.

Psychotherapist in Private Practice,
New York, New York

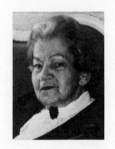
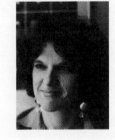

Margaret S. Mahler, M.D.   **Judith R. Smith, C.S.W.**

12

Margaret S. Mahler, M.D.:
Original Thinker, Exceptional Woman

When I was first asked to write a chapter about Dr. Margaret Mahler, I felt awkward about the assignment. Although I had known Dr. Mahler for ten years, I had rarely inquired about her personal life. I had produced five films for and with her, and she was my mentor, friend and teacher. I admired her greatly. When I told her about the assignment, Dr. Mahler said that she would feel honored if I wrote about her, and I felt challenged by her encouragement. This chapter was drawn from interviews that I did with Dr. Mahler during the summer of 1985 and from transcripts of interviews Dr. Mahler shared with me done by Dr. Bluma Swerdloff as part of the Oral History Project of Columbia University.

When she died on October 2, 1985, I had almost completed this piece. We had gone over the final draft together, and she had expressed her pleasure in it. I have left the piece in the present tense as originally written. As Dr. Mahler spoke to me about her early life, she hinted at many things that she did not elaborate on. It will be up to her biographers to fill in the details.

I dedicate this chapter to Dr. Mahler in gratitude for what she has left to all of us: parents, children, teachers, pediatricians and mental health professionals. My personal work as a psychotherapist and my commitment to preventive mental health via parent education and early intervention are continually inspired and supported by her example and her ideas.

I had ideas and I could think clearly. Before I

even embarked on my studies, I knew that I had to say things--that I had to contribute with my brain . . . that is why I went through thick and thin to become a doctor, to become a pediatrician and to become a psychoanalyst. . . . I had a kind of immodesty--a kind of conviction that I had it in me. . . . I had self-confidence that I had something to contribute.

Dr. Margaret S. Mahler is best known for her contributions to our understanding of childhood schizophrenia and her formulation of the separation-individuation process, which she has called the psychological birth of the human infant. In her work with both normal and psychotic children, Dr. Mahler realized that development occurs within the mother-child matrix. Her research has shown how the infant takes a leading role in adapting to the mother ("the lion's share") and that there can be inborn deficits in the infant's ability to respond to the mothering person. This insight helped dissipate the tendency in the psychiatric world of blaming the mother for the child's problems.

Dr. Mahler's research has given us a framework for understanding the steps by which the infant gradually develops a sense of self as separate from his mother. Her separation-individuation study was the first systematic research project done by psychoanalysts to be based on the direct observations of normal babies and their mothers. Her unique research project collected data on the same children three or four times a week from birth to age three years. She deciphered the preverbal epoch of life and showed how psychological birth, in contrast to physical birth, is a gradual process of growth--taking three years before the child is able to move from total dependence to relative independence. Her observations led to the formulation of four distinct but overlapping stages that now serve as an invaluable map of psychological and emotional development for mental health professionals and parents. She has written, "One could regard the entire life cycle as constituting a more or less successful process of distancing from and introjection of the lost symbiotic mother."[1]

Dr. Mahler has had a long and rich professional life as a pediatrician and psychoanalyst. She has done outstanding work as a psychoanalytic researcher, clinician, teacher and supervisor. She has received nearly every award given for outstanding achievement in the field of mental health. This chapter will look at some of the personal events that facilitated Margaret Mahler's individuation. How did she become so knowledgeable about psychoanalysis and mothers and babies? What events and people influenced this original thinker who created new ways of understanding the normal and pathological aspects of human development?

Margaret Schoenberger (Mahler) was born in 1897 in the small Hungarian mountainside village of Sopron, on the border of Austria and Hungary. Both her maternal and paternal family had lived in this agricultural, "but highly cultural town" for many generations. Her parents, Guztav and Jenny Schoenberger, were upper middle-class Jews. Her father was a doctor, the commissioner of health of the county of Sopron and the administrator of the local hospital.

When Margaret was born, her mother was only 19 years old and had been married for just 9 months and 10 days. Margaret's childhood relationship with her mother was distant and painful. She felt much closer to her father during her childhood, and only years later realized the deep love she had for her mother. Dr. Mahler describes her mother as having been unprepared to have a baby. Margaret's father engaged a wet-nurse to breastfeed Margaret, which was a typical custom for middle-class families--"either you (the mother) gave the breast or the wet-nurse did." What Dr. Mahler does believe was unusual, however, was that her family fired this nurse suddenly when Margaret was five months old-- forcing an abrupt and premature weaning from

the breast. The nurse had been caught stealing feathers from the family. Dr. Mahler realized, after many years of being a psychoanalyst, that this sudden separation from the nurse and the breast was a traumatic event in her life and led to her developing a sleep disturbance. At two years old she was described by a nurse as "a lynx--with wide eyes and ever watchful." In reflecting on this incident, Dr. Mahler says,

The thinking about babies was quite different then. The baby was there. It was put into the world like an egg with no needs of its own-- just to be handled properly and fed properly. There was no mutuality whatsoever.

When Margaret was about four years old, her parents had a second child. Now more mature, Mrs. Schoenberger could more fully enjoy and care for this baby. Dr. Mahler remembers watching her mother breastfeed her sister and listening to her mother cooing repeatedly, "My baby, my baby," whereupon Margaret exclaimed, "Und mich hat mein Papa geboren"--and I was born by my papa.

Throughout their growing up, Margaret felt that her parents had very different expectations for the two girls. Her sister was considered the pretty one and her dependency was encouraged. Margaret was considered extremely self-reliant, and she was constantly told that it was her job to look after her sister, Viola. During adolescence, Margaret and her mother constantly quarreled. She was upset

. . . that I wasn't dainty, that I wasn't household-oriented. On the one hand, she liked it that I liked the books and didn't interfere with her womanly and household pursuits; but then, she complained that I didn't do more.

At age fourteen, Dr. Mahler made an independent and unique decision for a girl of her era: she chose to venture away from her family and hometown in order to study. The academic high school in her provincial hometown was not open to girls for females were expected to attend finishing school. Margaret wanted an academic education. She was the second young girl to ever leave the town for further studies. When asked if she remembers feeling uncomfortable making this unusual choice, she unambivalently stated,

*I just knew that this is what I wanted to do . . .
I had a tremendous need to identify with my
father. I knew that I wanted to become a
doctor--I only did not know what kind of doctor I would be.*

Margaret's mother and father did not oppose
her leaving home at age fourteen but did insist
that she study in Budapest where she could live
with an aunt. Margaret's first choice had been
Vienna where her father had gone to the University. Dr. Mahler believes that her parents une-
quivocally supported her desire for an education
but were also relieved that her leaving would
bring an end to the constant fighting between
Margaret and her mother.

When Margaret was fourteen years old she read
her first psychoanalytic paper. In 1911, Alice
Kovaks, a classmate in the new high school,
showed her an article just published by the Hungarian analyst Sandor Ferenczi. During recess the
two girls avidly read the paper together. (Alice
Kovaks later married and became the psychoanalyst Alice Balint.)

Ferenczi, Freud's first disciple, introduced psy-
choanalysis and the theory of the Unconscious to
Hungary, making Budapest an important and
separate center of psychoanalytic thought. Mar-
garet met Ferenczi at the home of her friend
Alice whose mother, Vilma Kovaks, was one of
Ferenczi's first students and the leader of the
Budapest psychoanalytic group.

*Meeting Ferenczi sealed my fate. Right then
and there I decided I would become an analyst.
He was warm, brilliant, not afraid of being
relaxed about his position and he enjoyed
young people. He was fascinating and engaging
and asked me questions about myself. In looking back one could say that he was asking for
my free associations.*

The Budapest group exerted a very strong
influence on Dr. Mahler's development. They
were much more interested in the early mother/
child relationship than the Viennese group with
whom she would later study. "For the Hungarians,
the mother-child relationship was in their blood. I
am a living example of that." She considers the
understandings she developed with Ferenczi, Michael and Alice Balint and Vilma Kovaks equiva-

lent to "the mother's milk" of her psychoanalytic
orientation and most influential.

Dr. Mahler began her undergraduate studies at
the University in Budapest. In her first semester
she studied art and aesthetics. She avoided studying medicine, certain that her father would disap-
prove of her desire to become a doctor. She loved
art and painting but became restless as she realized that only through medicine could she make
the contribution she felt compelled to make. After
one semester, she decided that art would have to
be a hobby--something for her own enjoyment.

Even as a young child Margaret was interested
in her father's medical books. Yet she also remembers always having felt that something was
wrong with this strong interest of hers in her
father's field, as if she shouldn't want to know
what her father knew and shouldn't be interested
in the "dirty" human body. She had once heard
her father say that he thought ophthalmology was
an appropriate specialty for women doctors. Margaret interpreted this remark as his disapproving
of women in medicine. Assuming her father's
disapproval, she kept her efforts to get into
medical school a secret. Without anyone's knowledge of what she was trying to do, Margaret took
on the arduous task of applying to medical school
during World War I. The war made it very difficult for a woman to be considered as an applicant to medical school. That she was Jewish in an
increasingly anti-Semitic, Austro-Germanic world
made it nearly impossible. Yet she was accepted.
For the difficult task of breaking the news to her
father, over and over again she rehearsed how she
would say this. When she finally told him, she was
very surprised when he responded, "Darling, if
that makes you happy, I am all with you." Over
time, Dr. Mahler realized that her assumption that
her father opposed her medical studies was actually a projection of self-imposed taboo. She has
attributed part of her initial fascination with psychoanalysis to her early awareness of this inner
conflict over becoming a doctor.

Dr. Mahler describes her father and mother as
having had unlimited confidence in her ability to
achieve and to become self-reliant. Sometimes she
experienced their attitude as admiration, other
times, she felt perceived as an anomaly--a
neuter--and not like an ordinary woman. Most
families within her parents' circle typically invited
young men to the house to socialize with their
daughters. Margaret's parents, although they had

many opportunities, did not do this for her, but they did for her sister. In fact, on several occasions when Margaret spoke to them about a young man she was considering marrying, her father said, "What do you need that for? You can take care of yourself." Her parents' lack of support for her interests in men, coupled with their insistence that she look after her sister, made it difficult for her to marry until much later in her life. Dr. Mahler thinks that becoming a pediatrician was her way of integrating her feminine interests in children with her desire to be a physician.

Margaret Schoenberger entered medical school in Munich, Germany, sometime around 1917. The only school that accepted her was in a region that was controlled by the more liberal government of the Weimar Republic. The students however were reactionary. At times she was singled out and harassed for being a Jewess, at other times, she was persecuted for being a foreigner from Eastern Europe. Nevertheless, she describes herself as remaining relatively unaffected by the discrimination.

> There was anti-feminism, anti-Semitism, anti-Hungarianism. . . . I was doing what I had to against tremendous odds. I was a fighter and I didn't let anything deter me, absolutely not. I was challenged by difficulties all my life. If I knew I was right, I could fight to the finish. If I lost for a while, it didn't kill me.

When asked how she managed to study when surrounded by such hostility, she says that her primary concern was to learn the material thoroughly and "not be half-baked." As the political situation and discrimination worsened, Margaret had to continually relocate. Before graduating, she had transferred to four different universities in four new cities. In 1922, Margaret Schoenberger was one of two students in her medical school class in Jena, Germany, to graduate cum laude.

Margaret specialized in pediatrics. She chose to study with Professor Ibrahim, a foremost child neurologist who was interested in psychosomatic childhood illnesses, particularly spastic vomiting and rumination. She had learned of his work through reading his chapter, "The Nervous Diseases of Children," in the main pediatric textbook. She found him to be an inspiring teacher. He was also a special physician who understood that good medical care had to include attending to children's emotional needs. Margaret noticed that he would set time aside on the weekends to play and talk with the children in the hospital. She had also been impressed by what she had heard about Dr. Echerek, a professor of pediatrics at the University in Budapest who was said to spend time sitting in the park with mothers, trying to convey to them that being loving with their babies was more important than anything else. She sensed that something very important was being expressed in these physicians' simple but professionally unusual gestures.

Asked if she, as a young pediatrician, was particularly interested in understanding the emotional development of young children, Dr. Mahler replied, "No, it was not like I went after this or that. I did not plot a certain course. I only had ideas. Certain things made an impression on me. I had no sense that they were all part of the same thing until much later."

Dr. Mahler's first job was in Vienna with Dr. Ernest von Pirquet, a bright and charismatic pediatrician who first detected childhood allergies. Pirquet approached Dr. Mahler (then Dr. Schoenberger) and asked her to work with him. He would not give her a full assistant's title despite the fact that she was a licenced pediatrician. He said, "I shall never have a woman as my assistant. You are very smart, and I like you very much" but if one is a woman, and especially if one looks the way you do, one should marry and have children." Despite his attitude, Dr. Mahler accepted the opportunity to work with him. Though unwilling to give her the full assistant's title, he did give her a lot of responsibility. They wrote and published a paper together. Pirquet's primary interest when Margaret worked with him was statistical analysis of the nutrition and health of infants. Mahler found his approach totally unpsychological. "Pirquet saw only the child's organs--not the child." She was responsible for measuring the tonsils of 5,000 school-aged children. Although not interested in statistics, she saw the research value of following the course of a disease.

While she worked for Pirquet, Dr. Mahler also worked one day a week for Dr. Moll. Both Pirquet and Moll were treating children with intestinal bacterial viruses. The approaches of the two clinics however were very different. Pirquet's treatment focused on protecting the babies from infection, by keeping them in glass vessels where they could not be touched. At The Moll Clinic, treatment was based on the sense that infants needed mothering in order to survive. Dr. Moll assigned one nurse to stay around the clock with each sick infant and encouraged mothers to be with their babies as much as possible. The success rate at Moll's clinic was much higher than at Pirquet's.

> *At Moll, I saw that the babies who had the care of one special nurse or their mother thrived and were brought out of their comatose toxic condition--whereas the infants at Pirquet's clinic who were only receiving physical care were dying in droves.*

Although Dr. Mahler was affected by the tremendous difference between these two approaches, she did not challenge Dr. Pirquet.

> *One didn't dare to. One wouldn't be listened to. One would had to have had great prestige to suggest to Pirquet that Moll's successes might have to do with the mother's presence.*

She also felt that she still had a lot to learn.

> *I was dead set to get into analysis--that was my main goal. I was already analytically minded, but I wasn't analyzed yet. I could not yet have expressed my ideas.*

Margaret Mahler's early psychoanalytic training took place during the formative years of Freudian thought.

> *It was the birth of a new science. We all felt like priests. It was a new undertaking. . . . It was the Unconscious that I was interested in and the findings of Freud which were interpreted by Ferenczi. I was interested in a new paradigm. It wasn't a profession I chose; it was an avocation that I followed.*

Living in Vienna, she was part of the small group of people who had come to study and learn Freud's developing ideas. Among her colleagues were Heinz Hartmann, Ernest and Marianne Kris, Anna Maencher, Robert and Jenny Waelder, Jeanne Lampl-de-Groot and Grete Bibring. There were no formalized institutes, classes or specified procedures for training. Mahler attended several weekly informal seminars in which colleagues discussed the application of Freud's writings. One seminar conducted by Anna Freud in the Freud's house ("The Freuds lived in a very large house-- Anna had her wing and Freud his") focused on the treatment of children.

The first step in Dr. Mahler's analytic training was to begin her own analysis. Throughout her medical studies she had kept in touch with the Hungarian analysts--Alice Balint, Vilma Kovaks and Ferenczi. Ferenczi now recommended that Margaret enter analysis with one of the senior analysts in Vienna, Dr. Helene Deutsch. Margaret was in analysis with Deutsch for over a year, yet their relationship did not work out. Deutsch would cancel often, as many as three out of their scheduled five weekly appointments. After a year of working together, Dr. Deutsch said that she could not continue working with Margaret and recommended three other analysts whom she thought might be better able to analyze her. Dr. Schoenberger, upset from the abrupt termination of the analysis, did not accept Deutsch's referrals and searched out a new analyst on her own.

August Aichorn, who considered Margaret Schoenberger one of his most talented students, became her training analyst. She felt that she went from being treated as a second-class analysand to being prized and chosen by Aichorn. The Vienna Psychoanalytic Institute considered Dr. Schoenberger's analysis with Aichorn acceptable for meeting the requirements for graduation, even though, typical for the time, they had known and worked together prior to the analysis. After her work with Aichorn, Mahler wanted to go on to have a more classical analysis, which she did with Dr. Willi Hoffer. She describes this last analytic experience as one "where the transference was very benign and very positive. At that point there were not orthodox Freudian analyses. A good analysis included abstinence and transference, and there was friendship at the end."

Although Dr. Mahler was able to continue her training despite the rupture with Helene Deutsch, she felt that losing Deutsch's favor left its toll on her beginning career. Dr. Deutsch had a very great influence on the educational committee of the Vienna Psychoanalytic Society, and she could promote people if she chose to. Because psychoanalysis was in its nascent years, the educational hierarchy was only an informal system, leaving students vulnerable to the personalities of the elders.

Dr. Mahler credits Professor August Aichorn as teaching her "99 percent" of what she learned about the technique of working analytically with children. He was the director of a school program for juvenile delinquents and the author of the book, *Wayward Youth*. Mahler points out that Aichorn was unique for his time in his recognition that delinquent kids could benefit from psychoanalytic treatment. "At this point, there was no such thing as child psychiatry. There were only bad boys (not yet bad girls). These boys were considered the misfits. Aichorn recognized that these so-called delinquents were abused children or misunderstood children." He set up clinics in the public schools in Vienna, programs similar to what we now call child guidance clinics. With his encouragement, Mahler began to accompany him to these clinics, where she feels she learned "through osmosis," as she observed him work with the children, their parents and the teachers.

Mahler describes Aichorn's technique as his making himself available to these kids as an ego ideal, someone with whom they could identify. Slowly, through the very positive transference that would develop and the strong dependency that the kids eventually felt towards him, he would show them that their delinquent lives were chosen because of the abuse or lack of understanding they had felt in their earlier lives. Aichorn felt that if he could bring about this understanding, the kids would be neurotic rather than delinquent and therefore be treatable by psychoanalytic methods.

He was ingenious, he understood these kids better than anyone. He could talk their language. He could make them feel so much at home with him during an interview that they would tell him all their secrets. They felt that he would not betray them. The young person always knew that Aichorn was on his side.

When Dr. Mahler came to Psychiatric Institute in New York City, the staff was shocked at her ability to interview a child patient in front of a group of professionals, as this was not yet being done in the States. "I had the ability, which I learned from Aichorn, to make the child at home, to put him completely at ease." She describes how

her empathy for the child could make him feel as if there were no one else in the room except the two of them. She also feels that she was able to feel this same empathy for the mothers of her child patients and never felt vindictive or blaming towards them for their children's problems.

Of the many other supervisors and teachers she had in Vienna, Dr. Mahler remembers Drs. Grete Bibring, Jeanne Lampl-de-Groot, and Margaret Ribble as most meaningful.

Grete Bibring had the courage to talk about empathy. It was not called empathy at that time, but she shared her observations as a new mother--she told us that she could feel when her babies were uncomfortable, even if they were in another room.

She believes that Margaret Ribble's book, *Rights of Infants*, was crucially important to her and regrets that this book is overlooked in the literature. Mahler also states that she was strongly affected by the fact that there were so many more women than men in the pioneering generation of psychoanalysts.

Although there was much excitement in being a student of psychoanalysis in Vienna, Dr. Mahler also felt much tension due to the already established elitist and often suffocating hierarchy. Dr. Mahler never felt like she was a member of the inner group; she felt timid among the titans. She did not speak up in Anna Freud's meetings even though she had much to contribute from her work with Aichorn in the child guidance clinics. The elitism and the competition interferred with her independent thinking, and she did not publish any papers from 1928 to 1938. Mahler was not the only one who experienced anxiety in response to the Viennese hierarchy. August Aichorn felt it as well, even though he was in Freud's inner sanctum. Another colleague, Dr. Sandor Rado from Hungary, once told Margaret that the Viennese group was like the "camarilla"--the Austrian secret police who spied on Hungarians.

Later on in her career whenever she had a choice, Dr. Mahler opted for situations that were less hierarchical and non-elitist. Her most important and personally satisfying work was done within independent settings. She chose to commute to Philadelphia and establish her own child analytic training program. Her separation-individuation study was done as a separately funded, independent project, unaffiliated with any large institution.

Dr. Mahler was admitted into the Vienna Society for Psychoanalysis in 1933. Soon after this, she was married to Paul Mahler, a Viennese chemist with a doctorate in philosophy. When asked if her husband had supported her work, she replied, "Yes, although he was not directly involved in it." A few years after they were married, the Mahlers had to make plans to leave Vienna due to the growing Nazi threat. It was more difficult for Paul Mahler to consider going, because he was leaving behind a large and successful business which he could not take with him. Yet they had to move. Weekly round-ups of Jews were already taking place in Vienna's downtown. One day, Aichorn, who was not Jewish, saved the Mahlers' lives by phoning them and warning Paul not to leave the house to go to his factory that morning.

The analysts tried to help each other plan their escapes. Conferences were held at Freud's house with Anna Freud, Ernest Kris, Hartmann and Bibring. The Mahlers wanted to come to the United States, but they had no one in the States who could request a visa for them. It was suggested that they go to South Africa. Several of Dr. Mahler's non-Jewish patients spontaneously offered whatever help they could. It was a patient of Dr. Mahler's, the niece of a high British official, who secured exit visas for the Mahlers. She sent a letter to the Vienna Home Office of the British Embassy stating that she had invited the Mahlers to be her private guests in England while they awaited their final arrangements to go to the United States.

Margaret and Paul Mahler arrived in England in May of 1938 and came to the United States in October of that same year. In London, they were guests of the British Psychoanalytic Society and did what they could to help others get out of Vienna. Dr. Mahler also worked giving Rorschach tests and treated some British analysts' children. These child analyses were both an opportunity to do treatment and to quickly learn English--particularly slang. She remembers one child who said repeatedly, "I love you, you stinker"--and it took weeks before Mahler realized that the boy did not mean that she smelled bad.

Dr. Mahler believes that she might not have made the contributions she did if she had not come to the States. Leaving the constraints of the Viennese psychoanalytic hierarchical society opened up new vistas for her. She found Americans more open, more curious and more objective. "I dared to express my ideas here--however foolish they might have appeared at first."

In 1939, Dr. Mahler got her New York State medical license. She was one of the 5 percent of refugee physicians who passed the examination on the first try. She set up an analytic office in her apartment on 97th Street and Columbus Avenue, but soon learned that it was a faux-pas to have an office situated even one block north of the professionally circumscribed 96th Street border so she moved her office downtown to Central Park West.

In January 1940, Dr. Mahler gave her first paper, "On Pseudoimbecility--The Magic Cap of Invisibility," at the New York Psychoanalytic Institute. This paper showed how psychological conflicts can cause a child to appear stupid, and how the stupidity can be a device which enables the child to maintain a secret interchange on an affective level with his or her family. The paper was very well received. It was well-written on a new and important topic, presented at a time when the Psychiatric Institute affiliated with Columbia University College of Physicians and Surgeons was about to reorganize their children's service. Impressed with Dr. Mahler's abilities, the directors asked her to head their new service.

At the Psychiatric Institute Mahler worked with Teddy, a child with involuntary movements, i.e., tic syndrome. This case interested her greatly because of a previous interest in motility. After her work with Teddy, Dr. Mahler was given a grant to do an in-depth comparative study of several children with tic syndrome. She did follow-up studies for several years after treating children who had the disorder. The results showed that several of the children, even though they had lost their tic symptoms, became psychotic often during adolescence. This led her to recognize that the lack of control over motility, which the tic causes, creates such lasting assault on the ego that it often cannot be mastered and leads to adolescent pyschosis. Understanding the role of motility in the executive functions of the ego and its correlation to the subsequent development of psychosis was a turning point in Mahler's work.

A few years later in 1943, Mahler presented her hypotheses regarding the symptomatology of schizophrenia-like children. At the time there was much emotional resistance in the field to even consider diagnosing young children as psychotic. Dr. Leo Kanner was the discussant of her paper, "Malignant Cases of Childhood Psychosis," at the American Orthopsychiatry meeting. He called Mahler's work "a classic," and he said that it was the first attempt to dynamically understand the symptomatology of childhood psychosis.

It was a daring thing I had done--my first ideas on childhood schizophrenia were very new and very up in the air. One had to have chutz-pah [nerve] to come out with it at the Ortho-psychiatry meeting. I was more astonished than anybody when Kanner said it was a classic work.

Dr. Mahler continued investigating childhood psychosis during the 1950's at Albert Einstein College of Medicine. She and Dr. Manuel Furer got a large National Institute of Mental Health grant to study the natural history of symbiotic child psychosis in preschool children. They formulated a unique tri-partite design for treating psychotic children which included the therapist, the child and the mother. This method was a way of using the therapist as a bridge in establishing a missing bond between the psychotic infant and its mother.

At the age of 62, Dr. Mahler began the work for which she is best known, the study of the normal separation-individuation process. In her studies on psychosis, she had investigated the factors which interfered with the children's needed internal boundaries between themselves and their mothers. She then posed the question, "How is it that the great majority of human beings do attain a sense of individual autonomy and identity?" In 1959 the question, "How do normal children separate and individuate from their mothers?" became the basis for a pilot study on separation-individuation.

During Dr. Mahler's studies of psychotic children, she had already developed the idea that psychological birth does not occur simultaneously with biological birth. The separation-individuation study was to follow this idea and further explore the symbiotic nature of human existence--the steps by which children gradually emerge from being totally dependent on their mothers to attaining, more or less, a sense of independence and autonomy. Although Dr. Mahler had a general

sense of what she wanted to study, she was insistent about having a research project that remained open to discovery via the direct observation of babies and their mothers in a nursery-like setting. With a large grant from the National Institute of Mental Health, she created a naturalistic laboratory where a small group of neighborhood mothers brought their babies consistently, two or three mornings a week, for the first three years of their children's lives.

Mahler wanted to be able to observe behavior "in statu nascendi." She created a large staff of psychoanalytically trained workers (psychologists, teachers, social workers, lay people) who would be responsible for collecting the daily observations. There were weekly staff meetings where the data were gone over and discussed. In the very beginning of the project, Anni Bergmann joined the staff and a few years later, Dr. John McDevitt began working with them. Dr. Bergmann and Dr. McDevitt continued to be Dr. Mahler's primary research associates. Dr. Fred Pine helped to design the research methodology. Many others participated in the project which lasted for eleven years.

Dr. Mahler had the foresight to record some of the daily observations on 16mm film. As a result, many hours of filmed observations along with reams of written observations were collected. These data eventually led to the detailed formulation of the phenomena of the separation-individuation process. A detailed description of this research project and the states of the separation-individuation process can be found in the book, *The Psychological Birth of the Human Infant*, by Mahler, Pine and Bergmann.[2]

In looking back and trying to speculate on the influences that shaped her formulation of the psychological birth of the human infant as a process of separation-individuation, Dr. Mahler says,

I want to emphasize that it was deep down in my engrams, in my memory traces. I had this idea ever since I was a pediatrician, of psychological birth not being simultaneous with physical birth. I had the feeling that these normal babies who were brought by their mothers to the clinic were really in a twilight state of existence. It seemed to me that they were not aware of existing without the symbiotic orbit, the mother, who they seemed to sense, belonged to their own self.

When asked what role she felt her own relationship with her mother had on her life's work, she replied,

> *Only much later did I realize it had something to do with it. I thought the main influence had been the Budapest Group. But underneath, obviously, the very fact that I became a pediatrician, I was already interested in the mother/baby relationship and was very interested in how important the mother is to the baby--which was not the usual thing.*

When asked about her ability to develop such a thorough and original research project, Mahler said,

> *I was always a nitpicking perfectionist . . . when I saw something in my analytic practice or in the clinics, I always had the need to formulate a hypothesis . . . then I went about making my observations more explicit, more extensive and so on--to see and match my observations and my hypotheses. I think that the sudden loss [of her nurse] at five months, promoted my tendency to be hyper-alert and watchful. I had a real need to be vigilant and to look and to see and to understand. This necessity was a great liability in my personal emotional life, but it certainly was a great asset to my scientific life.*

Dr. Mahler is now 88 years old. Although semi-retired, she remains interested in analytic issues, particularly preventive mental health. She recently organized a seminar to investigate the impact that daycare has on children who spend so many hours away from their mothers. She believes that understanding the daycare experience is essential for the mental health of the nation.

Dr. Mahler has also applied her psychoanalytic eye to the aging process. She describes the stresses that result from "too many losses and too many longings," and how the ego is taxed by the demands of the failing body. At times she feels the despair of being a "survivor's survivor," having mourned the death of so many colleagues, family members and friends. For this writer, Dr. Mahler's tremendous life-force, her unique ability to think clearly, to observe, hypothesize and learn from experience continue to be inspirational.

References

[1]Mahler MS: "On the first three subphases of the separation-individuation process." International Journal of Psychoanalysis 53:333-338.
[2]Mahler MS, Pine F, Bergmann A: The Psychological Birth of the Human Infant. New York, Basic Books, 1975.

(*Editors' Note:* Judith R. Smith, C.S.W., is a psychotherapist in private practice in New York City and an independent film producer. She has been a research associate and friend of Dr. Mahler's for the past ten years. She has produced several 16mm films for The Margaret S. Mahler Psychiatric Research Foundation which are based on the research data recorded during the separation-individuation study.)

13

Hilde Bruch, M.D.:
A Seeker of Truth

Paul E. Garfinkel, M.D.

Psychiatrist-in-Chief,
Toronto General Hospital; and
Professor and Vice Chairman,
Department of Psychiatry,
University of Toronto,
Toronto, Ontario, Canada

The author gratefully acknowledges the assistance of Mr. Randy Sparks of the Harris County Medical Archives, Houston Academy of Medicine, Texas Medical Center Library, for making available documents on Dr. Bruch, and of Mrs. Rita Gouett for her technical assistance. Drs. Gary Rodin, David Goldbloom and Molyn Leszcz provided useful comments on earlier drafts of this manuscript.

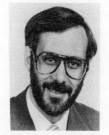 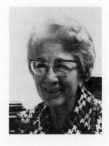

Paul E. Garfinkel, M.D.   Hilde Bruch, M.D.
                          Courtesy of the Harris County
                    Medical Archive Photographic Collection

13

Hilde Bruch, M.D.:
A Seeker of Truth

Throughout her life, Hilde Bruch displayed great personal strength together with a deeply humanistic view of life. Her views on personality development and serious psychopathology reflected her overriding interest in human identity and the authenticity of the individual: "Anything that means superimposing on the patient or on the child or on a person would offend me."[1]

Anecdotes reflecting her personal nature and style abound, both in her professional and personal life. I knew her on a personal level only from the mid 1970's, but on repeated occasions I was struck by her firmness, honesty and outspoken manner. On one occasion, my wife and I dined with Bruch and the Sadovoys at an elegant Toronto restaurant. She ordered an avocado vinaigrette to begin the meal, and when it arrived, she found it too firm to eat. She summoned our somewhat haughty waiter, who removed the offending dish; moments later he replaced it with a carefully diced avocado. After tasting it, Bruch immediately recognized it to be a carved preparation of the avocado she had just rejected. She recalled the waiter and informed him in no uncertain terms that she was not deceived, nor would she be coerced by his haughty manner and dishonesty. She often attributed her sensitivity to coercion even in such trivial matters to her early encounters with Nazis in her German homeland. Throughout her life she stood out against authoritarianism and rigid dogmatic views and often found herself to be alone in criticizing existing theories in medicine and psychiatry.

Bruch once described the creative process to Jane Preston and Hanna Decker; her description reveals features of herself which enabled her to become a productive and innovative academic clinician. She emphasized the capacity for independent thinking, courage and perseverance as important for creativity. She herself had an unusual gift for independent thinking, manifested in early life; she liked to recall her high school experiences when the teacher would ask her to explain why another student could not understand a math problem. Bruch could usually point to some unstated misunderstanding underlying the questions, but not directly related to the problem.[2] This ability to step outside a problem and draw her own conclusions was repeatedly evident in her career, whether in debunking the endocrine hypothesis of childhood obesity or in identifying why a trainee might be blocked in the psychotherapy of a patient.

Her courage was an important component to her creative abilities. Years before it became fashionable she recognized the limitations of drive theory in psychoanalysis and emphasized a broader interpersonal learning theory. She found that her questions "were not only unwelcomed but were immediately branded as indicating something unfavorable about the individual who asked them . . . I felt as if I were back in my small-town high school where independent thinking had been equated with misbehavior."[2] Nevertheless, she consistently continued to display the courage to ask these troubling questions in spite of the rejection that may have resulted. At 16 she selected a maxim from a page of sayings which reflected her attitude: "Damaging truth, I prefer it to advantageous error. Truth heals the pain which perhaps it evokes."[2] She maintained this attitude throughout her life.

Bruch also emphasized the importance of perseverance: "I put stock in a certain degree of stick-to-it-ness."[1] She alone of 10 students from her town completed the high school course work. An example of her perseverance is apparent from her use of the literature in her academic manuscripts. She insisted on quoting only those articles she had read herself since she noted that errors were frequently passed down by misquoted secondary sources. This same perseverance enabled her to pursue an area of inquiry for nearly 50 years. When this attitude was matched with her confidence in her abilities to make accurate observations and draw valid conclusions, it becomes apparent why Bruch courageously stepped outside the existing scientific theories of the day and added fresh new insights.

Bruch's academic work covered many areas over 50 years--eating disorders, schizophrenia, endocrinology, historical subjects and parent education; but she considered the eating disorders to be "the red thread" that goes through her writing from 1938. They attracted and sustained her interest for so many years because of the relationship of eating to so many aspects of living: sociocultural, transactional learning, growth, endocrinologic and drive disturbances.[1] She repeatedly cautioned against simple recipes as solutions for complex problems, whether it was developing an understanding of anorexia nervosa or the supervision of a resident in the psychotherapy of a patient: "In a way the teaching of psychotherapy is very parallel to what I try to write in the book on parent instruction--that you can't prescribe a cookbook of childcare and you can't prescribe a recipe book of psychotherapy."[1]

Biographical Data

Hilde Bruch was born in Duelken, Germany, on March 11, 1904. Duelken was predominantly a Catholic, industrial town about 10 miles from the Dutch border. Her parents, Hirsch and Adele (Rath) Bruch, operated a successful livestock business. She grew up as the third child of seven; she had four brothers and two sisters. Her early

remembrances involved such things as the use of the first electric lights in the family home, the acquisition of the first family telephone, and the day the entire town gathered to see the first zeppelin flying by.

Bruch began school in 1910. There were about 10 Jewish families in the town, and the school was literally a one-room school. From early on she was attracted to learning. Before she was old enough to go to school herself, she bribed her older brother and sister to forget their sandwiches so that she could follow them to school with their missing lunches. By the time she was in the fourth grade, she was a disturbing student because she asked questions; while she was well-behaved, she never accepted what others said uncritically, even then. She recalled Germany's celebration of Wilhelm II's twenty-fifth anniversary on the throne in 1913. The celebration was focused on the many years of peace the country had enjoyed and the "peace emperor" who was responsible for it. The following year the country went to war. Bruch was convinced that the celebration had been set up so that Wilhelm could receive the accolades for having been the peace emperor and then go to war. She later recalled her awareness of this deception as her first conscious criticism of authority.

Bruch's early childhood goals were in keeping with her place and time. When asked what she wanted to be when she grew up, she replied, "A mother." But her parents supported her in her efforts to obtain the best education possible (R. Sparks, unpublished). Serendipity played a role, however, in her going on to high school. In 1917, the winter was so cold that the schools had to be closed. One day the students were all taken to a frozen lake to skate with other children from the area. Bruch saw other girls there with red berets; they were part of the uniform of girls who attended school in Gladbach, just a few railway stops from Duelken. Transferring to this school allowed her to study Latin and mathematics and then go on to University.

Bruch's father suffered from diabetes before the discovery of insulin and died at age 55; she was 16 years old. He had been a wealthy man and left a considerable amount of money for his children. However, relentless inflation rendered the money worthless, and Bruch was able to attend medical school only because of generous allowances given by her uncles. She had enjoyed studying mathematics in high school and had planned on becoming a scientist. However, under the influence of a maternal uncle who was a physician, she decided to enter medical school in 1923. This uncle regarded her as his intellectual protege and took her on his rounds. He convinced her to "study medicine and you can do anything you want." Although Bruch was ambitious, it was the "maternal aspect of medicine" that eventually appealed to her.[1]

After graduation from medical school in Freiburg in 1928, Bruch interned in Dusseldorf. This was followed by a year at the Physiological Institute in Kiel, a leading place for physical chemistry. Her work there dealt with the behavior of electrolytes in semi-permeable membranes and led to an interest in electrolytes which continued during her pediatric residency. From 1930 to 1933, Bruch was a resident in pediatrics at the University of Leipzig. During this time, she wrote on cerebrospinal fluid and acid-base balance.

Bruch completed her residency in October, 1932 and immediately opened a private office in a suburb of Dusseldorf. She closed her office in April, 1933 because of Hitler's ascent to power. "Unable to blind myself to the gravity of the situation or to accept the status of a second-rate citizen, I decided within a few months to leave Germany."[2] She went to London with characteristic reasoning: "Everybody went to France...so I didn't want to go to France."[1] She spent one year in London, where she worked in Emmanuel Miller's Child Guidance Clinic and sat in on staff conferences at the Tavistock Clinic. This provided her with an exciting view of psychiatry, quite different from her German medical school training. However, she did not feel comfortable in England and left for the United States in October, 1934.

On the trip to America, Bruch met a biochemist who worked at Columbia Presbyterian Medical Center. He introduced her to Dr. Rustin McIntosh, chief of Pediatrics at Columbia, who offered her a position at Babies Hospital in New York. McIntosh was impressed with her training at Leipzig and her interest in electrolytes. However, many years later he confessed to Bruch that although hundreds of refugee doctors came to see him, she was the only one who said she wanted to learn something.

In 1935, Bruch was assigned the job of developing a pediatric endocrine clinic; the vast majority of the patients were obese children because obesity was thought to be primarily a hormonal problem. Over the course of five years more than 250 obese children were studied and followed. Less than 10 percent of these suffered from a primary hormonal disorder, usually congenital hypothyroidism. She became aware of how easy it was to distinguish hypothyroidism from other causes of childhood obesity. During this time she described why a diagnosis of Frohlich's syndrome was being incorrectly applied, based on erroneous assumptions regarding Frohlich's original report and misapplication of the basal metabolic rate test.[3,4] At the same time, she began to turn her attention to the broader world of the obese children.

Her interest in the family was sparked by her observations regarding the difficulties that parents of obese children encountered in attempting to comply with a treatment plan. While treatment was directed to reduce eating and increase activity, she began to recognize that the obesity was related to more complex issues. Out of 160 families in the clinic at the time, 40 were selected for detailed study. Bruch observed that many parents were themselves obese, but surprisingly, she found that it was the non-obese parents who displayed more obvious psychopathology. There was much evidence of severe marital discord in these families, and the "child would be treated as a personal possession who was supposed to compensate a parent, usually the mother, for his or her own frustration."[2] The results of this study were published in 1941 in a paper titled, "The Family Frame of Obese Children."[5]

While her work at this time drew her more closely to the field of psychiatry, this paralleled her personal experiences. She was naturally concerned for her own family in Germany and became preoccupied with her helplessness in being able to assist them. In fact, her worry and perhaps feelings of guilt about her family's fate seemed to lead to a depression in 1935. "Guilt for having left and greater guilt for not being able to do more" (Sparks, unpublished). Her oldest brother's children were taken for safety to Holland, and when the Germans invaded Holland, her nephew was taken to England, while her niece was returned to her parents and perished with them in Auschwitz. Bruch eventually brought her nephew, Herbert, to America and adopted him. She assisted her mother and two brothers in escaping, but other relatives died in the Holocaust. Bruch's mother came to New York in 1941, where she lived with her youngest son until her death in 1943.

Involvement in Psychiatry

Bruch gained an informal introduction to psychiatry through her friend Janet Rioch. At that time, the medical staff of Presbyterian Hospital ate together in one large formal dining room. Bruch and Rioch were the youngest on staff and were usually together at lunch. Rioch was working with Flanders Dunbar on her early psychosomatic theories and shared these with Bruch, together with news about the work being done on the psychotherapy of schizophrenia. Rioch was also in psychoanalytic training at the time and began taking Bruch along to her classes. During this time Bruch's work on obesity began to move toward family dynamics, and she felt she required help from a psychiatrist. Rustin McIntosh spoke to Nolan Lewis about this, and Florence Powdermaker was assigned to work with Bruch. This resulted in a helpful collaboration and a close personal friendship.

By 1940 Bruch recognized that "I didn't want to be a pediatrician who was interested in psychiatry because you do it always apologetically."[1] She decided on becoming a trained child psychiatrist to enable her to further her interests in the family of the obese child. She applied for a Rockefeller Foundation Fellowship, and the day after she applied she was phoned by a Mr. Lambert of the Foundation. He expressed interest in her proposal and recommended that she go to the Johns Hopkins Hospital. She left New York in 1941 to study psychiatry at the Children's Psychiatric Service of the Johns Hopkins Hospital and the Henry Phipps Psychiatric Clinic. In Baltimore she began to study with and develop friendships with Frieda Fromm-Reichmann, Harry Stack Sullivan, Edith Weigert, Olive Smith and Theodore and Ruth Lidz. Jerome Frank was chief resident during her time at Phipps. Dr. Lawrence Kolb once said to Bruch: "Hilde, I feel sorry for the young people. They don't have the teachers the way we had."[1]

While a resident at the Phipps Clinic, Bruch began a psychoanalysis with Frieda Fromm-Reichmann. This initiated her subsequent association with her two most significant mentors: Fromm-Reichmann and Harry Stack Sullivan.

Fromm-Reichmann served as both psychoanalyst and teacher to Bruch. One day in 1943, Fromm-Reichmann asked Bruch to present a case of a compulsive disorder to a guest teacher who was conducting the psychoanalytic seminar that day. Much later Bruch was told she was selected since she was the only resident who did not know enough to be overawed by Sullivan's reputation.[6] She was so impressed by Sullivan's suggestions about that case that she asked him for regular supervision of a young male catatonic schizophrenic who apparently recovered with their combined effort. Bruch felt that she learned from Sullivan "how to understand the schizophrenic mode of communication and also how to use it as a guide towards exploration of the reality entanglements that had precipitated the schizophrenic's withdrawal."[7]

Bruch considered Sullivan to be her most important supervisor and teacher.[8] While it has been said that Sullivan took Freud's concepts and attached new terms to them, Bruch felt that his major contribution lay not in his ability to agree or disagree with one or another aspect of psychoanalytic theory, but rather in his use of a conceptual framework which derived from physics; he felt that older views in which the individual was considered in isolation were inadequate, and that a change in approach was needed, in which people and their behavior had to be considered in terms of multiple interactive forces. Bruch felt that Sullivan's formulations of the concepts of the importance of interpersonal processes were in good agreement with what she had previously observed in her studies of childhood obesity. While greatly impressed by Sullivan's theory, such an interpersonal model did not help her understand how bodily functions, such as hunger and fullness, could misdevelop in such a conspicuous fashion. Nor did she find that the therapeutic approach was useful for her obese patients. While they developed insight, it did not aid them in better adjustment or weight loss.

In spite of her reservations about Sullivan's theoretical model, she found his supervision extremely valuable in dealing with patients with schizophrenic and obsessional disorders. She had regular supervision from him for about 5 years, almost until the time of his death in 1949. She also attended almost every seminar and lecture course he gave in the New York and Washington area. In 1945, with the war over and Bruch's nephew, Herbert, alone in London, it was Sullivan who arranged for the State Department to immediately secure a visa for the boy, and Fromm-Reichmann who personally brought Herbert back to the United States.

While in Baltimore, Bruch had regular supervision from Sullivan. She and Olive Smith would drive together to Rockville, where Bruch would have her 4 p.m. analytic session with Fromm-Reichmann. Then at 5 p.m. Smith would begin her analytic session with Fromm-Reichmann while Bruch would be supervised by Sullivan. He often prepared a brandy for himself and a martini for her. At 6 p.m., she and Smith would return to Baltimore.

Bruch felt a common bond with Fromm-Reichmann since both were refugees from Nazi Germany. She first met Fromm-Reichmann socially. When Fromm-Reichmann heard that Bruch was in Baltimore, she arranged a dinner party for her to meet 6-8 other women psychiatrists who lived in that area. This led Bruch to begin attending her seminars. When the United States entered the war, Bruch began an analysis with Fromm-Reichmann. She found this to be very useful. Eventually the two women became close friends. Given their relationship, it is not surprising that they also shared a common attitude toward therapy, in which the essential work is done by the patient, and the therapist "at best is a guide." Bruch often used this to describe not only therapy, but learning in general. To her, a teacher should not indoctrinate or "train" the student, but rather develop the particular assets the student possesses so that he may use himself more effectively.

But Bruch's understanding of human development and psychopathology moved further under the influence of work by Piaget and Bateson in the 1950's. Piaget's book, *The Construction of Reality*, had a great impact on her. He emphasized conceptual development, not merely the vicissitudes of drives and effects, in the individual. Bateson and his group were describing the double-bind in interpersonal communication. This impressed on her that disordered thinking was not necessarily due to inner processes, but rather requires learning. Similarly, her close involvement with Theodore Lidz had an impact. His formulation for schizophrenia concerned the idea that one has to be taught crazy thinking, the transmission of irrationality. Bruch began to draw

upon these theories to view the disordered conceptual and perceptual development in people with serious eating disorders as central to their psychopathology. But she felt that the faulty learning which led to these disturbances--in thinking style and in misrepresenting feelings such as anger or depression or frustration as hunger-- had to be learned from early experiences.

During this time Bruch became increasingly outspoken in her criticism of classical psychoanalytic views. The past emphasis on drive disturbance to her reflected a view that the individual was "conceived of as a passive result of what happened to him." For anorexia nervosa, psychoanalytic explanations for the food refusal included unconscious fears of oral impregnation. But it became "increasingly difficult for me to conceive of these various unconscious conflicts as 'causing' these disorders."[2] She also conflicted with Fromm-Reichmann during this period. By then Fromm-Reichmann had become the most respected proponent of Sullivan's ideas, and she was concerned about Bruch's new interest in and emphasis on "the body." But it was precisely this aspect which Bruch felt Sullivan's conceptualization lacked: the individual's experiences of his or her body, which she thought are the outcome of particular interactional patterns. In this regard, there was an affinity between Bruch's thinking and that of Margaret Mahler. Mahler studied the separation-individuation process between mother and child, and in so doing, integrated interpersonal experiences into psychic development, much as Bruch was doing. Nevertheless, there were basic differences. While Mahler felt that individuation begins around the 8th or 10th month of life, Bruch was convinced that the important elements of that process start from the moment the mother receives the infant and in the manner she nurses him. In this sense, Bruch's views presaged much of the current research findings on early infant development.

Bruch returned to New York in 1943 to begin the private practice of psychoanalysis and an affiliation with the College of Physicians and Surgeons at Columbia University. She was appointed a clinical associate professor in 1954 and a clinical professor in 1959. In 1964 Bruch accepted Shervert Frazier's invitation to become professor of Psychiatry at Baylor College of Medicine in Houston. At the time, she was concerned about the relatively severe winters and the increasing urban violence in New York. Before moving to Texas, she purchased a Rolls-Royce, saying that she would not "kowtow to Texas Cadillacs" (Sparks unpublished). It was during her time at Columbia, and later at Baylor, that Bruch began seeing increasing numbers of patients with anorexia nervosa and formulating her theories about the disorder. The initial referrals of anorexics were based on her experiences with the psychotherapy of obese adolescents. Bruch, who had always opposed tyranny and authoritarianism, now became involved with a group of young women who, in a search for personal worth and control, became tyrannized by starvation.

Theories of Anorexia Nervosa

During the late 1950's and early 1960's, Bruch formulated her main theories on the pathogenesis of anorexia nervosa. In 1961 she began to publish her observations and deductions, initially based on a sample of 12 patients, which was a relatively large number at that time.[9] As her reputation for treating the problem became widespread, and as the illness became common, the number of referrals mushroomed.

Diagnostically Bruch made an important contribution by emphasizing the need to distinguish between "primary" anorexia nervosa and others in whom the weight loss occurred because of depression, schizophrenia or conversion hysteria (atypical anorexia nervosa in her terminology).[8] This precise separation of a specific syndrome occurred at a time when anorexia nervosa was a term applied to all emotionally determined causes of weight loss. Bruch's recognition of a core subgroup with a "relentless pursuit of thinness" enabled more careful observation of their psychopathology.

Bruch first described a group of three interrelated "perceptual and conceptual" disturbances in anorexia nervosa: 1) body image disturbances; 2) interoceptive disturbances such as an inability to accurately identify internal sensations such as hunger, satiety or affective states; and 3) an overwhelming sense of personal ineffectiveness.

Bruch[10] distinguished the use of the term "hunger" in its purely physiological sense from the recognition of particular sensations and cognitions that are experienced and associated with food deprivation. She used the term "hunger" in the latter sense to refer to a series of learned

behaviors. According to Bruch, normal "hunger awareness" evolves when the mother's reactions to the child's state of food deprivation are congruent with his or her internal experiences. Initially the child requires clear signals from outside to confirm the knowledge of when it is time to eat and when to stop. The child's labeling of internal experiences needs to be confirmed by his or her environment. Faulty "hunger awareness" results in "perceptual/conceptual confusion," and Bruch recognized components from both mother and child in producing this. The mother's role was thought to be related to her failure to respond to her child's bodily needs and to the tendency to superimpose onto the child her perception of his or her needs. Bruch, like Piaget, differentiated behaviors that are initiated by the individual from those that occur in response to external stimuli. For healthy development, both are important. Bruch felt that anorexics have serious deficits in self-initiated behavior. Bruch proposed that lack of recognition of inner processes extended to other areas of functioning so that the child becomes unable to differentiate feelings and sensations originating within from those which occur in response to external events.

Bruch first emphasized body image disturbance to be an essential characteristic of anorexia nervosa, but she considered it to be related to a general misperception of internal states. Specifically, it involves the patient's inability to recognize her appearance as abnormal. The misperception reaches "delusional proportions" and is manifest in the lack of concern about, or stubborn defense of, an emaciated shape." While others had described aspects of the body image in anorexia nervosa, Bruch clarified its important role to the distorted drive for thinness and linked it to inner deficits in self-awareness. As a result of these observations, a growing body of research literature has begun to explore the perceptual and conceptual dimensions of anorexia nervosa.[12]

Bruch viewed these distortions in body image and internal perception to be closely tied to a third ego disturbance--a sense of ineffectiveness. Her central theme was that the search for self-mastery and autonomy is maladaptively pursued through control over one's body. Bruch herself had experienced ineffectiveness in helping her family escape from Nazi Germany. Later she recognized the central role of helplessness in the development of anorexia nervosa in her patients.

One aspect of the illness which was puzzling to her was its prevalence among individuals who, according to families and school reports, have been unusually good, successful and gratifying as children. The onset of the illness is accompanied by marked changes in behavior, in which previously compliant girls become negativistic, angry and distrustful. Bruch observed that in therapy, behind this self-assertive facade, they experienced themselves as helpless, as acting only in response to demands coming from others rather than from themselves, and at times, experienced their bodies as not being their own.[8] Bruch's description of the disturbed sense of self and of parental empathic failures have much in common with more recent work by Kohut and others in the psychoanalytic school of self-psychology who have described similar disturbances in patients with narcissistic disorders.

More recently, Bruch[8] focused on the cognitive style of the pre-anorexic child. She suggested that in such individuals their conceptual development does not advance appropriately. In Piaget's terms, anorexics do not pass into the abstract phase of development but remain with the style of thinking of earlier childhood, preconceptual and concrete operations. The egocentrism that is characteristic of this phase is manifest in behavior, morality and relationships. It is this failure in conceptual development together with the deficit in a sense of self that makes them both overly compliant in their pre-teen years and vulnerable to anorexia nervosa in adolescence with its demands for autonomy and separation.

Over the years, Bruch maintained her interest in the role of the family in eating disorders. In addition to her emphasis on mother-daughter interactions, she observed certain parental characteristics in anorexia nervosa.[13] She felt that in these families there is competition between parents about who is making greater sacrifices for the child, with the concomitant expectation that the child will accede obediently to the parents' extreme demands. These demands were thought to be for appearance, behavior and success in achievements. Bruch[11] felt that the fathers of anorexics were especially concerned with external appearance. She thought that despite considerable personal success, the fathers tended to feel they do not measure up some way. She observed that they were very preoccupied with physical appearance, proper behavior and performance, both

in themselves and in their children.

Bruch believed that the increased prevalence of anorexia nervosa in the 1970's was due to cultural change. But she strongly objected to the common argument that the cultural emphasis on increasing slimness was the determining factor. Rather, she felt that the usual teenage dieting was related to the pressure for slimness, but that anorexia nervosa was related to other cultural factors. In particular, she felt that changing expectations for women plays an important role: "Girls whose early upbringing has prepared them to become 'clinging vine' wives suddenly are expected at adolescence to prove themselves as women of achievement."[8] This, she felt, created a basic uncertainty for which anorexia nervosa provided a maladaptive solution.

Bruch also argued that the illness was likely to become rare again when its widespread prevalence diminished the sense of "specialness" associated with it. "We might even speculate that if anorexia nervosa becomes common enough, it will lose one of its characteristic features, the representing of a very special achievement. If that happens, we might expect its incidence to decrease again."[14] However, she also later observed, "I probably will not be around to learn whether my prediction is correct, though I should like to be kept informed."[8]

Bruch's major achievements related to her developing both a psychological framework for understanding people with anorexia nervosa and an approach to treatment. Early on in her work, she became very critical of traditional psychoanalysis in the treatment of people with eating disorders. She thought that when they received interpretations in a traditional setting, this might represent a painful re-experiencing of being told what to feel and think. This would confirm their sense of inadequacy and interfere with their development of self-awareness and trust in their own psychological abilities. She therefore set out to treat these patients in a way that encouraged the anorexic to search for autonomy and self-directed identity. The framework involved a setting in which what the patient said was listened to and made the object of repeated exploration. In this situation, the patient then becomes an active participant in the treatment so that she can grow beyond the passivity of her illness. While she was critical of the popular behavioral approaches to therapy as being mechanistic,[15] she did recognize the need for nutritional rehabilitation for the patient to properly benefit from psychotherapy. In doing so, she set the stage for current multi-faceted treatment approaches.

Throughout her life, Bruch rebelled against rigid authoritarianism. This was evident in her stance toward developing a novel understanding of anorexia nervosa but was also apparent in everything she did. Her book, *Don't Be Afraid of Your Child*,[16] stressed a common sense approach to child-rearing at a time when parents often felt paralyzed in dealing with their children because of multiple rules of so-called experts. This same emphasis on personal observation and common sense made her an outstanding psychotherapy supervisor. Her emphasis was on an appreciation of the uniqueness of the individual patient, and she fought hard against jargon in psychiatry. For this reason she often enjoyed teaching medical students who knew little of psychiatric terminology. Her book, *Learning Psychotherapy*,[7] is an excellent example of her clarity in thinking and teaching about the subject. At times, she regretted not having a school of followers, but she also recognized that this was "nearly incompatible with my style of thinking," with its emphasis on the uniqueness of the individual and the encouragement of students to build on their own strengths rather than following the rules established by others.

By the time she died on December 15, 1984, Bruch had lived a full life. She saw her nephew reach adulthood, treated many grateful patients, taught several generations of psychiatrists and gave readily to her many friends. She was a prolific author--about 200 scientific articles, six books and a seventh will be published posthumously. She also received many important awards. Moreover, while often feeling an outsider because her theories were not widely accepted and because of her outspoken nature, she lived to see a time when her views on psychotherapy and anorexia nervosa became part of the mainstream of psychiatry. "Probably the happiest discovery was that psychoanalysis has revealed itself as more flexible, less rigid and dogmatic than I had feared during the early 1940's. Since I went my own way, I have often felt like an outsider; I now feel that I again have a home."[8]

In an autobiographical sketch appropriately entitled, "The Constructive Use of Ignorance," Bruch[8] noted: "There is probably no lonelier feeling than 'Everybody is out of step but me.' "

How fortunate for all of us that she had the courage to endure this loneliness.

References

[1]Preston J and Decker H: APA Interviews of Hilde Bruch, M.D., 1975.
[2]Bruch H: The Constructive Use of Ignorance, in Explorations in Child Psychiatry. Edited by E. J. Anthony, Plenum, New York, 247-264, 1975.
[3]Bruch H: Obesity in Childhood I. Physical Growth and Development of Obese Children. Am. J. Dis. Child. 58:457-484, 1939.
[4]Bruch H: Obesity in Childhood II. Basal Metabolism and Serum Cholesterol of Obese Children. Am. J. Dis. Child. 58:1001-1022, 1939.
[5]Bruch H and Touranine G: Obesity in Childhood V: The Family Frame of Obese Children. Pyschosom. Med. 2:141-206, 1940.
[6]Bruch H: Interpersonal Theory: Harry Stack Sullivan, in Operational Theories of Personality, Edited by A. Burton, Brunner-Mazel, New York, 143-160, 1974.
[7]Bruch H: Learning Psychotherapy. Harvard University Press, Cambridge, 1974.
[8]Bruch H: Four Decades of Eating Disorders, in Handbook of Psychotherapy for Anorexia Nervosa and Bulimia, Edited by D. M. Garner and P. E. Garfinkel, Guilford Press, New York, 7-18, 1985.
[9]Bruch H: Conceptual Confusion in Eating Disorders. J. Nerv. Ment. Disease 133:46-54, 1961.
[10]Bruch H: Hunger and Instinct. J. Nerv. Ment. Disease 149:91-144, 1969.
[11]Bruch H: Eating Disorders: Obesity, Anorexia Nervosa and the Person Within. Basic Books, New York, 1973.
[12]Garfinkel PE and Garner DM: Anorexia Nervosa: A Multidimensional Perspective. Brunner-Mazel, New York, 1982.
[13]Bruch H: Anorexia Nervosa, in Nutrition and the Brain, Edited by R. J. Wurtman and J. J. Wurtman, Raven Press, New York, 101-115, 1979.
[14]Bruch H: The Golden Cage: The Enigma of Anorexia Nervosa, Harvard University Press, Cambridge, 1978.
[15]Bruch H: Perils of Behavior Modification in Treatment of Anorexia Nervosa. JAMA 230:1419-1422, 1974.
[16]Bruch H: Don't Be Afraid of Your Child. Farrar, Straus and Young, New York, 1952.

14

_____

Leadership in
Child Psychiatry

_____

Helen R. Beiser, M.D.

Clinical Professor Emerita,
Department of Psychiatry,
University of Illinois College of Medicine;
Supervising and Training Analyst,
Institute for Psychoanalysis,
Chicago, Illinois;
Psychiatric Consultant,
Jewish Children's Bureau of Chicago; and
President, American Academy of Child Psychiatry 1983–1985

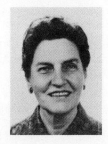

Helen R. Beiser, M.D.

14

Leadership in
Child Psychiatry

When I was elected to the office of president-elect of the American Academy of Child Psychiatry the year after I was retired to emerita status on the faculty of my medical school, I was surprised, to say the least. This is not out of false modesty, but because such recognition of a person who was "present at the creation" of the Academy almost 30 years before is rare. I had no burning goals I wanted to accomplish at this point, and only agreed to run because it seemed wise to have one woman on the slate. Marion Kenworthy and Anne Benjamin had preceded me in the office, but when the Academy was much smaller.

Being asked to write this essay led me to think more deeply about leadership, and what goes into it. Literally, the leader is one who goes first, with others following, toward a common destination or goal. Kracke,[1] in an anthropological study, states that leaders mediate between persons and their social environment. Gutmann,[2] in a study of age and leadership in cross-cultural studies, found that great exploits, wisdom, and spiritual power were aspects of older leaders. The old men were able to link the past to the present and the mundane to the unordinary. This certainly is different from the idea that leaders are simply stronger or smarter than followers. The leader has to know enough to be able to reach the goal, but a more important attribute may be to know how to use the talents of others. Some leaders may aspire to their position out of a need for power, and achieve it by inspiring fear in their followers, but

this can be a very shaky base. A more solid foundation is to be seen as of use to the followers, which is more likely to inspire loyalty. In my case, I hope I have a degree of wisdom and knowledge, and I certainly link the present to the past. Although I am aware that the women's vote was instrumental in getting me elected, I think my strength lies in my ability to link seemingly diverse strands of professional interests into a common goal, the welfare of children.

The literature on political leadership does not seem pertinent to the present topic. There are a number of psychological studies on the attributes of leaders, and on the comparison of male and female leaders. In general, leaders are creative, intelligent, generally competent, warm, expressive, and supportive. The studies I found did not test physical strength or quantitative intelligence. Qualitative differences in personality were found between male and female leaders. Hollander and Yoder[3] found men to be more exploitive, competitive, and task oriented. Women had more concern for interpersonal relationships, were more accommodative and tension reducing. Using various terms, other studies have come up with similar findings. Koralish[4] found that characteristics were related to the sex role rather than the biological sex, and that females often put passive males into leadership roles. Masculine style is initiating whereas feminine style is considerate. Adams and Hicks,[5] in a study at West Point when women were being put into leadership positions, found no difference in the ability of men and women to accomplish missions, but that women were more sensitive to the welfare of subordinates.

In early studies, women were perceived as less dependable than men. I would guess that this related to the cyclic physiological changes in women, which no longer seem to interrupt women's lives, and to the time needed in caring for children and home. Modern technology and changing attitudes have allowed for less time needed for home care, and the assistance of fathers and acceptance of day care have supported other methods of child care. However, the modern, energetic, conscientious woman does need to be reminded that there are only 24 hours in a day, and she may not have time for everything she can and wants to do. On the whole, it seems that men and women are each capable of leadership, although there may be different styles depending on the mix of characteristics. I doubt if any one style is clearly superior to any other, and it is more likely the balance that is important. A certain amount of power is necessary, but not to the point of exploitation. Competition between persons aspiring to leadership can be desirable, but it is more important to get competitors to cooperate to work toward the common goal. The ability to accommodate and compromise is necessary to bring diverse groups together, but not to the point of the loss of integrity. Sensitivity to interpersonal relationships is essential to getting cooperation toward the common goal, but not at the price of losing task orientation. My own study[6] of men and women psychoanalytic supervisors confirms other studies that the men were more task oriented and the women more concerned with the supervisory working relationship, but both were considered good supervisors.

Leadership roles may be by designation or by selection by the group. Leaders may be designated by an accident of birth, like kings, or the oldest in a sibship. Of course, if they are unable to lead, they can be deposed. Leaders may also be appointed by others in power. This would include administrators and teachers. Selection by the group may be formal or informal, and certainly produces a much different relationship between leader and led. In small groups that are deliberately formed without an appointed leader, the group eventually chooses one of their number to assume that role, and may shift with time. One person seems to talk more, or have interesting ideas, but this may not be enough. The leader is more likely one who can mold the group toward a common purpose by stressing similarities of goals rather than differences.

Election to office in a professional organization is a more formal process, but still on the basis of how well the stated goals of the candidates match the goals of the voting members. There are also significant differences in groups to be led. They may be uniform or mixed as to age, sex, educational background, or other characteristic. The leader may be the same as or different from the group. Teachers are almost always older, or at least more knowledgeable, than the taught. Administrators may or may not be. They have more power, and their job is to see that the group performs a task. They may or may not teach in this process. The group has little or nothing to say about the selection of teachers or administrators, but may be instrumental in their removal. A professional organization has a common educational background and should have common goals. The leader is one of the group, chosen for a limited period of time.

I bring these points up because I think there are different issues of leadership dependent on these variables. In other words, followers form transferences to leaders, and they are much more likely to be negative if the leader is designated. Women leaders produce interesting transferences. Perhaps because they are so easily related to mothers and the teachers of the early childhood years, there may be a reaction against them as leaders of persons of mature years, making followers feel immature. This may be particularly apparent among men, but not limited to them. I have seen that women have a harder time accepting women as ministers than men do. A negative counterreaction can escalate the problem. Women administrators tend to encounter such negative transferences more than teachers, and elected officers least of all. There the problem is to get elected in the first place. This is easiest in organizations wholly or largely composed of women.

An area that needs study is how leaders cope with failure. It is not possible to achieve all goals. I doubt if leaders quit when they get angry or depressed, nor simply knock their heads against stone walls. I would predict that they either consider new methods or alter the goals to something more achievable. I would call this flexible persistence.

There have been some studies on the family backgrounds of leaders. Frequently, they have been the oldest children or have been accustomed to leadership by right. Then there are families in which a number of leaders can be found, although it is also difficult for the child of a famous parent to feel competitive in this regard. It might be useful, then to give some idea of my family background and experiences to explain my having achieved my present position.

My family had its share of leaders, although not in the professions. My father was the president of a small corporation and held a number of offices in his national business organization. Although usually the treasurer of that and other organizations to which he belonged, he was also president one year. My mother was never gainfully employed outside our home after marriage, but was very active in charitable organizations. Although she shunned office, she was frequently the chairperson of various charitable drives and was a remarkable fund raiser. Perhaps there was some significance in her choice of the president of a local women's political club to be my godmother, although this woman was always too busy to have anything to do with me until she learned that I had graduated from medical school. My sister was very active in the same charity organization as my mother and was elected president of the board for several years, and also served as president of my father's business after his death. Of course, she was the oldest, as were both of my parents. My brother tried to be president of the business for a while, but did not have the personality characteristics necessary.

How did I, as the youngest by many years, achieve leadership roles? Becoming an aunt at a young age and having considerable responsibility for the care and training of my six nieces certainly helped. Except for usually being a patrol leader in the Girl Scouts, I showed no early leadership qualities. I was often second in command, a position I was used to as the second daughter. Until medical school, my intellectual competence had pushed me ahead so that I was usually one of the youngest of my classmates. It is rare for peers to choose someone younger to be leader. In college I was the treasurer of a failing sorority and actually influenced its closing down in the face of much more prominent people wishing it to continue. I also achieved some leadership positions in the athletic area, although I had given

that up as a career goal. Working for a couple of years after college, in the process of finding medicine as my life goal, both gave me more focus and put me up into a somewhat older group. This plus my strong academic standing put me in the running for office in my sorority, and I was elected secretary of Alpha Omega Alpha, the honor medical society, in my senior year. World War II started during my internship, and I found myself being pushed into positions of responsibility before my training warranted it. I started training in pathology with the idea of a career in research, which seemed to suit my intellectual abilities. I had worked for a master's degree in bacteriology, which I received simultaneously with my medical degree. With men so scarce during the war, I found myself pushed into teaching, and with a faculty appointment, as pathology residencies were declared unnecessary to the war effort.

While pursuing my research interests, I discovered that I became allergic to any animal I touched and had to rethink my career goals. Settling finally on psychiatry, I found myself in my first serious discrimination against women, as so many returning veterans were also looking for psychiatry residencies. This required that I receive training in an old-fashioned state hospital, which I shortened by shifting to child psychiatry at the state-run Institute for Juvenile Research. I simultaneously started psychoanalytic training, and the combination was a good one. The dynamic point of view together with my teaching experience immediately put me into positions of leadership, and I was early given administrative appointments to go along with it. I was also elected secretary of the psychoanalytic candidates' organization, and became involved in the necessary changes in the Institute's structure produced by the sudden postwar expansion of its student body. I met Dr. Irene Josselyn through my child analysis training, and she recommended me for the position of director of a mental health clinic she started in the north shore suburbs of Chicago. Although I showed excellent clinical and organizational abilities, I was not good at working with board members at this time, and returned to the Institute for Juvenile Research as training director.

During the fifties the local Chicago child psychiatrists and a national group who wished to split off from the multidisciplinary American Orthopsychiatric Association formalized the profession of child psychiatry, which attained board certifi-

cation in 1959. I became acquainted with the
leaders of the field, and concentrated my organizational efforts in both the local and national organizations. Locally, I was elected president in
1961, and found myself in the middle of a political battle with some of the most powerful psychiatrists in the state. During the sixties I found
myself in one struggle after another, trying to
conserve services for children as well as chronic
mental patients, and unsuccessfully pointing out
that freedom and money are not necessarily therapeutic and do not guarantee mentally healthy
children. I served on many state-wide committees,
learning to use coalitions of psychiatric and
medical organizations for political purposes, which
culminated in the state medical society nominating
me for appointment to the state Medical Disciplinary Board. Here I learned something about the
law and how to be a hearing officer.

Nationally, I served on many committees of the
Academy, as well as on the Editorial Board of the
Journal of the Academy, and was elected to the
Council. I was on the By-laws Committee which
structured the new Academy to an organization by
application rather than by invitation, and was
chairperson of the Membership Committee which
brought in all those new members. After this, I
seemed to be taking a new role by being elected
to the Nominating Committee repeatedly, with
several terms as chairperson, so that I was involved in selecting the leaders of the Academy.

Just as I was thinking of myself as a senior
citizen, whose last contribution to the Academy
was to start an art show at the annual meeting, I
was surprised to find myself elected president. It
has given me much food for thought, as well as
hard work, and I have decided that my value is
my ability to understand the importance of research, or private practice, of the care of the
chronically ill as well as of the neurotic who can
use psychoanalysis, of the problems of funding, of
the impact of legislation, and of the relationships
to other organizations and other professions. If
there is one aspect of child psychiatry that is
unique, it is not only our ability to communicate
with children, but also to integrate information
from many sources and to deal with the many and
diverse persons in a child's environment. From
this standpoint, even though I do not actually see
children any more, I feel like a child psychiatrist
and hope I can adequately represent them as a
professional group.

My work has not been limited to child psychiatry, although my medical school teaching and
supervision have largely been in that area. I have
always maintained a private practice of adults in
psychoanalysis and psychoanalytic psychotherapy,
and used to do the same with children. Now I
only consult on children with a social agency.
With the Institute for Psychoanalysis in Chicago, I
have taught in the Child Therapy Program as well
as in the program to train psychoanalysts. I have
been a supervisor of both adult and child cases
and directed the child analysis training program
for a number of years. I have served on a number
of its educational committees and have been a
training analyst and on the editorial board of its
Annual. I always have a few research projects
going, presently related to the effects of various
types of parent loss on children, as well as studying the supervisory process.

However, one's life cannot be all work. I have
not had homemaking and child care responsibilities, but found other outlets. Even in medical
school, I went to a weekly sketch class, and I have
continued to devote time regularly to artistic pursuits. I was even president of the American Psychiatric Art Association one year, but prefer not
to exercise my leadership abilities in that area. An
occasional sale gives me much more pleasure. I
enjoy traveling, which started because of my allergies and has aroused interest in archeology and
anthropology. I have also served on the board of
the same charity as my mother and sister and
taken a leadership role in church activities. I
enjoy both music and sports as a passive participant, and I keep up my early athletic interests in
walking and swimming when possible.

As I look back on my career, I have wide experience in different kinds of leadership and in
different settings. I wonder if I could have gone
farther earlier. Physical limitations changed my
career direction several times, and that is beyond
control. I have often thought that the one attainment I might have liked which would have been
more possible if I had been a man, would be to
head a university department. However, there is
nothing I can do about that now, either. This goal
may be more available to women in the future.
Sometimes a strength may turn out to be an
obstacle. For example, being skipped through
elementary school seemed something to be proud
of, but being the youngest in the class for so
many years can interfere with early achievement

of leadership roles. Similarly, my ability to transform a problem or a disappointment into something positive, such as broadening my interests through travel necessitated by hay fever, may have interfered with the intensity necessary to pursue leadership goals. On the other hand, I enjoy the breadth of my interests and have never been that interested in top leadership roles. When they have offered themselves to me, however, as in the accident of war or politics, I am happy that I have been able to fulfill them. The values I have found to be important in my work are quality, but with the acceptance and tolerance of individual differences, flexibility, with maintaining personal integrity, and just plain hard work, but without needing to take all the credit. Delegation of duties is something I had to learn and am still learning. I hope I combine the seemingly masculine trait of getting a job done and the seemingly feminine trait of sensitivity to the feelings of those doing the job. Recently George Tarjan, past president of both the American Academy of Child Psychiatry and the American Psychiatric Association, paid me the ultimate compliment. He said, "Helen, you are not just a leader of women, but of men, too."

References

[1] Kracke W: The complementarity of social and psychological regularities: Leadership as a mediating phenomenon. Ethos, 8(4), 273-285, 1980.
[2] Gutmann D: Age and leadership: Cross cultural observations. Psychoanalytic Inquiry, 2(1), 109-120, 1982.
[3] Hollender EP and Yoder J: Some issues in comparing women and men as leaders. Basic and Applied Social Psychology, 1(3), 267-280, 1980.
[4] Koralish K: Sex-role orientation and leadership style. International Journal of Women's Studies, 5(4), 329-337, 1982.
[5] Adams J and Hicks JM: Leader sex, leader descriptions of own behavior, and subordinates' descriptions of leader behavior (Project Athena West Point). International Journal of Women's Studies, 3(4), 321-326, 1980.
[6] Beiser H: Studies of supervision related to child-analysis training and the gender of the supervisor. The Annual of Psychoanalysis, 10, 57-76, 1982.

15

———

Medical Practice and
Medical Politics: One Route

———

Dorothy Starr, M.D.

*Private Practice,
Washington, DC*

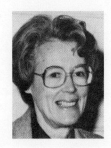

Dorothy Starr, M.D.

15

Medical Practice and
Medical Politics: One Route

I do not know how I came to announce at an early age that I was going to be a doctor, and I have even less an idea why it was always taken so seriously, but it was all settled before I was out of grade school. So much revolved around illness in my family. Family lore had it that my mother had wanted to go to medical school and even had been accepted, but then the family doctor said she was too frail. My father, a very good mechanic, came out of a brief stint in World War I with a chronic ear infection and it was his illnesses rather than his unemployment that prompted the family move from the Bronx to upstate New York. My older sister was the bright one but she was also sickly and somehow dropped out. I was the only healthy one who could, should, would grow up to be a doctor, and even in the Depression, doctors were needed. In high school I planned to be a doctor and I went to college to take a pre-medical course. I never considered any other career, and I had no talents to distract me.

My age cohort was born in a boom (the twenties), raised in a bust (the great Depression), and came of age in World War II. One paradox of the Depression was that it was easy to get into college--all it took was money--and being a working student was easier than getting a real job. We had the alphabet soup of government agencies to absorb the army of unemployed before the war solved that problem. Our fathers could earn a pittance that looked quite substantial then on PWA (Public Works Administration) and WPA (Works Progress Administration). The National Youth

Administration (NYA) paid students 35 to 50 cents an hour "for useful work for which no one would otherwise have been hired" to keep them in school. Young male dropouts could go off to the Civilian Conservation Corps (CCC). There was no equivalent program for girls, but then we could always find work as live-in domestics.

In the thirties and forties, most of us were not very questioning when it came to inequality, not that we didn't note its existence but that we, or at least I, took it for granted. In high school, I secretly wept when I saw M. scrubbing and powdering her face in the girls' washroom and suspected she at that moment secretly hated being black as much as I secretly hated being Catholic in this white Protestant town, but these were not things we could change.

I went back to New York City for college because it was familiar and cheap. New York University let students pay on time with an NYA job, i.e., a government check. NYA paid 50 cents an hour for a maximum of forty hours per month. Twenty dollars times ten months added up to almost half the total tuition and fees.

In college we were preoccupied with and pragmatic about getting into medical school. The Washington Square College of NYU was reputed to have over one thousand pre-medical students enrolled that fall of 1939. We were all very determined, and we and our advisors assessed our liabilities and our assets and plotted our courses accordingly. It was better to be male than female, but a Jewish boy from New York City had more like-competitors than a Catholic girl from a small town upstate. I stopped mentioning that I was born in Manhattan and raised in Highbridge. A sensible advisor also astutely predicted that I would have an uneven academic record and had better cultivate a well-rounded image, get into activities and take some non-science courses. Getting into medical school was the deadly serious business in which most of my friends were engaged. Apparently none of us was brilliant enough to expect to get in on honors and scholarship. Almost anything was fair although we all disapproved of the young man who had a scheme to get better grades--he studied for and took half of his examinations and then pleaded illness so he could cram separately for the other half at a later date. Despite the part-time jobs, studying and no money, we had a marvelous time, most of which we spent talking. We spent an inordinate amount of time talking and everything was a grave issue although I do not remember what the issues were.

In the end, I did what any aspiring student might do--I worked my way through college, cultivated contacts, fenced with the women's team and, when I graduated, enlisted in the Army. When I finished, I had no funds to go to medical school, and, in the midst of a war, I probably couldn't have gotten in anyway.

The Women's Army Corps was not a risky enterprise; women might be stationed in combat zones but never at any great risk. For me, it was a welcome change of pace, and I travelled more than I had ever done before or since. In twenty-eight months I was stationed in Florida, Massachusetts and Georgia; I went to Australia via California, north via New Guinea to the Philippines to return via Biak and Hawaii to California to go to Iowa and finally mustered out at Foster Field, Texas. When I came out of the Army I had the G.I. Bill and renewed enthusiasm for medical school; all I had to do now was to get accepted.

Returning veterans were very popular after World War II and there were not a lot of returning women veterans applying to medical school. I went back and got a job at New York University while I applied to medical schools. I went to my old professors and I took the medical aptitude tests. I had kept in some touch with two good supporters, Dr. Harry Charipper and Dr. van der Merwe. I had gotten to know Dr. Charipper, chairman of the Department of Biology, when I took an honors course he taught: with most of the

men gone we women stood out. I had worked for Dr. van der Merwe's Physics Department in an NYA job dismantling pinball machines for the parts. Both encouraged me and either interceded or wrote strong recommendations to offset my undistinguished academic record which included an F in organic chemistry. Incidentally, I did not know what mentors were and if there were any "role models" around, I don't remember them. I did know that people could be very helpful and they usually were. By the time I was at the Long Island College of Medicine, I recognized that with the luck of the Irish, there always seemed to be someone who supported me when I most needed it.

In medical school, I worked as a laboratory technician in a nearby hospital at night, and when I had some academic difficulties, one of the doctors on both the staff and the faculty interceded for me. Medical school was exactly what I had bargained for, totally engrossing and overwhelming. I worried and prayed for four solid years that I would graduate. We were the first post-war class and probably more paranoid than most--many of us had been out of school for three years and wondered if we could keep up. Most of us believed the rumors that they accepted more first-year students than they had room for in the second year. Thirteen women started and ten of us finished together, one dropped back a year, one dropped out, and one, I think, got married and left to have a baby. Women medical students were not the only ones banned for pregnancy. Later, when I was interning, I found a nursing student on permanent night duty for the last few months of training as a compromise between letting her graduate and kicking her out after her secret marriage was revealed by her not-so-secret pregnancy. Maternity uniforms were not made then for any field.

It must be remembered that singly and collectively women did not then challenge the established order. Nobody went to court in those days. I can remember some discussions about discrimination and, in New York City, we were usually talking about anti-Semitism. The military had made me aware of segregation. I finally noticed that there were separate companies and facilities for black troops. More painfully, my travels had shown me that separate was rarely equal. I can still see the bus station with three restrooms, "Ladies," "Men," and "Colored." Those black men and women stood quietly in that line and women tolerated sexist jokes and the absence of facilities for women.

I finished medical school broke, just as I had left college. In 1950, as now, the military offered substantial financial inducements during training years. At that point they were the only ones who paid interns. Failing to obtain a military internship, I applied for a sponsored one. The small St. John's Episcopal Hospital in Brooklyn paid fifteen dollars a months plus a meals' allowance; the Navy gave me the regular pay and allowances of a lieutenant junior grade, a bonanza! House-staff quarters were for men only in those days. We women got rooms in the adjoining Episcopal Home for Elderly Ladies. It did not occur to us to expect other arrangements. The hospital had a good program: there were a busy inner-city emergency room, some terrific residents and a lot of staff babies to deliver. This was before the technological explosion and the development of tertiary care facilities, so small hospitals were mostly just smaller. I don't know how much different the training was in the more prestigious hospitals--I suspect not a lot--but it would have made a crucial difference had I not gone on in the military in terms of getting a residency in a surgical specialty like obstetrics and gynecology. The military probably offered some reverse discrimination: they tended to send the women to the major teaching facilities, which got us into accredited training programs.

On completion of the internship, I reported for active duty at St. Albans Naval Hospital, Queens, New York. A group of us reported in en masse, and we were asked our preferences and reminded that the needs of the service came first, and then each of us was sent off to the service of his or her choice. As reserves, we were not entitled to training, but St. Albans was an accredited training hospital and we were henceforth treated as residents. Ten months later, the needs of the service intervened and I was ordered to Bainbridge Naval Training Center in Maryland, to take over the WAVE medical ward; an epidemic of children's diseases among the recruits had hit the WAVE detachment. Here, too, an effort was made to give me what I wanted. I was encouraged to work on both services, and the chief of OB-GYN wrangled a consultant so that we would get some kind of credit toward required training time.

It was a good experience. I was also working with two good psychiatrists and renewed my interest in psychiatry. They had more answers for a lot of the problems I saw than my other two specialties. Also, and perhaps more powerful, I had turned thirty, and I could not envision combining any semblance of family life with the way I expected to practice OB-GYN. There was a lot of enthusiasm for psychiatry, and the Navy offered six months' training for reserve medical officers at Bethesda. I applied, reasoning that it would be useful if I stayed in OB-GYN and a start on approved training if I switched to psychiatry. Dr. George Raines, Chief of Navy Psychiatry, approved, and I was ordered to Bethesda in April 1953. I later learned that the department had never had a woman trainee and did not want one.

They were all very genteel or else I couldn't tell a cool welcome from a warm one. To their everlasting credit, when I did not turn out to be a problem, or ruin the service, or turn off the patients, or upset the troops, they could not do enough for me. Within a few months, they offered me a promotion to staff at the end of the six months so that I could start in the program and complete an accredited residency. They even gave me one of the few air-conditioned offices. So isolated were we few women physicians that I never met Dr. Elizabeth Crisp, an obstetrician-gynecologist and the first woman assigned to a residency at Bethesda. I also may have been distracted by my other goal, to find a husband. When I got married in August, they continued me in the program. This may be commonplace now, but it was special then. When I became pregnant and duly submitted my resignation, they took their time processing it and I had completed fourteen months of residency and six months of the pregnancy before I was discharged.

The civilian world was a rude awakening. I could not even give my services away and it was several months after the baby was born before I restarted residency training at St. Elizabeths Hospital in Washington, D.C. There was not nearly as much to learn back then: residency was largely on-the-job training, and psych residents had no night duty and few weekends when they had to remain in the hospital. It was an exciting time in a growing specialty with a bright crowd. We were enthusiastic and so was everyone else. It was a great time to be starting out in medicine in any specialty.

Some people still insisted that women leave

work weeks to months before their due dates, so juggling pregnancies was still tricky. I learned not to be definite about the dates, worked till I went into labor and then took off whatever accrued leave I had as a matter of right. I was much impressed and a bit envious of another resident who had somehow sold the idea of a part-time residency to the administration and only worked half days. Most of us needed all of the $4400 to $4800 a year we earned to pay for child care. Help was a lot more available and a lot less expensive. We paid our first housekeeper less for a five and a half day week in 1955 than we pay a day worker for six hours in 1985.

After residency, I stayed on as staff for four years developing a service for outpatients at the hospital and building a private practice at home. My first office was the spare bedroom in the large old apartment we had fortuitously rented, sight unseen. Chas., my husband, took care of the babies while Ma had office hours. We bought a dishwasher with the first check I collected. Then we took the plunge, and I rented an office across the street at 3000 Connecticut, an address well-known in Washington for its concentration of psychiatrists. It was a two-office suite and Max Boverman came along almost immediately to rent the other office. We got along fine but I am not sure if we were there much at the same time. That was the heyday of psychoanalysis, and everything was so confidential that patients sidled in and out, and so did we.

Subsequently, we bought a house and, having learned nothing from my earlier experience, I moved the office back to the home. We thought that there were all manner of tax advantages--it said so in all the articles I read. The tax benefits are illusory, but it certainly was cheap office space providing low overhead when I took months off for school vacations. The down side is that I spent the next ten years silently wincing when I detected shrieks overhead and praying for the day when I could decompress between work and home and vice-versa. I must say it got me and the patients off this sidling in and out bit; I was no good as a "blank screen," and patients and their children ran into me and mine all over town. They usually introduced themselves to my children. One time I was discretely not recognizing a patient in a crowded museum elevator, and she called out, "Dr. Starr, don't you remember me from St. Elizabeths? You were my doctor." I

finally decided it was we, not the patients, who were so secretive.

Before the fourth daughter arrived, I had moved from the hospital to the city's Adult Mental Health Clinic. I was so naive at that time that I thought I could improve communications between the hospital and the clinic in the transfer back and forth of outpatients if I was at the clinic. I did not know then that when "we" becomes "they" the perspective changes and the problems don't. But, it was a good job, and I learned a lot. We had a generally outstanding multidisciplinary staff, a good boss downtown and we were on the threshold of the great community mental health movement. At the clinic, as at the hospital, some professionals kept looking for the "good treatment cases," and I made myself unpopular by insisting that anyone who was sick was a good case, or there was something wrong with our treatment. One man blew up one day and stormed that I had made this clinic a dumping ground, that all the worst cases were sent to us. I guessed that meant the public clinic was doing its job.

Four years later it was time for me to move on into full-time office practice. Community mental health centers were now big business. One of our consultants had given me a new theoretical framework; Murray Bowen's family systems theory seemed not limited to selected patients. I had not applied for analytic training partly because of ideological reservations. The techniques didn't seem right for multi-problem inner-city patients and their psychoses and personality disorders. I cannot assess how much of my reluctance was a rationalization for my unwillingness to invest the time and money in the training and in supporting the training. Being a juice-mother and a lunch-room mother and attending activities at two or more schools and professional society meetings took rather a large chunk of time already. Getting active in the medical community is a good way to make contacts; establishing oneself in the community and establishing a practice are the same operation. It was easy to build a practice in those days. This is a one-company town and the company, the federal government, offered equal coverage under its employees' health insurance for out-patient treatment of mental illness. In fact there was general expansion in the medical community. We had a sophisticated population demanding the best in health care and a government funding an increased supply of specialists and multiple training centers to turn them out. Expectations were high all around, too high.

The cash registers down the street were off on another trend--health care is now an industry, we are providers, patients are consumers and insurance companies are in business to cut costs and make money, profit and non-profit alike. Even as I write, university teaching hospitals, like the industries around them, are negotiating mergers with, or sales to, the for-profit sector. Residents and professors are paid decent salaries, but they have to earn them, and programs are tailored accordingly.

But, as I said, getting established then was easy. I attended a lot of meetings of all kinds and soon discovered that an organization with a thousand members was unlikely to see even a hundred of them at any one time. In fact meetings are mostly attended, as one colleague put it, by "office seekers and office holders"; thus it is not only a small group but an influential one. If you want to join the leadership all you need do is show up regularly and speak up, preferably usefully. A large percentage of the membership also does not vote, but, if they vote, most people vote on name recognition. Writing letters to the leadership also tends to make you well-known. Obviously both speaking up and writing letters is easier if you are concerned about issues and causes. It is my impression that a lot of people who are equally concerned about matters stay home, don't vote, and complain about the leadership instead of going down and getting into the action. It is ironic that the leadership sits around talking to itself about membership apathy and the membership is grumbling somewhere else.

Through interest and energy devoted to organized medicine, I have enjoyed my terms in office, including being elected as the first woman and first psychiatrist to serve as president of the Medical Society of the District of Columbia.

As I look back I was very busy juggling interests, work and family but I was not alone. Superwoman USA was not just out in the professional work forces, she could be found in suburbia and exurbia as well. If she didn't have the talent to write books at night when everyone else was asleep, she was starting a little home business or making everyone's clothes. At the least she was running a transportation system that would boggle Metro's general manager. As we lived through this era, I did not think that we were following any role models; I thought that we had all been fired up by the criticism heaped on American women during World War II. As I remember it, American mothers were alleged to have raised a bunch of weaklings unfit to serve, and younger women were being told that all the American men were bringing home foreign war-brides because, unlike American wives, they weren't spoiled and knew how to work and take care of a man. The contradiction between these escaped me somehow, but I certainly had the impression that we were all trying harder. I remembered forever, though I thought it a bit much, a medical schoolmate's wife who signed out of the hospital within hours of delivering their second baby to go home and get his supper. Remember, those were the days when women were hospitalized for five to seven days after a normal delivery.

The emerging professionals, the baby boom bunch, are a new ball game. Their world is smaller and their egos bigger. A group that can take on a hierarchy like the AMA and ask as a matter of right for a seat on the Board of Trustees is not going to have any trouble holding its own. For the first time ever, women physicians are more in demand. Organizations are falling over themselves to elect their first women presidents and I believe they will all find a way to deal with the physician surplus, if there is one. We had a good time, and I expect our successors will have an even better time.

16

An Interview with
Stella Chess, M.D.

Leah J. Dickstein, M.D.

*Associate Dean for Student Affairs
and Associate Professor,
Department of Psychiatry and Behavioral Sciences,
University of Louisville School of Medicine,
Louisville, Kentucky*

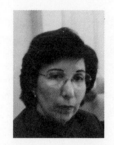 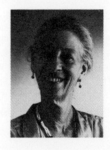

Leah J. Dickstein, M.D.   **Stella Chess, M.D.**

16

An Interview with
Stella Chess, M.D.

Stella Chess was born in New York in 1914 and graduated from New York University College of Medicine in 1939. She has taught child psychiatry since 1945 and is now Professor of Child Psychiatry at New York University Medical Center.

Let me start with my maternal grandmother. Incidentally, I look very much like my mother, age for age, as my mother looked very much like her mother. I don't know whether physical features and other features went hand in hand. I was selected to teach this grandmother to read English. My mother told my grandmother I could not read, but my grandmother didn't believe her. I was teaching her to read from my older sister's first grade books, and my mother proved it--she put her hand on the third word, and I said the first word. She put her hand on the fourth word, and I said the second one, but it didn't matter, because as long as we started from the beginning I had the right words, and I taught my grandmother how to read.

My grandmother came over to this country from Russia with those of her children who were born there, including my mother. Some were born in this country. I know that she bore eleven children, but eight grew to maturity. I do not know when the other three died, probably in early childhood. They just never were mentioned as people. There were four girls and four boys, of whom my mother was the second child. I remember my great grandmother only as a ninety-year-old lady who was senile. She only spoke Yiddish,

and I only knew enough Yiddish to know when my parents were talking about us, and whether it was good or bad. Sometimes they would talk in Russian with each other--I could catch on by tone of voice. I don't know which languages my grandmother spoke, but she learned English, and she, as her children grew up, wanted to learn to read. We moved on with reading as my sister moved on, because I memorized my sister's books.

It wasn't until I was finishing second grade and couldn't read that my mother took me in hand and taught me. I remember that at the beginning of the summer it was torture. She brought me in three times a day for lessons, and somewhere in the middle of the summer I caught on. I remembered that when I was a child psychiatry resident, because I had a child who had real dyslexia, and I said to my mother, "Did I ever have trouble reading?" I will never forget her gesture as she said, "Did you have trouble reading?" Then she told me that I ended the summer reading fast and accurately. That was during the "whole word" era, and she taught me phonetically. Perhaps I learned better that way; perhaps I was just in the developmental spurt. I always thought of myself as an accurate and fast reader, as someone who loved to read, and I never could understand why I could never spell. I still can't spell properly. It wasn't until I was a psychiatric resident that I understood why I couldn't spell even though I studied. I also never understood why I was such a dud at foreign languages.

I don't know how much my grandmother qualifies as a pioneer, but I think that coming to a new country and having eight living children, all of whom went to college, should count. My grandfather must have been unusual too, because the girls went to college as well as the boys, although they all became schoolteachers. Two of the boys became physicians, another became a chemical engineer, and one went into my grandfather's business.

I did not know until the day I changed my college major from chemistry to pre-med and came home with the news, to my father's distress and my mother's saying, "Let's see, I have some insurance I can borrow on," that my mother had wished to be a physician. She never mentioned it; I have combed my mind to see--did I know this unconsciously--really I didn't. She said, "If you want to be a doctor, you are going to be a doctor." In our family we had to go to work as schoolteachers. Uncle Sam became a doctor, and Uncle Harry became a doctor; we had to help support them through medical school. She didn't feel victimized as a young woman. She went to Hunter College in New York City and graduated in 1902. Her next two sisters also went to Hunter, and her very youngest sister went to Barnard. The oldest child was a boy, and he was a physician. I don't remember what schools he went to. I know the other physician went to Harvard. I don't remember where the chemical engineer went--in the City somewhere. They were a bright family. But it was unusual in that generation for the girls to go to college, even though the four daughters went to the traditional normal school and became schoolteachers.

My father also came from Russia, although they didn't know each other there. My mother came to America at eighteen. I think she was unusual. She picked up the language rather rapidly, I gathered. She'd go to one school, and they'd put her in whatever elementary grade they thought she belonged in. She'd zip through that. Since they didn't keep good records at the time, she'd take herself to another school and tell them what class she belonged in, which was two classes above, and by the time she finished what would be high school, she was where she belonged, and then she continued with her age group without an accent. She moved herself through school and through knowledge, and I always remember her as an avid reader. My father, who was fifteen when he came here, always had a slight accent.

My mother taught the lower elementary school grades. She was interested in becoming a high school mathematics teacher and was good at mathematics but never became that because, when she became pregnant with my sister, she refused to resign. There were no maternity leaves in those days. My father was a plodding lawyer, slow thinking, undoubtedly bright, because he put himself through law school as a Singer sewing machine salesman. He took her case, and she lost it. But it was a court battle that made history, and when it was clear she was losing it and would be fired with this against her record, one of her friends put her on his school roll as a teacher and marked her as leave of absence. So when my sister was ten and my mother went back to teaching, she had her entree, but she couldn't make waves by taking the examination for teaching high school mathematics, not because she didn't have the capacity, but because she gave that up in order to take on this fight. She was a very quiet and unassuming person in manner, but she carried things through. She must have known when she started this that she was going to take her lumps somehow or other.

I would ask my mother any question, and she would catch on to the issue, answer what I wanted to know, leave it open for any further exposition. If she didn't know, she said so. I read voraciously and at one point she caught me reading *Lady Chatterley's Lover*. And all she said was, "Your father will be upset; don't let him see you reading it." As far as she was concerned, I could read through anything. If I asked her, she would explain what I didn't understand, and if I needed more explanation two years later, I'd ask her the same question. There was nothing closed.

There was an extensive library in our house. And it was my mother's library that I read through, because my father enjoyed biographies. There was a period in my life in junior high when I read from morning until night.

I had a younger brother who had the mumps, I think mumps encephalitis. His early development was quite normal, then he was terribly sick and finally he disappeared into an institution. My mother would visit periodically, and she took me along once. He was retarded and then died of an intercurrent infection; that situation was also a drain on their money.

In those Depression days schoolteachers could have charge accounts. So when we bought anything we would run through all the charge accounts. If I needed a winter coat, we decided what department store would have it, and since she was always two months in arrears, she'd pay up for that department store, and then we'd go buy my coat. We went through childhood without realizing that this was anything unusual, very parsimonious on ostentation and clothing, but there was never any dearth of books, and we went to a private school because there was always money for books and education. I was on a half-scholarship as was my sister.

At one point we moved to Brooklyn, and I went to public school for two years because my mother thought I was too young to travel on the subway. I hated the school for good reason--it was the kind of rote material that I'd been through already. I heckled to go back and, finally when I was nine, I did and I traveled by subway. I never knew you weren't supposed to travel by subway when you were nine years old. Once I had to change trains, and on the platform there was a man who would sidle over to me and push against me in the crowded train. I told my mother about it, and she said to me, "The next time he does it, wait till he gets close, spot the people around you, find some middle-aged woman and say to her in a loud voice, 'This man is bothering me.'" I did, and that ended it. My mother didn't gasp, she thought. She never said it was dangerous, just an annoyance, and this is how to do it. And it worked. I didn't worry. I didn't know you were supposed to be in danger in subways. So I just went on about my business. It was years later that I found out that people were horrified that a nine-year-old traveled alone on the subway.

I went to Smith College and so did my sister on half-scholarships. I moved after my first year to an endowed self-help house so that two-thirds of the cost of living was taken care of by our doing all the work in the house except cooking, to reduce the cost. I took a job at college, too, and earned my spending money. Every once in a while I wonder if there were things I took for granted because of the atmosphere at home. I took piano lessons. There was one point when I wanted to quit, and I had to fight to quit. My mother thought I was giving up piano and I wasn't, I was giving up this teacher. I didn't realize it. I just knew I was bored and I didn't want to do it any more. When I got to college I took lessons again. Occasionally, my mother would send me a couple

of dollar bills in a letter toward these lessons. I was also in the dance group and in the "Y" Club. It was a liberal club, and at one point I was president. At certain points, I had to make choices. I gave up my piano lessons because the dance group was more interesting. Since I couldn't come every time because I was pre-med, I made an arrangement with the head of the dance group. The teacher understood, and I really worked when I was there. As a matter of fact, I got into the dance group in the spring of my freshman year which was very unusual; one usually got in as a sophomore.

It's been nice because my appreciation of dance and of piano is qualitatively different than my appreciation of symphony. When Alex buys tickets for piano concerts, he always tries to get them on the left side so I can see the hands. I haven't played for about fifteen years now because I have arthritis. Not terribly bad, but when you start getting arthritis in your thumb and you're trying to play Chopin an octave plus one or two, fortissimo and then you listen to Rubenstein, you don't play any more.

At college I took a job for a teacher who was doing a book. She was clipping subjects from all papers, and I'd clip them out. I had to make decisions about where the important facts were which she wanted. After a while she just left it to me. I had run out of everything she had marked. One day I came and looked, and nothing was marked, and she said, "But you're not working, and I know you need the money." I said, "But you haven't marked anything. Why don't I mark, them and then you look at them and see if I've marked the right things?" When they were all marked, she still hadn't looked. She said, "Just clip them." So I had this job which was really very interesting because it was on comparative economics of Russia, the United States and one other country. I was making money and learning some economics.

At the house where I lived, the house mother wanted to make sure we didn't get sloppy, so wearing a little apron, we learned how to wait on tables properly, which was very good, because when there were dinner parties given by the faculty, they called our house for waitresses because it was known that anyone who lived at Lawrence House knew how to serve properly. Whoever answered the only phone in the hall either took the job or hollered, "So-and-so needs a waitress for such and such a night." We also had the spin-off that there were a certain number of usher places for Lawrence House people, so we got to go to the visiting symphonies without cost. We had about three evening dresses between us-- and we lent them to each other, because you had to usher in an evening dress. It was a good place to live because everybody there was semi-poor; they were there because they needed the jobs.

The only thing that got us very angry was that, when the final results of cumulative averages came out, house by house, we were always second. One of the quadrangle houses which was inhabited by wealthy girls was always first.

I don't know how I chose Smith. My aunt ran a summer camp that was 20 miles from there, but I don't think that was a factor. I picked it before my sister did, and she was two years older; I think from the high school talk. I'm not a bit sorry I did. It wasn't a cloister; it's in Northampton, and there was a lot of interaction. I mean, there were Williams, Amherst and the University of Massachusetts. It might just as well have been co-ed except for the classes.

I learned early in my college career, partly from my sister, that you didn't have to follow prerequisites. You could take what you wanted if you could prove that you were a good student. I was rotten at languages but I was good at everything else. When I wanted to take Cultural History of the United States, I had not taken freshman history but I had taken freshman economics and philosophy. I showed the teacher my marks in sociology and in whatever else I took as a freshman, and he said, "Fine," and signed my petition, and I took it and had a marvelous time with a great course.

I took freshman physics and got terribly interested in physics of sound. By some luck my section was given by the head of the department, who was a musician, and there was a course given on physics and sound. It was a second semester course, and the prerequisite was freshman physics. I went to him and I said, "Is there any possibility of my taking physics of sound this second semester?" He said, "Yes, what we need to make sure is that the section of first-year physics on sound has been given before the second semester begins. The curriculum now schedules it for second semester, but I'll just reorganize it." So he moved the freshman physics of sound, and the second semester I took the rest of freshman physics and physics of sound. And so I learned very early that

you could really do what you wanted if you're ready to put in the work.

To a great extent I tried out things. I took art and history of art, because I wanted to, though art is not one of my fortes. And psychology turned me off. In those days it was all rats and mazes and color wheels. Kafka was interesting, so I read about Kafka though it wasn't part of the course. With languages I was terrible, though; I didn't realize it was because of my dyslexia. I could read but not write well in French, so I took literature in French and I can still read it. I had to take Latin to get into Smith and I managed it somehow. I had to take another language, so I took scientific German and had a very funny incident. There was a particular chapel--you only had to go to certain chapels--and, this one was required because they read aloud the Dean's list, which included those above a certain average, and the Registrar's list, which included those in trouble. I was on the Dean's list, and as I was walking to the door of Freshman German after the chapel, one of my classmates was walking to the door opposite me, and she said to me, "Congratulations, I heard your name at chapel." Behind me came the teacher's voice, and he must have only heard, "I heard your name in chapel," and not the congratulations. And he said to me, "Oh, Miss Chess, I'm so sorry. I know you work hard. But I couldn't give you anything better than a D." And I said, "You don't have to worry about me. I was on the Dean's list, not on the Registrar's list." He said, "Oh, you must be mistaken." I said, "No, look, I got an A in Physics, an A in Chemistry, and an A in Sociology and I was really on the Dean's list." He looked puzzled. I could just see that the poor man couldn't understand how somebody so dumb could be on the Dean's list, and that somehow they must have gotten my name mixed up with somebody else's. It was like spelling; I simply could not understand German.

I did things I didn't realize until later that if I hadn't been good friends with enough people they might have thought that I was trying to curry favor but I only did them because I wanted to. In comparative anatomy there was a science demonstration being given for alumni day, and I suddenly discovered that our class was giving nothing. So I went to the teacher and said, "Why not?" And he said, "Well . . . " as if he were talking from years of experience, "I didn't think anyone would be interested." I said, "Look, wouldn't it be fun to take a dogfish and a frog and so forth and get colored ribbon and lay them out through the comparative organs with a legend?" He said, "Would you really want to do it; would it be too much work?" I said, "No, it won't be too much work. I'll get a bunch of people to do it." And I got five people, and we worked together. I don't know whether that was after the marks were in or not, but it never occurred to me that this was the way people curried favor; I just did it because I wanted to.

I do happen to be persistent. Apparently my math level at age 5 was so impressive that I got my half-scholarship. Later on I realized that some things happened that I was mad about and then forgot about and later, as I was trying to put them together, I realized that male chauvinism had been in there pitching. I remember I saw all the boys pouring out of class with slide rules in their hands. I said, "What are you doing?" They said, "It's a slide rule class." I said, "Oh, great!" They said, "Oh, but we've already had four sessions." So I said, "Well, how did you get into it?" They said, "The teacher asked us." I was a top math student, but they never asked me. Matter of fact, I was one of the few girls who took carpentry.

In other subjects I wasn't so great. In history I was terrible. I could lose or gain 1000 years in Egyptian history without any trouble at all. And I had to learn dates, such as when they fenced in the Commons. Somebody in college showed me a marvelous book called *1066 and All That*, just what I needed. So that's the one date I remember, 1066. Once in chemistry we were going to have a test on atomic theory. Something hit me about that one, and I said, "I've got to sit down and memorize names and dates because they are going to be on this test." I walked up and down memorizing the dates, not the theories. I had heard them; they tucked themselves into my brain and they were there. I got 100 on the test and forgot the dates a week later. But if I hadn't done that I just would have been lost. I remember one time when there were dates and I didn't know them and I got a poor mark. The instructor came to me and said, "What happened to you?" I said, "I can't remember dates."

I was more interested in chemistry than in math and I was a chemistry major. But then I took physiology. I never had elementary biology because in high school I had to choose between chemistry and biology. In college my adviser

never noticed because everybody had had high school elementary biology. When I wanted to take physiology, I discovered I didn't have the prerequisites. By that time I was an old hand at arranging matters. I went to the teacher, she asked me a couple of questions, signed my petition, and I had no trouble with it. Though I never knew about fruit flies, I discovered that the biologic sciences were terribly interesting. I had in fact already had comparative anatomy just because it struck me as being something interesting. I hadn't thought of medicine at the time. It was in the middle of my junior year that I decided. I officially changed my major, and when I came home from vacation, I announced it to my parents.

My father reacted badly. By this time, I had mixed feelings about my father. Apparently I used to adore him. He was great with little kids. By then I had gotten to learn not to ask him important questions because he would never stop talking. I had learned that, in fact, his knowledge of literature was very limited because he wasn't interested; he had no ear for music and no palate for food. It wasn't till I married Alex that I developed a palate. My father would always tell my mother the food was too spicy, and all it had in it was a grain of salt. My mother was a marvelous teacher, but she was a terrible cook.

I think my father's reaction to my medical school plan kind of sums him up. He said, "It's too hard a life for a woman. You can't do it; you have to give up too much." I said, "No, it won't be too hard a life for me. And it's what I want to do." He gave me his opinion but he did not put a block in my way. He said, "We can't afford it," but my mother said, "I can borrow on the insurance." And I had summer jobs. I saved every penny I could. Medical school cost $600 a year, and I knew I could only apply to New York City medical schools.

I had unfortunate advice. The college pre-med advisor didn't know her business. She said, "When you get to medical school you will have only science, and you had better get all the culture you can now." When I got to medical school, I found that the other students had had much more preparation. Our medical school's two-week course in embryology for me was totally new, but it was review for everybody else. I studied and really hardly did anything else. At the end of the year, one-third of the class had to take the final examination, and I was in that third.

By that time, I had made a number of friends and had gotten a room downtown just to study for this crucial examination which terribly worried my father. I had promised him I'd go to the Martha Washington Hotel. I got there, took a look at the lobby and saw that there were a lot of young women talking to a lot of young men and I said to the woman, "Can't you have men in your room?" She said, "No." And I said, "Well, I can't stay here." I went up the block, found a rooming house, got a room, and my friends, mostly boys who didn't have to take exams, organized themselves into a core. Each took a subject in which to coach me, and the landlady had tea and cookies and the right number of cups and cookies; she was even ready to phone and reassure my father.

It was a horrible first year. When I went back to college for a reunion that year, I told everybody. The advisor brushed it off and said, "Oh, we've heard about NYU; we tell our students not to go there. It's not made for them." So I told the other instructors I had gotten to know, "Please for goodness' sake, if anyone is planning to go to medical school, tell them." And I gave them a list of the subjects. I said, "They'll only get two weeks on them, and it's going to be terribly rough." One of the girls who was in my class had gone to NYU and dropped out. She was also given the option of taking this final examination to make good and she failed it, but I was not going to give this up. Although most of the students had gone through an enormous struggle to get there, once they were in, there was no dog-eat-dog atmosphere; everybody was enormously helpful.

NYU Medical School really took people on merit. It happened that there were ten girls to 100 boys, but it was not a closed system. They told you at the first lecture, "Look to your right, look to your left. One of you three will not be here next year." I wasn't going to be one of them. Once I got through that first year, I had all these wonderful facts, they were part of me.

About my father, once it got through his head--he was hard at learning, and now that I know about temperament, I think he was a "slow-to-warm-up" kind of person--he had to get used to ideas and, once he did, he didn't make as many dire predictions. I got my first refusal from Cornell, then on its heels, a second one. He hit the ceiling that any school should dare to turn down his daughter. So he started going through all the people he knew, visiting them and getting letters

of recommendation. I didn't want them, didn't need them, but I couldn't stop him. And then I said, "I had better put in another application because I only had NYU left. So I went and put in an application at what's now Downstate, and when I did, they said, "Oh, are you related to our Dr. Chess?" It turned out they had two relatives of mine on their faculty. I came back and I said, "Who are Dr. Samuel and Dr. Rudolph Chess? They're father and son." My father went through the family tree and figured out who they were, got on the phone, and they said, "Come and visit us." The morning of the day I visited them, I was accepted to NYU. I visited them, and while I was there, I said, "Look, I have this acceptance; what do you think I ought to do?" Dr. Samuel Chess said, "I think you ought to go to NYU; it's better than my school." So that was it. I got in on my own merits, and my father was as glad as everybody.

Then somewhere in my third year, Alex and I, he was in his fourth year when I was in my first year, decided that there was only one time we could get married, when I had one month off between my third and fourth year. He could take a month's vacation from his internship, so we announced that we were getting married. My father went into the doldrums. I said, "What's the matter?" He said, "After all your hard work, you're giving up medical school?" I said, "I didn't say anything about giving up medical school." He said, "You're getting married." I said, "I'm getting married, but I'm going on with medical school." It took him a long time to get this idea, and when we had our first child, he went through the same--I mean, he had these concepts that came in packages. By this time I was used to the idea that he was always against something important that I wanted. He liked Alex, and I thought for a minute, "My God, did I choose the wrong person?" because he liked him. Then I decided I hadn't chosen the wrong person because he was simply against our marrying.

In medical school we had no psychiatry lectures. However, the Department of Psychiatry here at NYU was a very unusual one. Paul Schilder, Lauretta Bender, Walter Bromburg and Frank Curran were in the department among others. On their own they gave a series of lectures every noon and at 5:00. I had gone to one of Paul Schilder's lectures and I went to another, and it was a good show, but I thought it was for the birds.

People had asked me, "What do you want to be?" But they didn't ask it that way. They said, "Do you want to be a pediatrician or a gynecologist?" I said, "Neither." I didn't know what I wanted to be, but I didn't like this sexist tracking. They said, "Then what?" I said, "A surgeon." I didn't want to be a surgeon, but it was the most shocking thing I could think of, and after that they left me alone.

One day as treasurer I was adding up some Student Council receipts, and a student came over and said, "Why don't you come--Bender's giving a lecture," I said, "Psychiatry's for the birds." She was the only person in the class with a car and she lived near me. She said, "I've got my car here. I'll give you a ride home." I said, "All right, I'll go." So I went to this lecture and I was astounded. In my life I had been a camper, a camp counselor, and a camp head counselor. As a head counselor I had been a trouble shooter and had really had a knack to help get to the root of the problems of kids who were unhappy. I'd move into the bunk and work it out, getting scapegoated kids into the spotlight, with the rest of the bunk helping, but I didn't realize where it was leading. And here was Lauretta Bender giving a lecture that sounded absolutely splendid and sensible. So I said to my friend, Olga Francel, "This is great stuff." She said, "Well, why don't you volunteer to work on a ward?" I said, "Work on her ward? She doesn't know me from a hole in the wall." She said, "All she can say is no."

I went to the lecture the following week with this in my mind and by the end of the lecture, I was sure this was what I wanted to do, so I went up to Dr. Bender and said, "Do you take volunteers?" Typically of Lauretta Bender, she didn't say yes or no. She said, "There are two things I demand of volunteers." I said, "What?" She said, "That they figure out when they can come and let me know and that they come when they said they would come." I said, "By next week I will have figured out when I can come and let you know." So I went through my schedule, figured it out, leaving time enough for studies. That was junior year. It was the fall, and through the fall of my junior year and all of my senior year, I spent all the possible time I could on PQ6 with Lauretta Bender. I didn't need to study so hard because in the clinical years it was easier; I didn't have so much to memorize and clinical material seemed to sink in without effort.

By the time I was in my fourth year Dr. Bender said to me, "You know as much as the residents, so just sign up and take a case and work it up. And whenever you feel you are ready for the next one, put your name down next to another case." So in my fourth year, I had already begun to do the work of a resident. When I finished I applied for one-year internships, a pediatric one at Brooklyn Jewish Hospital and a one-year rotating at Montifiore. I got the Montifiore one, but it was a January start, and I arranged with Lauretta to have a full six-month externship. So before I even had my rotating internship, I'd had these two years plus a full-time externship and then after the internship, I was able to get a residency in White Plains. This was after getting a lot of rejection letters, which I threw in the wastebasket. They literally said things like, "We are sorry, we have filled our quota of women." I should have saved those but I didn't.

I got a part-time job with what was then called the Colored Orphan Asylum, but the name was changed. The original name was left over from the Quaker years when children lost in the underground railroad were cared for in a group home. I worked mornings for agencies after I had finished my residency, so I could have a few hours of private practice after school time. So I was really doing full-time child psychiatry with a few adult patients.

Alex and I eventually had four children. The oldest are adopted. I've always said of Len, who was the third, that he was either five years late or one year early because we had just decided that the third adoption was going to be when Rick was two years old. Suddenly I discovered I was pregnant. So Len was fourteen months younger than Rick, and then I lost the next pregnancy, and the fourth one was very uncomfortable. I prolapsed actually, and I knew I couldn't go through another pregnancy. I had wanted six kids to begin with so I was terribly grateful that I already had the first two.

Alex and I were really quite troubled about psychiatric realities. We had gone through psychoanalytic training, clinical training, and I had this splendid experience from Lauretta Bender, but there was just something missing. Little by little we worked out psychiatric theory which had failed to take into account individual differences in children and we set out to figure out what they were. Then Mike Rutter came to the United States for a year. He had heard Herb Birch speak at the Maudsley Hospital and decided that he wanted to spend time with us during a fellowship to the United States. He worked half time with us; the other half he traveled around learning about child psychiatric research. His name is on one of our early papers because he wanted to explore a particular issue. Also he was the one who gave us the name temperament. He said, "Why are you using this burdensome, complex term 'individual' differences in behavioral individuality in childhood? There's a perfectly good English word for it and that's temperament." We decided he was right.

Alex with adults and I with children could see that there was a quality that kids brought to their interactions that hadn't been accounted for in our psychiatric theory that we were taking into account in our practice and with our four kids, who were obviously very different. When Joan had a little scrape, she'd holler bloody murder, and I'd take my time getting to her. When Len would come in with the corner of his mouth down making no noise at all, I'd hop, because I knew that something dreadful had happened to him. For her the noise didn't mean anything; in fact, once she came in all bloody, and it hadn't sounded any different than a scraped knee. One of our kids was a high active kid, and I learned a trick when I went to his school. I'd wait until the teacher had her mouth open, but before she would say anything, I'd say, "Has he been giving you very much trouble?" She'd close her mouth because then what she had intended to say didn't fit. Then we could begin to talk about cooperative functioning.

As a fourth year student, when I had gotten interested in language and had asked my mother if I had trouble reading, Lauretta Bender said, "Change cases with so and so because his kids have a language difficulty, and there are a couple of other kids I can remember whose charts I'll get, and maybe we can get them back. You obviously are somebody who is going to do some writing so you might as well start now." When I was working on this language problem, I had gone to Orton's book reporting his new ten-year study. He had this theory about the right and left hemispheres that didn't work out with the kids that I had tested. I came to Lauretta in despair and said to her, "Can you give me some time?" She reacted typically and said, "Right now." Fortunately the first time I was ready for her and

after that I learned to get everything ready before I'd say, "Can I make an appointment with you?" Because it would be that minute. And I said, "Well, here's the data that has come out. And I've done the aphasia tests with them, and I've checked laterality. I haven't used a telescope, I've used the piece of paper with a hole so that the handedness didn't interfere. I've done this and I've done that, it doesn't work out." She said, "Well, what's your problem?" And I said, "This disagrees with Orton's theory." She said again, "Well, what's your problem?" And I said, "Well, who am I to disagree with Orton?" She said, "You'll say who you are, and you'll say what you think." She left me with my mouth open, but with a basic principle to follow.

She helped me get that first paper on the program in orthopsychiatry, which at that time had one session in one room. By that time I was an intern, and the paper had been delayed because I hadn't finished it, although she and Schilder had gone over it with me. Then I went into my internship and was so busy that I had to put it aside. One night I finally felt on top of things and I sat down to do it when the phone rang, and it was one of the people who had been on the children's unit with me, and he said, "Have you listened to the news tonight?" And I said, "No, I'm working on something." He said, "Schilder was just killed." Absent-minded as Schilder was, nobody doubted the truck driver who said that Schilder suddenly had stepped in front of him and was killed instantly. I put the paper down and couldn't look at it. It was months before I could make myself get to it. And then, of course, I didn't get to any writing for awhile because I was busy getting trained.

You got interested in something and pursued it, and then after you came to a conclusion, it had to be put in the public domain. Rotten as I was at writing, that's the only way you do it. And I struggled with it myself for awhile and then I got Alex to correct all my spelling. Matter of fact, it was Alex's fault that I wrote my first textbook in child psychiatry. In my psychoanalytic training, I was put on the faculty to teach child psychiatry. Alex said, "Someday somebody is going to take the notes they took from your lectures and publish them." Then he added, "No, you're going to write that book." So I looked at him and realized that when he said things in that voice it was like Lauretta saying, "As long as you are going to write you might as well start now." It would be easier to write the book than to tell him 'no.' Before each lecture, I arranged for a secretary to help. I would give the lecture and say, "Take down every word that I say, and when I get ahead of you, just leave a gap. So I had it typed out and I worked from that as a first draft. That was the first book, *The Introduction to Child Psychiatry,* and the other things just got written because they had to go in the public domain, not because I enjoyed writing. I was very fortunate in that Alex would cheerfully correct my spelling and my grammar and go through my writing and say, "Explain what you mean by this." And I'd say, "Well, it's obvious because blah, blah, blah." Then he'd say, "Now sit down at the typewriter and type out just what you said to me. It's not so obvious to everybody, it's only obvious to you." This is the way we have worked. Alex enjoys writing. He thinks things out. He does the first draft in his head. And then when he writes it down, it's virtually his last draft, and then he gives it to me. I do my first draft on the typewriter or in writing and let it lie for a week and then I throw it in the wastebasket, and it's gotten me off the ground at least. Sometimes it's worse, sometimes it's easier. It's never been easy, but the ideas have to be put in writing, there is no getting around it.

There have been times when I've known that because I was a woman I have lost some opportunities. Occasionally I've been asked to run for office because they wanted a woman candidate, and each time I lost. I didn't do much campaigning, so I don't know how to count that. If you hold an office you have to give the time, and I needed all the time I had.

When the kids were young, I didn't get around very much. It was a choice. For example, I had been invited to GAP (Group for the Advancement of Psychiatry). I was working on the committee on nomenclature, and one of the meetings was at a time when one of our kids had a family weekend at his boarding school. I wrote and said I couldn't come, and they wrote me a very nice letter, saying, "You know the GAP rules are that you give GAP precedence over everything else. You ought to know that if you want to become a member of GAP because it will be important." So I thought this over and wrote back. "I have four children, so, obviously, four different conflicts could come up. And in thinking over other things

in my life, there are a couple of others, so let's say I've got seven things that I would put before going to GAP. If it means not being a member of GAP, then the other things are really more important." When the booklet was put out on nomenclature, the committee was listed but I was listed as a consultant. Dane Prugh had written back to me and said, "Thank you for your candor," without saying he was going to put me down as a consultant. In the booklet I was even more prominent than if I had been on the committee. That was not female/male business except that, being a mother, I didn't want to be tooting off from home. Actually, as things are now, I don't think I lost very much.

Alex made sure, except when we went on vacation, that we weren't both off at the same time, and when he came home from the army, we already had two children and pretty soon a third. He said, "I'll get up at night from now on." And pretty soon the kids stopped calling, "Mommy," when they woke up at night. Mommy never came; Daddy came. We never made a bargain or wrote a contract; Alex took the lead in sharing the caregiving.

When I had my total hip replacement ten years ago, I really had very bad arthritis. I was in charge of the liaison with pediatrics, and I couldn't get over there, so I had to become amazingly organized. I'd wait until I had an errand in the psychiatric building and an errand in in-patient pediatrics so that one trip would do for four purposes. The orthopedist who refused to operate asked, "Why don't you retire?" I was speechless, and Alex was fit to be tied. He wouldn't have said that to a male colleague. So we researched to find somebody else and we found Dr. Lanzansky. Alex went with me, and he said to Dr. Lanzansky, "I want to let you know that Dr. Chess is the most important child psychiatrist in the United States, perhaps the world, and her clinical work is very important." Dr. Lanzansky examined me and said, "You do have more passive motion than one would expect." And I said, "I used to be a dancer, but you know, I don't have active motion, it hurts. I can't go more than a quarter of a block." He said, "Well, how about December." I said, "December, my God, I've got a final report due on the Rubella Study. I haven't been able to sleep for a year, so it is late and it's due by the end of December." He said, "All right, January."

There were certainly rotten men, and I did not have the support in general of my male colleagues. But I have had the support of enough individuals. I have made some very, very good friends, male and female, who have helped out. What did I lose aside from having that hip operation deferred? I didn't want to be president of this and that. The New York Longitudinal Study we did on our own time for the first year; then we got a small grant, $2,000 from NIMH, to analyze the data. We got a small grant from the Gralnick Foundation to do some more work, but the NIMH has been very generous from that point on. We had to prove ourselves first. They had seen too many longitudinal studies that started out well but ended up not being analyzed. The Rubella Study was initiated by the Department of Pediatrics here at New York University because they were doing work on physical birth defects and they found that behavioral issues were coming up and asked me to look into it. What used to be called the Maternal Child Health Section supported me for the Rubella Study. We didn't get a grant for the adolescent part of the New York Longitudinal Study; we used our own funds. We've used our own funds for other things at times because children don't stop growing while we look for funding.

Some young women have gotten caught in the ambience of the time. I remember one discussion I had on a ride from Monterey Peninsula to San Francisco with two young psychiatrists. One of them had a boyfriend interested in emergency medicine who was going to take training and go elsewhere. She was feeling that she should break off with him. I said, "Well, are you in academia?" She said, "No." I said, "Are you a San Franciscan?" She said, "No." I said, "Are your friendships here valuable?" She said, "No." I said, "Do you care where your private practice is?" She said, "No." I said, "I don't understand why you are not going where he is going." She said, "But women shouldn't . . ." I said, "Don't be a fool. If you want to, do it. You're not giving up anything. Don't get stuck in as much of a cliche as the old days. I was lucky. I didn't have so many choices to befuddle me!"

17

An Interview with
Cornelia B. Wilbur, M.D.

Leah J. Dickstein, M.D.

*Associate Dean For Student Affairs
and Associate Professor,
Department of Psychiatry and Behavioral Sciences,
University of Louisville School of Medicine,
Louisville, Kentucky*

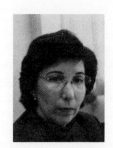 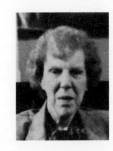

Leah J. Dickstein, M.D.   Cornelia B. Wilbur, M.D.

17

An Interview with
Cornelia B. Wilbur, M.D.

Cornelia B. Wilbur, M.D., has been the foremost leader in the diagnosis and treatment of multiple personality disorder. Her creative alertness, adopted from her research chemist father's similar characteristic, led her to "pay attention to details" which she always did throughout her years of schooling. She did what too many students read about but ignore in practice--she paid attention to facies, skin qualities, patients' smells and so forth.

In April 1986 Dr. Wilbur received an honorary doctorate degree from Eastern Michigan University for her contributions over the past four decades to educating a variety of people--medical students, residents, nurses and many others.

I was raised in a family of pure scientists. My father was critical of physicians, not anti-medicine. He said that physicians did nothing except develop empirical treatments that had no scientific basis. However, as a chemist, he was interested in medicine and felt that chemists eventually would develop specific treatments for illnesses and that medicine would progress through chemistry. He was right; if we had had more scientists in medicine, we might have progressed faster.

My father was born in 1866 and didn't encourage my going to medical school but bowed to my mother's dictum that I attend college. My mother simply insisted that as a woman I get the best and most education possible because, even if I married, my husband might leave me or die and I might need to support myself. She insisted that I

at least get a college education and she helped me as I earned my master's degree and encouraged me to go to medical school. My mother was a very forward-looking person for someone born in 1877. She worked as a secretary when it was considered not very nice to do so and had become private secretary to the president of a large company when she met my father who was a chemical researcher and they married in 1898.

My father was trained to pay attention to phenomena and to all details. He obtained his Ph.D. in chemistry in three years under Dr. Fittig at the University of Strasbourg. Dr. Fittig was half of the Wurtz-Fittig duo who discovered the chemical reaction named after them.

Early in his career my father had to use this observing technique. He was called to the Texas oil fields to solve the problem of why Texas retorts lost their bottoms while those in Pennsylvania didn't. He tested and smelled the mixture, realized Texas oil had sulfur in it which converted to sulfuric acid and hence demolished the bottoms. Telling them to add ground-up limestone to the mixture, he solved the problem!

Father taught at Western Reserve Medical School at a time when students were all brought together by learned, frock-coated men of wisdom. They all stood around the live patient who was very sick, or around the dead patient and the clinician said what was the matter with the patient, the chemist discussed the chemistry, the physiologist discussed the physiology and the anatomist discussed the anatomy. This was the way medicine was taught before the turn of the century. I think in a way Father felt frustrated about not being more powerful in the medical field.

My paternal grandfather was in the insurance business and my grandmother was a lady of the house but I knew them only very slightly. I was their only granddaughter and the only girl child of their two sons. I am told my grandfather thought very highly of me.

My mother was the oldest of three girls in a German family. Her father was apparently quite successful until he developed and died of cancer in his older years after his marriage broke up. Her mother was described as very strong-willed and shrewish in many ways. The parents felt that everyone should get an education and so my mother and one sister attended college. My grandmother lived in her own home until she died and I would visit her.

I never knew my Schade (maternal) grandparents well until I was grown. My mother had six brothers and sisters; three were engineers and my mother's sister married an extremely successful chemist. I didn't know them until I was nearly grown because my parents left their home town of Cleveland and went to Montana before I was born.

My parents were older than most parents at that time. I had a brother seven years my senior who was injured during his breech delivery in 1902. My mother was given chloroform and this brother was a very troubled and troublesome child. My younger brother and I were very close; he has done very well as a chemical engineer.

Both sides of the family held the attitude that education is valuable, fun and brings satisfaction. Father was a voracious reader. I remember that at seven I found an embryology book. I asked my mother about the book and she sent me to my father. I climbed on his lap and he told me all about an embryo's development.

In 1922 at fourteen, I mentioned to my mother that I'd like to be a doctor and she said, "Women are not doctors." Then I said I would simply be a nurse and she explained the unpleasant side of nursing--bedpans for example--and I agreed that I did not want to be a nurse. At this time there were no antibiotics but infections were discussed. Father kept saying that if people would use chemicals, they could solve such problems.

I have no idea why I decided very early to be a

doctor but I was discouraged by elders. When I was about finished with my master's degree in chemistry, I went and saw the medical school dean and told him that I wanted to enter medical school. He told me to have my transcripts sent over. I had not taken sufficient physics or any zoology or botany so once again I began as a freshman at age 23 with a master's in chemistry and took all of these requirements and was very successful.

I attended the University of Michigan Medical School which had admitted women students since the late 1800's. There were eight women in my class. The school had a policy of admitting a few outstanding women but these women didn't feel they were pioneering at the time.

We had many chauvinistic teachers, but I had little difficulty; only one was really nasty to me personally. There was a Scotsman who liked women and was very happy to see them in his anatomy laboratory because he thought women weren't so clumsy or in a hurry and made better dissectionists. Another teacher, Elizabeth Crosby, taught neuroanatomy and in fact was world reknowned because she wrote the neuroanatomy section of *Gray's Anatomy*. But the chauvinism showed up--she was not made a full professor until after I was graduated and she had been there for fifteen to eighteen years. The school didn't do much for women but it always tended to be proud of the women graduates.

I thought Michigan was an extremely fine school and I got a wonderful medical education. In my freshman year, I came in contact with Dr. Robert Dieterlie, who had been analyzed by Freud. After he graduated from the University of Michigan, he entered psychiatry, but he wanted to be an opera singer, so he went to Vienna to study singing and to be analyzed by Freud. He became so fascinated with what Freud was doing with human psychology that he returned to Michigan and taught at the medical school and I met him then. At the end of my junior year, he arranged the first female externship in a Michigan state hospital for me. The hospital was required by law to have a woman psychiatrist, but they had never had any women externs before. So I went to the Kalamazoo State Hospital. Michigan state hospitals, in comparison to others, were absolutely marvelous. Kalamazoo State Hospital had about three thousand patients, on an enormous campus with beautiful elm trees. As many patients as possible were accommodated outside the buildings. Patients also worked on farms. They were given jobs; their self-esteem was encouraged. We had wards, of course, with disturbed people. We had nine ward psychiatrists who held classes during the summer for externs, interns, and new young doctors. The other extern and I were given the job of Dick and Schick testing and giving everybody in the entire hospital typhoid shots. We had two typhoid carriers in isolation. That job meant that I came in contact with half the patients. The patients knew who I was through the grapevine, and I got a stack of letters a foot high from patients telling me they were glad I was there and asking if I was going to stay in psychiatry.

I was asked to help in the treatment of an agoraphobic, hysterical girl. Not being even a senior medical student, I was delighted. The assistant superintendent told me what to say and what to do. I was the first one to take the girl out in the open. That summer, she got well. I have received a Christmas card from her for forty-two years. I learned from that experience that one should treat the hysteria and not the symptoms. After I graduated from medical school and entered psychiatry, I dealt mainly in the treatment of hysterics for the obvious reason that one of them had enhanced my life even before I got out of school.

I was offered a job which I accepted at the University of Nebraska with A.E. Bennett, M.D., who was both a neurologist and a psychiatrist. I was very much interested in neurology because there are so many neurological symptoms in hysteria. I operated three epilepsy clinics doing EEG's and learning neurology, and I apparently got half the hysterics in the state of Nebraska! The first was a girl sent home by the local ENT man; he said she had nothing wrong, but was unable to talk. I was doing some research with pentathol. I gave her some, and she started crying. I asked her what was the matter, and she told me why she couldn't talk and she recovered. The same doctor sent me another woman who hadn't talked for three years. She was tougher, but I got her to talk after about two weeks.

I treated several interesting neurology patients in Nebraska. Penicillin was not generally available at the time and I called Charles Keefer in Chicago who had penicillin flown to me in six hours in a single engine plane from Chicago to Nebraska through a blizzard for a comatose patient who promptly recovered in two days. The patient was the first recovered case of a special form of thrombosis. Another interesting patient I diagnosed was a young male heir with a foramen magnum meningioma who recovered completely after surgery.

I also used pentathol to treat a beautiful young woman who was paralyzed from the waist down. She was able to talk about herself and her personal conflicts and recovered completely.

In 1948 after World War II, I went to New York because I realized that if I were going to be as good a psychotherapist as I wanted to be, I would have to get analytic training. Shortly after I got to New York, I was ready to take my Boards; I decided to take double Boards and passed both Neurology and Psychiatry in 1945. When I finished my psychoanalytic training, I was certified in analysis in 1959, so I had all the proper pieces of paper. I also co-authored a book on homosexuality with Irving Bieber.

Florence Powdermaker invited me to be assistant chief of the Veterans Administration Outpatient Service in New York City, its biggest unit at the time. There were hundreds of patients and we could do what we felt was necessary for their treatment but this lasted only 2 years and then I entered private practice and taught part-time at Columbia University, Department of Psychiatry while I was in analytic training.

The first time I saw Sybil, she was nineteen; then I saw her ten years later--that was when I discovered she was a multiple. She came to New York when I was there with the idea of getting her master's degree at Columbia, which she did, but her real reason for coming to New York was to find me. I had told her when I first saw her to go to Chicago, where there were two women analysts, but her father wouldn't let her. I think I learned as much from treating Sybil as I learned from any other single thing. I met the original personality first. She kept losing weekends. She knew that once she lost two years, and she was scared about it. She was very fearful about what happened during these missing times.

I wrote eleven papers, and three of them were published by a doctor who was editor of a small journal. The other journals just turned the papers down. In 1952 (I saw Sybil in 1954), they discovered Thorazine, and the journals were filled with psychopharmacology articles and behavior modification was coming in. Analysis was passe.

I'll never forget the first patient I gave Thorazine to: she turned yellow in one week. I took her off the medicine and treated her psychoanalytically for five years and she got well. And she still had her liver!

At one point I decided to give a paper on transference in multiple personalities at the Academy because the Academy publishes all the proceedings. About two months after the meeting, I got a call from the editor. He said that the publisher had just told him about space limitations and that he was leaving out my paper. I presented three papers at my psychoanalytic society, wanting some feedback. Nobody was the slightest bit interested. I discovered later that a lot of people thought it was a freak case or a hoax.

The executive of the National Association of Private Psychiatric Hospitals, of which I was treasurer, vice-president, and president later, got a lot of publicity and got Flora Schreiber to write about us. She came to interview me on homosexuality for *Science Digest*. I had had difficulty before with reporters leaving things out or changing the meaning, but she got things right. I decided that the case of Sybil was important and would appeal to people, and I asked Flora to make a story of it. They met, and Flora was enchanted with Sybil. Flora wanted to wait for Sybil's complete fusion to start the book, and this occurred soon after their meeting. We finally got a contract with Cowles Publishing, but they sold out and sold our contract to another publisher. Cowles had assigned an editor from *Look Magazine* to help Flora write the book. Flora didn't need any help writing books, and the editor kept telling her to write 30,000 words on this and 30,000 words on that. Then they sold the company and the new company turned down the book. We went to other publishers, but nobody wanted it. In the meantime, Harvey Plotnick, who had bought the Cowles contracts, took it home and gave it to his wife. She started reading it without doing the supper dishes, and at 2:30 in the morning she dropped the manuscript on him and said, "You'd better publish this." So he wrote to say he wanted it.

Flora spent ten weeks working hard and at the end had a manuscript that was practically complete. We got hold of Sybil, and she went over the manuscript to make sure there were no mistakes. We went out to dinner in the country, and on the way back I said, "What are you girls going to do

if this is a bestseller?" And they said, "We'll think about that when it happens." I said, "Look, I went to the opening of *No Time for Sergeants*, and Roddy McDowell asked Andy Griffith, 'What are you going to do if this makes you a star?' And he said, 'I'll think about that when it happens.' 'No, you won't, you'll think about it now. What if Jack Warner comes in and offers you an $80,000 contract?' He said, 'I'll take it.' Roddy said, 'No, you won't. Somebody might walk in with a $90,000 contract.' " At a New York literary auction the rights sold for $425,000 and *Sybil* was published in 1973. The hardback sold 400,000 copies, the paperback seven million. It was translated into eleven languages. The movie was sold and seen in twenty-two countries. I travelled all over the United States and Canada to publicize the book because I knew there were many people with Sybil's illness.

I decided I had to give Sybil's story to the public, because, if they were interested, they would force psychiatrists to do something about this disorder. Eventually, that happened. People who suspected that they had multiple personality insisted on receiving help. At a meeting in 1976, the prize-winning essay was "The History of Multiple Personality," but one psychiatrist got up and said, "I don't believe multiple personality exists." The chairman looked at me and asked, "Doctor, would you like to say something?" The young man who gave the paper didn't know I was in the audience. I said, "I don't believe in multiple personality either," and everybody gasped. I said, "It is not a belief system. I was brought up in a family of pure scientists, and I was taught to observe phenomena. We were taught that if you have enough observations, you try to put them in order. When I saw Sybil, I decided she was a hysteric. I followed through, and I saw one personality after another. I had the information that they were different people and said different things. I was very surprised when they appeared. You can call it abracadabra if you want to; you don't have to call it multiple personality. I called it multiple personality because that seemed to describe what was going on. I have decided that people who do not observe this phenomenon are poor observers." I sat down. I have never been challenged since.

After twenty-three years in New York City I came to the University of Kentucky at the invitation of Dr. Parker, the chair at the time. I remained on the faculty until I retired at age 65 as professor emerita and served as acting chair for one year shortly after I arrived.

I still treat patients who have been abused as Sybil was and I continue to devote considerable energy to the problems resulting from child abuse as well as other childhood antecedents of multiple personality.

The interest in multiple personality disorder has in fact broadened and deepened our concept of dissociative states in general.

My feeling about "living" is that life is for living and that women carry the germ plasm of our immortality. If they don't have children, they aren't immortal. So they may want to have children, maybe two, three, four. But children are a very limited experience: they are born, they are infants for six years, they are children for six more years, then they are teenagers. They do need some support, but my mother worked almost all the time after I was ten, yet she was a very real support. I think women can be extremely successful mothers and still be very fine physicians. If they want to go to medical school, they should go to medical school. Let them have their babies when they're supposed to be taking their OB exam, like one girl who did just that at Columbia!

18

——

A Psychoanalyst
and Women's Liberation

————————

Alexandra Symonds, M.D.

Associate Clinical Professor of Psychiatry,
New York University School of Medicine; and
Training and Supervising Analyst,
American Institute of Psychoanalysis, Karen Horney Center,
New York, New York

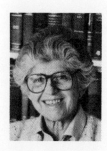

Alexandra Symonds, M.D.

18

A Psychoanalyst
and Women's Liberation

I was asked to write about those experiences in my personal and professional life which influenced my becoming a psychiatrist and psychoanalyst, interested and active in women's issues. With this in mind, I have noted what I think are some of the most pertinent facts of my background.

I was born in New York City at a joyous time, two weeks after the armistice of World War I. I was told that they called me the "peace baby." I was also the first girl in my family with two older brothers. So I believe that the first few years of my life were good. When I was four years old, the second brother died in the post-war influenza epidemic. This produced a permanent change in the emotional climate of our home. My mother told me many times that she never got over this loss. There were two more children added to my family, a girl and a boy, but I distinctly recall the sadness of those years. From that time on, I remember my mother as depressed in varying degrees. My father was a businessman who was preoccupied with his work and paid little attention to his children, except to see that they were taken care of in material ways. When my mother was able, she was warm and caring.

The structure in my family was traditional. My father was definitely the person in charge, while my mother was a housewife who took care of home and children. My father was concerned about the education and future of my brothers, but did not think it was necessary for girls to be educated beyond a commercial course in high

school. He felt that this would prepare them to find an office job until they married.

No one ever spoke to me about my schoolwork or discussed plans for my future. I did well in school and graduated from high school at age 16-and-a-half. A few weeks before I graduated, my father discussed with me how I would get a job. This was the first time my parents realized that I had taken a general course and therefore had not studied typing or shorthand. At this point I told them that I wanted to go to college. My father was completely taken by surprise. Both my parents were immigrants and neither had completed grade school. They wanted an education for their sons, but to send a girl to college was a completely novel idea. However, I was eager and resourceful, and was able to convince my father that we could manage the finances. I was to work for my meals and he would pay for room and tuition. I went to the University of Wisconsin in Madison since I was determined to go away to school, and I had met someone who recommended it highly. Wisconsin was a state school, and in those years tuition, even for out-of-state students, was very low.

I enjoyed college and especially liked sciences. A friend of mine was pre-med and she urged me to consider medical school. I had never known any girl who planned to go to medical school and had never met a woman doctor, but as soon as she suggested it, I felt it was an excellent idea. It appealed to me. In those days, my concept of being a doctor was not primarily out in the world taking care of patients, but rather studying and learning in a separate, secluded environment, wearing a white coat and somehow conveying my knowledge to help people.

I discussed it at home, but my father absolutely, positively ruled it out. College, yes, but medical school was completely out of the question. It would be terribly expensive, and why bother? After all, I would get married anyway and all this education would go to waste.

In my third year of college my father died as a result of an accident. From this time on, I made my own plans for education and personal life. With several lengthy interruptions during which I worked at various jobs, I was able to finish college and medical school. Early in college I had given up the possibility of going to medical school, but a friend encouraged me to pursue my original goal. With some help from my family and working summers, weekends and nights to augment my finances, I succeeded. I had to go back to college for some additional pre-med courses, and in doing this, I earned a Master's degree in psychology.

Getting into medical school was not easy. It took two years and applying to 40 schools. The years were 1942-44 during World War II. There had always been a small quota of women accepted, but during the war there were even fewer because most of each class was taken by the Army and Navy, who sent selected men to medical school to fulfill the military's needs. I applied to almost every medical school which was listed in the book and finally was accepted at Hahnemann Medical School in Philadelphia. I transferred after two years and graduated from New York Medical College, Flower-Fifth Avenue Hospital in 1948. There were seven women in my class of 110 at Hahnemann, and a similar proportion at New York Medical College. In my third year of school I married Martin Symonds, who was also a medical student.

In all those years I never felt discriminated against because of my gender. This does not mean that I was not discriminated against. Of course I was, but I never thought of it in those terms. From childhood on, I had made up my mind that I had to make my own life, and I accepted as a given the various obstacles along my way. It wasn't until recent years, when my consciousness was raised by the women's movement, that I began to see this aspect of my life in its proper perspective. The women's movement raised my consciousness to issues of gender and has caused me to see everything in a different way; not only my life, but the lives of my patients and, in fact, the entire world. I have looked back on my early life, wondering how it happened that a little girl with my background became a professional woman. No one in my family guided or encouraged me. I had no role model. Whatever expectations there were for me were the traditional ones for women. However, nobody in my family tried to stop me either. There was no ridicule or active rejection of my goals. In fact, I hadn't shared them with anyone until absolutely necessary.

I believe that my father respected my efforts on my own behalf, although he never said so. He himself had achieved a great deal as the result of his own energy and struggle, rising from a penniless, uneducated immigrant to owning a modest business and supporting his family well. My mother found me a total mystery and it seemed we had little in common. I definitely did not identify with her. I see now that as I was growing up, I absorbed what the culture considered to be male values. Very early on, I recognized that women were second class citizens and were not given much respect. I did not want to grow up to be like my mother, or any of the other housewives and mothers whom I knew. Marriage and homemaking did not appeal to me. As far as I was concerned, boys had much more fun than girls. Furthermore, they had more freedom and could do more interesting things.

As a child, I liked to read and was a tomboy. From an early age, I tried to be self-sufficient, and I was able to accomplish this. These interests set me apart from other girls and young women, and I think that in some ways it also protected me from consciously recognizing any personal effects of discrimination. To admit that to myself would have been equivalent to saying I was a second class person, at least in the eyes of the world. This would have been too painful. Without consciously saying that to myself, I was determined to prove that I was not. This accounts for why so many professional women of my generation reacted to the women's movement by saying, "It's not my fight. I have nothing to do with this movement. Each person must prove herself on her own. After all, I did."

I found medical school difficult, but tremendously satisfying and exciting. Each clinical subject was so interesting to me that every few months as I went to a new service, I mentally changed my choice of future specialty. Even though I was interested in psychiatry from the very beginning, I could also have done medicine, obstetrics, dermatology, pediatrics, even surgery. Psychiatry, however, held my interest most deeply. People had always fascinated me. I had a background in psychology and found that the psychiatric conferences during my internship and medical years were most absorbing.

I spent three years in the Public Health Service. My internship was at the U.S. Marine Hospital, Staten Island, N.Y., and I had two years, one in medicine and one in psychiatry, at the U.S. Marine Hospital, Ellis Island, N.Y. The Public Health Service supplies the medical needs of various federal agencies which include the Coast Guard and the Merchant Marine. Therefore, all of the patients at these hospitals were male. They were either members of the Coast Guard or Merchant Marine, and all of the doctors were male, except me.

During my internship, in July 1949, the war with Korea broke out and we automatically became part of the armed forces. I wore a uniform, the same as the WAVES, except for the Coast Guard insignia. The patients and staff were all very proper in their attitude towards me as the only woman on the medical staff and I was not aware of any discrimination, except from the head of the G-U (genito-urinary) department. He did not allow me to rotate through his service and he also insisted on having only male nurses. These were the days before widespread use of sulfa and penicillin, and complications of gonorrhea and syphillis were very common, especially in that patient population. However, this exclusion did not bother me.

What did bother me was something that occurred with the government in my third year of service. One day on Ellis Island I was called down to the office and told that I must refund $1245 in cash within 24 hours because I had fraudulently received this amount in my monthly paycheck. When I had first joined the Public Health Service, I filled out a routine form which asked if I had any dependents. I said yes, as my husband was then in medical school. It later evolved that this form was for male officers in the Service. Any male who was married received an extra stipend,

regardless of whether his wife worked or was at home. The wives of my male colleagues worked at the hospital while they received a dependency stipend. A female officer, however, was required to prove that any dependent whom she claimed was not able to work. Thus, a nurse or WAC or WAVE officer could receive extra pay for minor children, or an elderly parent. Of course I was angry at this blatant discrimination, but I refunded the money and filed for dependent pay. Eventually, however, this was disallowed because although my husband was a medical student, he was considered able-bodied and capable of working. His status as a medical student did not allow for an exception. This procedure took months of aggravation and reams of paperwork. At one point I was referred to a woman lawyer who offered to take my case without a fee if I promised to follow through with it as she felt it was sure to go to the Supreme Court. It seems that women officers had protested this injustice for years and years, and this lawyer was interested in having a test case. I regret to say that I did not accept her offer. At that time I did not appreciate the importance of the issue in regard to women. This policy was not reversed by the Supreme Court until the early 1970's!

I entered psychiatry at a very exciting time. I started my residency in the Public Health Service at the U.S. Marine Hospital, Ellis Island, and did 2 years at Bellevue Hospital. New York City in the late 40's and early 50's was a fortunate time and place to be exposed to new ideas in psychiatry and psychoanalysis. Psychiatrists were just discovering that one could make sense out of the talk of schizophrenics. Frieda Fromm-Reichmann's work at Chestnut Lodge, where she and her staff spent months and even years in psychotherapy with one psychotic patient, was revolutionary. When I started my residency in 1949, the treatment modalities we had available for psychotic patients were ECT (electroconvulsive therapy), insulin shock, sedation and restraints in the form of cold packs and strait jackets. In 1950 and '51, they started to use Thorazine for the first time. This produced a dramatic change in the atmosphere of the wards, and patients were much more available to talk to. The studies at Chestnut Lodge were extremely challenging to me and I thought that I would like to work with schizophrenics. However, I felt the need for additional training in the treatment of psychoneurotics, and I became interested in psychoanalysis. In those years in New York City, a large percentage of psychiatrists went on for psychoanalytic training. We had our choice of five psychoanalytic training programs, each with a different psychoanalytic theory. There was the New York Psychoanalytic Institute which was the traditional Freudian school; the William Alanson White Institute which taught the theory of Harry Stack Sullivan; the American Institute of Psychoanalysis which was founded by Karen Horney; the Columbia group which was headed by Sandor Rado; and the Psychoanalytic Program of New York Medical College, Flower Fifth Avenue Hospital which we called the Flower Group, headed by William Silverberg and Bernard Robbins, which was electic.

The field of psychoanalysis was in ferment. In 1940, Karen Horney, who was a training analyst at that time, had been forced to leave the American Psychoanalytic Association because of her outrageous idea that cultural forces influenced developing character structure. She had just published her first book, *The Neurotic Personality of Our Time*, in which she discussed the role of culture. She also had other differences with Freud, including his concepts of feminine psychology. While she had originally presented her ideas with the hope of broadening the horizons of psychoanalysis, she was bitterly attacked for being critical and disloyal to Freud. Horney, along with a group of analysts left to form another psychoanalytic institute which was to be less rigid and more accepting of new ideas. This group eventually divided again: one part to join the William Alanson White Institute, another to form the Psychoanalytic Program of the New York Medical College. Some of the original group remained with Horney to form the American Institute of Psychoanalysis.

The effect of all this activity produced many interesting and stimulating meetings, with passionate discussions of the various new viewpoints in psychoanalysis. I went to as many of these as I could manage. During my college years I had read Freud and I could not accept many of his concepts. Even then, I sensed the traditional, patriarchal attitude of condescension which Freud had towards women. I distrusted a theory that reinforced the cultural stereotype of femininity, assigning to women a passive dependent role which was immutable and biologically predetermined. I felt torn between the schools of Harry Stack Sul-

livan and Karen Horney, finding both interesting and stimulating. Eventually I joined the American Institute of Psychoanalysis which had been established by Karen Horney.

I joined the Institute as a candidate in 1950 and Horney died in 1952. However, I had heard her speak numerous times in the years before I joined and her presentations at meetings were influential in my choice. No matter how large the audience, it seemed as though she spoke directly to each person. At all times, she was compassionate towards her patients, and demonstrated an attitude of openness and searching for understanding. She did not use theoretical jargon. All of these qualities appealed to me. I felt, at these meetings, that we were talking about human beings, not pathological specimens.

In spite of Horney's early interest in feminine psychology, her unique contribution to psychoanalysis was not specifically in that area. She went on to develop her own theory of character structure which is not gender related. However, she stressed that the development of neuroses is the result of negative forces in the environment which prevent the individual from evolving into his or her potential. Horney's stress on constructive forces and her concept of the "real self" as the source of our authentic, spontaneous feelings struck a chord in me and has always been important in working with patients. No matter how depressed or resigned, there is always a spark of the constructive which keeps us going towards growth. Our job in therapy is to identify these forces and help remove the blockages.

Horney wrote 20 articles pertaining to feminine psychology. Some of these were published recently in a collection entitled *Feminine Psychology*. As early as 1922 she expressed reservations about Freud's theory of feminine psychology. It was these doubts which eventually led her to question many other aspects of his theory. Her work must be understood in two main phases. The first when she was strictly Freudian (approximately 1923-1936) and the second when she gradually freed herself from the rigid confines of Freud's thinking and developed her own ideas and her own vocabulary. Her early papers were written in the context of Freudian theory and language dealing with penis envy, libido, id, masochism and castration complex. Later, starting in 1937 with the publication of her first book, *The Neurotic Personality of Our Time*, we see a change of language, and a recognition of the importance of cultural factors. People are seen not as male and female, and therefore basically different, but as human beings with similar needs, desires, impulses and potentialities, each one struggling for self-realization and self-fulfullment. She saw that men as well as women can be dependent or aggressive or envious or spiteful. Masochistic suffering is not "enjoyed" by healthy women as Helene Deutch stated, but is the only alternative for certain neurotic individuals. Sadism is the end product of hopelessness, not an inborn instinct. Horney also saw that people could change throughout their lives, they were not fixed in early childhood. She recognized that the sexual drive was not the source of life's energy but only one of our needs. Creativity is not sublimated sexual energy, but a positive constructive force pushing to be expressed. The driving force in each of us is growth and self-realization rather than sexual instinct. These are some of the basic principles which Horney eventually evolved and upon which she developed her theories of character structure. Her last book, published in 1950, was entitled *Neurosis and Human Growth* and was subtitled, *The Struggle Towards Self-Realization.*

All of these were refreshing and exciting insights at a time when psychoanalysis was burdened by the mechanistic and pathological traditions carried over from the 19th century. However, because they challenged some of Freud's basic tenets, the traditional analysts of the late 30's and 40's were greatly disturbed by these concepts. I attended many psychoanalytic meetings in New York City where the atmosphere was charged with emotion. Ideas which we take for granted today were labeled heresy and quackery, ending eventually in the resignation of Horney and her colleagues.

The three analytic schools which formed in New York at that time are still in existence. From this original division, important and creative developments in the areas of interpersonal psychiatry and humanistic psychology emerged. Thus, looking back we can see that feminine psychology played an important role in the history of psychoanalytic theory. As a result of the early questions by Horney, vast new horizons were opened up by her, Eric Fromm, Clara Thompson, Abraham Maslow and others, leading to the humanistic understanding of human nature and the entire neo-Freudian body of knowledge.

After training at the American Institute for Psychoanalysis, I remained in New York and, in addition to my practice, I was on the faculty of New York University College of Medicine and the Institute. I also taught at the New School for Social Research. I was in charge of the adolescent wards at Bellevue Hospital for a number of years and treated many adolescents in my private practice, which was not all psychoanalytic, but included a broad range of patients.

I became interested in issues pertaining to women around 1970, and became active in 1973. The first writing that stirred my emotions was Simone de Beauvoir's book, *The Second Sex.* But it was not until 1973 that I became personally involved in an active way. In that year a group of women members of the Academy of Psychoanalysis started a study group to discuss recent literature on women. Shortly after we formed, we discovered that the Academy was planning a panel at its next meeting on "The Effects of Feminism on Campus," and there were no women Academy members consulted or selected to speak. We first brought this to their attention in a very calm way, but when we were brushed off by the all-male program committee, we became galvanized as though an electric current had suddenly run through our group. We circulated a petition of protest which was signed by many members and presented it to the Executive Council. Eventually, after a few years of persistent effort, the Academy became receptive to our ideas and we now have items of interest to women on each program. I became chair of the Committee on Women and we now have a semi-annual workshop on Psychoanalysis and Women's Liberation. This committee was stimulating and productive, leading to many interesting articles and meetings by people such as Ruth Moulton, Rose Spiegel, Anne Turkel, Esther Haar, and others.

The group of women analysts in New York City, in which I participated for several years, still exists, although last year they added some men. Among the early members were Rose Spiegel, Marianne Eckardt, Anne Turkel, Rosa Lenz, and Esther Greenbaum. This group experience was a crucial one for me, and one which I recommend to all women professionals. Originally we met to discuss literature, but almost immediately we began to exchange experiences we had as women, as girls growing up, and as members of a small minority of women in medical school, hospitals and in our profession. What came out was a torrent of feelings in all of us, a mixture of anger, tears, and frustration. Memories of personal experiences of discrimination, humiliation, exclusion and rejection, in the family and in the world, flooded our awareness. Voicing these feelings among friends, as I did then, was a tremendous experience. By finally acknowledging what it felt like to be an object of discrimination, my outlook on everything changed. Ventilating the anger and sadness relieved me of a weight which I did not even know I was carrying. It was as though new aspects of myself were being opened up, and fresh air came in. I felt different. I had more energy, and I soon began to get deeply involved in other issues.

The most important one was the campaign to try to get the American Psychiatric Association not to have its annual meeting in New Orleans in 1981 because Louisiana was one of the states which had not passed the Equal Rights Amendment. In 1980, with Jean Bolen as co-chair, we formed Psychiatrists for ERA (PFERA). Boycotting states which did not pass the ERA was part of the effort of the National Organization of Women to exert financial pressure over those few male legislators throughout the country who were frustrating the will of the majority of the country. The activities of PFERA brought me in contact with many women psychiatrists throughout the country. A strong network developed, and though we did not win our point, I believe we all learned a lot. Many men became interested in the relationship between discrimination and mental health as a result of the literature in our campaign. With Matilda Rice and Anne Turkel as co-editors, I revived the newsletter for women in the APA. It is still being published as "News for Women in Psychiatry." A group of us also started the Association of Women Psychiatrists to provide a network and support group for women in psychiatry. In addition to these concrete products, I know that my work with my patients has benefited immeasurably from my understanding of the effect of discrimination on women and on me.

In looking back, I can see that my interest and involvement in the women's movement made a permanent change in my life. I feel younger and more alive now than I did 10 years ago. I became freer after personally dealing with the issues of discrimination and less worried about being too aggressive for a woman. I stopped worrying about whether men could call me "a castrating female" or use other sophisticated ways of putting women down. As a result, I have been able to use my energies more effectively and have obtained tremendous satisfaction from doing so.

I look forward to many more developments in theory and action which will relieve both women and men from the rigid confines of spirit which have been produced by the sexual stereotypes of the past.

19

Women in Forensic Psychiatry

Kathryn J. Ednie, M.D.

*Unit Director,
Center for Forensic Psychiatry,
Ann Arbor, Michigan*

Gail Farley, Ph.D.

*Associate Director, Evaluation Unit,
Center for Forensic Psychiatry,
Ann Arbor, Michigan*

Elissa P. Benedek, M.D.

*Director of Training and Education,
Center for Forensic Psychiatry,
Ann Arbor, Michigan*

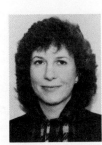 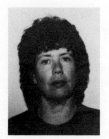 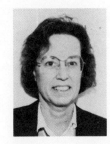

Kathryn J. Ednie, M.D.   Gail Farley, Ph.D.   Elissa P. Benedek, M.D.

19

Women in Forensic Psychiatry

For many years, society believed that women did not have the mindset to operate well in adversarial situations. This belief excluded women from medical school, law school and forensic psychiatry until the late 60's and early 70's. Traditional and lay literature alike stressed the socialization process of women which encouraged negotiation and conciliation and extinguished aggression. The subject of aggression/assertion in women has always been an enigma.[1] Aggression was thought to pose a threat to women's sense of self-esteem. To acknowledge the existence of aggression/assertion and to use it directly suggested that a woman was seen as a failure, inadequate and inferior both to herself and society. In addition, it was thought that most women could allow aggression to exist and made it available for us as long as it was being used in the service of another.[2]

Aggression, assertiveness and independence, which are supported and reinforced in men by society, have been seen as less desirable in women. Aggression is necessary to survive in the forensic system. The courtroom has been likened to a battlefield. Metaphors describing forensics focus on aggression. Each soldier takes advantage of whatever tools, weapons and skills are available. The courtroom is designed to be adversarial as is the whole forensic system. To succeed, one needs personality traits which are generally assigned to males, i.e., ambition, courage, aggressiveness, self-confidence, independence, forcefulness, clear-thinking and lack of emotionalism. Qualities more characteristically assigned to females include consideration, quietness, unselfishness, superstitiousness, excitability, tempera-

mentalness, anxiousness and neuroticism and do not serve one well in court. We speculate that increased numbers of women in the professions and the effect of the women's movement supporting increased assertiveness and nontraditional career choices have helped women professionals to assess themselves as possessing the stereotypic male qualities of self-confidence, autonomy and aggression. Unfortunately, although individual women professionals may display these personality traits, society at large has not changed in its reaction to a woman who displays the traits necessary to succeed in forensic psychiatry: especially aggression, autonomy, assertiveness, etc.

Recently we were again reminded of the persistence of sex role stereotypes in forensics and of the fact that they have changed little in two decades. We were also reminded that society continues to view men as forceful, independent and stubborn and women as more mannerly, emotional and submissive, and that when there is role incongruence, people are uncomfortable. One of the authors testified as an expert witness in an extraordinarily complex case revolving around the insanity defense. The prosecutor commented favorably about the testimony, complimenting the witness and mentioned that she performed articulately and was even professorial! Despite his glowing reviews, he felt constrained to comment that several of his colleagues and "courtroom watchers" suggested that the witness was perhaps "too argumentative and bitchy." We were reminded how difficult it is yet for the criminal justice system to tolerate an assertive woman, a woman with a strong professional opinion which she felt comfortable in articulating in the face of extensive and hostile cross-examination.

In addressing the problems and pleasures of women in forensic mental health and forensic administration, there are two caveats. The number of women forensic psychologists and psychiatrists is still extremely small, and the number in administration is smaller yet. We attempted to survey women forensic psychiatrists and psychologists before writing this chapter. By diligent searching we were able to identify approximately 100 women involved in forensic mental health. Of these, perhaps five were involved in forensic administration. Our chapter is a commentary about the issues that have surfaced in the survey as well as our personal experiences in forensics and forensic administration. We warn the reader that it is not backed by statistics or survey data. It is impressionistic and based on our personal experience and our extensive contact with the forensic system.

What Is Forensic Mental Health?

What is a forensic clinician and what does a forensic clinician do? A forensic clinician is a mental health professional who has subspecialized in that area of psychiatry, psychology or, in some jurisdictions, social work which deals with the interaction of mental health and the law. Subspecialization involves rigorous training, including a background in psychology, an M.D. or Ph.D., and subspecialty training in forensic issues. The forensic clinician has been trained to perform a variety of specialized examinations including examinations for insanity, child custody, termination of parental rights, malpractice, workmen's compensation and personal injury. The nature of the forensic evaluation, although similar in many respects to standard clinical evaluations, differs both in technique and purpose. Forensic examinations may be carried out in a variety of settings including an office, a court clinic, state hospital or a forensic center. As our experience in forensic administration was in a maximum security forensic hospital, those issues germane to work and administration in that setting are the ones we shall primarily address.

The forensic examination and forensic treatment differ from the more standard clinical evaluation in regard to agents or agencies. The treating clinician's allegiance is always to the patient although he/she also has had an obligation to protect the public. The clinician is primarily the patient's agent, hired and contracted for the work of therapy. As in other consultative roles during the forensic evaluation and forensic treatment, the clinician's allegiance is divided between the patient and the consulting agency, court or attorney. Gutheil and Appelbaum[3] have noted that the forensic clinician serves more than one master. On occasion, the results of the forensic evaluation may be detrimental to the psychiatric best interests of a defendant/patient. For example, little literature supports incarceration or execution as a treatment modality. In this regard, Pollack[4] has distinguished between psychiatry and the law and forensic psychiatry. Pollack defines forensic psychiatry as the application of psychiatry to legal issues for legal ends, i.e., for the purpose of legal justice. He expands his discussion on forensic psychiatry and suggests that it is "not primarily concerned with the medical and psychiatric treatment of the individual." Thus, according to Pollack, the clinician's allegiance in the forensic evaluation is not mixed and is solely to the legal system. Gutheil and Appelbaum believe the forensic clinician is in a situation in which the clinician "merely shares employment with the patient, with another party or institution."

Training and Employment

The woman entering the forensic system enters a profession which is almost completely male dominated. A brief anecdote about one of the author's entries into the forensic system prior to assuming the role of an administrator at a forensic hospital might be illustrative. The author had left a purely clinical position. She had no training in forensic psychiatry and took the job for personal and professional reasons, making clear that an extensive period of training in forensic psychiatry would be necessary before assuming an administrative role. The first professional memory associated with training was a court trip with a senior mentor as a part of the training experience. It was surprising and disconcerting when both the prosecutor and defense attorney assumed that this Board-certified psychiatrist was a secretary accompanying "her boss." There was an unspoken hint of a nonprofessional relationship between the secretary and boss. The mentor never did identify the trainee/psychiatrist as a colleague physician psychiatrist. Looking back at the incident, it appeared to us that the insecurity and discomfort accompanying a new situation, the first time in a courtroom, were apparent to all. In reacting to anxiety, the woman fell back on old defenses with quiet compliance--she never identified herself as a professional. Though she had been in leadership positions before, old coping techniques surfaced. The male mentor fostered the ambiguity. In addition, those in the courtroom noted anxiety but used stereotypic defenses in translating anxiety into "problems in a relationship." No one in the forensic system was accustomed to seeing a woman in the courtroom in any roles other than those of wife, secretary or girlfriend. Since that first time in the courtroom, the author has never had the role of secretary, messenger or girlfriend ascribed. That is not to say that we have always been recognized as professionals, but more about that later.

Training in forensic psychiatry is difficult to achieve. There are very few training programs in the country and, as a consequence, very few training positions. Those positions are often unadvertised, and students interested in forensic mental health learn about fellowships through word of mouth. In our own training program, we have a higher proportion of women trainees because the training director is a woman, and the informal network has provided information about trainee positions through the network to other women.

After learning about forensic psychiatry, one is confronted with finding the best way to practice it. For women, some obstacles to full private practice in the forensic field remain. In the private practice of forensics, one is dependent upon referrals from a non-medical field, which is also predominantly male. Thus, getting oneself established with a referral network may be limited for a woman by not being part of the "good old boy" system. In some communities, criminal, high profile cases are jealously reserved for the established practitioners and not readily shared with the "new girl on the block." Breaking into both the male-dominated legal and medical referral system can be doubly difficult.

Those seeking employment in clinics or inpatient settings face other drawbacks. Many opportunities occur in penal-like institutions which remain heavily male dominated because of concerns for security and because the majority of forensic patients are male. Up until the present time, the infrequent presence of women in roles of authority in these settings have presented little challenge to the idea that these settings are "naturally" male. Women working there are confronted with the lack of other women professionals for alliance and support. There may even be a lack of facilities (such as restrooms) reflecting the lack of women working there.

Women interviewing for such jobs are questioned closely, as they are often seen as having handicaps based on their sex which may influence their work. Though men as well as women may have difficulty dealing with certain types of crimes or situations, women are more often questioned about how they will deal with possible problematic situations. For example, a woman may be routinely questioned about her expectations of how she will feel interviewing a rapist or child molester or dealing with predominantly male patients. Yet men also have countertransference difficulties. In many situations, male practitioners deal predominantly with patients of the opposite sex (e.g., gynecology). It is seeing males as the norm that leads to such questioning, not recognizing that similar clinical situations can present difficulties for men also.

Interactions with Institution and Hospital Staff

The presence of women in institutional settings may lead to more awareness of areas of concern which have previously been ignored. Women can express concern more freely for the safety of themselves and others and pinpoint potentially dangerous situations. However, a woman's observation may be discounted because of her gender. A female presence allows a different viewpoint with which to examine patient care, ethical issues and to offer new solutions. Research has demonstrated that the presence of female personnel can model a more nonprovocative stance towards violent patients, leading to a decrease in violent behavior.[5,6]

Gender expectations of women's competence can impact in many ways on their work. First, women are seen primarily as women, then as clinicians, coloring their interactions with other mental health professionals, ward staff and secretaries. Our previously mentioned informal survey uniformly revealed that conflicts between secretaries and female clinicians were more frequently a source of concern to female clinicians. Gender awareness leads to clinician performances being viewed primarily in the context of expectations of their sex. The limited number of women professionals in the field also contributes to this. As the numbers of women professionals rise, stereotypes may become harder to maintain. But for now such stereotyping continues. For example, when questioning the clinical decision of one of the authors, the hospital director reminded the woman that the patient was "known for his ability to manipulate women." Such a statement implied that her clinical decisions were based on her feelings as a woman, not that her clinical decisions were based on her clinical judgment. This was particularly striking as the primary women that had been manipulated by this patient/man had been his victims.

Others in an institution or courtroom may have difficulty in acknowledging a woman's competence. Her presence may be dismissed as being a "a token" or required by affirmative action. This does not recognize the woman's efforts, training or skills and dismisses her accomplishments as "luck" or her presence as required because of her obvious handicap (her sex). For example, two of the authors were involved in opening a new unit. When this new treatment program started, its success was dismissed as "luck." Despite the fact that several patients had presented serious management problems on their old units, all the patients were now characterized as "good patients." Allusions were also made to a "honeymoon period," implying some kind of sexual reason for the relative calm and goodwill between patients, treatment staff and clinical staff. This characterization of "luck" was maintained despite a history of testing and power struggles when other such clinical units in the same hospital were opened. The possibility that clinical skill and hard work contributed to the new unit's success was never raised. No wonder women have difficulties attributing their successes to their own abilities and efforts! They are not getting such feedback from the environment.

Professional organizations are still male-dominated in both membership and leadership. One of the women in our survey noted that at a professional meeting, the location of a forthcoming conference was touted as being a good place because "tricks were cheaper and more easily available." There was no recognition that such "humor" might be offensive since female members in the organization are a minority. Continu-

ing medical education in regard to topics of special interest to women is limited or relegated to a position of lesser importance on the program. Female judges, attorneys and mental health professionals are rarely on the program either as members or invited guests. Planned programs for spouses are of limited interest to husbands of professionals. It is not surprising that women continue to show little interest in joining these male-dominated professional organizations.

Interactions with Lawyers and the Judiciary

One might anticipate many occasions of difficulty and conflict in interacting with attorneys and the judiciary because they are rather traditional male professions. Rather surprisingly, many of our respondents indicated they did not experience many difficulties with sex role stereotyping as it applied to themselves. In this context, the survey was surprising in that all the authors experienced many traditional problems in this regard. Informal conversations with colleagues have revealed consistent patterns of sexism in the courtroom. There appears to be a distinct tendency to discount women as professionals and to disregard consultations, advice or testimony that they may give. Such stereotypes may also impact on a witness' perceived credibility as "an expert." When psychiatrists are consistently fantasized as men with beards who smoke pipes, a woman clinician may frequently be confronted with "but you don't look like a doctor." Such expectations may have been involved when a judge recently queried of his secretary, "Is the doctor here yet?" while looking past the expert in an otherwise empty waiting room. From the witness stand, women have to take a firm stance to appear skilled and competent. In an adversarial setting, a woman must defend her position. This goes against the stereotype of woman as mediator and compromiser. Although the authors have had the experience of going to court with a male colleague in a training capacity, we have all been surprised at the difficulty the court has in believing that the female of a dyad is the supervisor and the male is a student. So marked is this tendency that on occasion it continues even when other clues such as style of dress would suggest otherwise. One of the authors had occasion to be called to testify at a complex competency hearing. She dressed appropriately in conservative business attire. The male student who accompanied her was casually dressed in slacks and crew-neck sweater. Despite constant corrections and these obvious sartorial clues, the lawyers in the case persisted during the pre-trial conference in addressing questions about the evaluation and the opinion to the male student. Such discounting presented itself in a similar way on another occasion when one of the authors arrived shortly before a hearing and sat alone in the gallery portion of the courtroom. As the hearing commenced, the prosecutor turned and surveyed the gallery and then indicated to the judge that the "doctor was not in the courtroom." It was apparent that it seemed to him quite statistically unlikely that the female in the gallery might indeed be the expert witness. Even when that witness stood up to indicate to the bench that she was present, so powerful was the stereotype that the prosecutor in question turned and responded, "Are you sure?" Although incidents such as these occur infrequently, they are sufficiently dramatic and disconcerting to increase areas of stress when functioning as a forensic examiner.

Sexist commentary, both on and off the stand, also occurs with some degree of frequency. Quite regularly, psychologists and psychiatrists who happen to be female are addressed by all parties as Ms. or Mrs. or even Honey or Dearie. Again, this often occurs despite corrections by the woman about the proper professional title of address. While some of this may be strategically done by attorneys to discommode an opposing witness, it occurs with sufficient frequency that it appears to reflect not only a conscious strategy, but also an unconscious assumption. Allied to this is a tendency to question female experts about irrelevant aspects of their personal lives both on and off the witness stand. Areas of inquiry include marital status and the combining of professional career and family responsibilities without shortchanging either. These kinds of questions have, in the experience of the authors, rarely been addressed to male professionals and would cause consternation, surprise and fury were they to be presented. Commentary about one's dress or physical appearance again more frequently occurs when the witness is a woman. On one occasion, one of the authors was involved in a jury trial involving a lengthy testimony. The witness had been subject to thorough, direct and rather rigorous cross-examination and was preparing to descend from the stand, silently congratulating herself for

having presented comprehensible and professional testimony to the jury. As she stepped from the stand, the judge from the bench and on the record commented, "You sure have nice legs, Doc." This casual and inappropriate comment may well have successfully undercut hours of professional work by reframing the witness as simply a sex object and not as a professional. No one in the courtroom formally questioned the appropriateness of this remark.

Outside the courtroom, problems may also arise. There appears to be a greater tendency to assume an illusion of intimacy with women professionals. Being addressed as Sweetheart or Honey does little to enhance professional relationships between lawyers and mental health professionals. Another area of difficulty is managing the courtroom lunch break. Traditionally, expert examiners and the lawyer who is presenting their testimony may lunch together. These lunches serve an important function in terms of discussing the case in question, in reconnoitering testimony and, in traditional male ways, provides social bonding, as informal conversation about sports and professional matters may take place. When the examiner is a woman, the aura of a shared meal carries a different set of social assumptions, and sometimes in a disconcerting way has a tendency to slide into a "pass" rather than a professional conversation.

Interaction with Patients

Lastly, one must consider the impact of being a woman on one's relationships with forensic patients. This appears to make itself apparent in three general areas: First, the kind of behavior a patient may display and how one deals with it; second, the attitudes and transferential feelings patients demonstrate, and; finally the attitudes that the therapist will experience and countertransferential matters that arise when the therapist is female.

Dealing with patient behavior centers around assaultive acting out and sexual inappropriata of one sort or another. Being a woman is both an asset and a liability when dealing with assaultive acting out. On the one hand, gender alone may provoke certain patients to anger and violence. Additionally, a woman may be physically handicapped by reason of height and strength in dealing directly with the assaultive patient. On the other hand, the very fact that women are not accustomed or usually equipped to physically defend themselves may function as an asset. Male professionals often display the wish and intent to indeed defend themselves in such circumstances when it might more appropriately be left in the hands of experienced and trained security personnel. Female professionals are more likely to ask for such help without loss of "face." Being a woman also appears to act as a protection when dealing with forensic patients. Many patients have been socialized to "never hit a woman." This old learning comes into play even in situations of great psychological disorganization.

The other area of patient behavior which may present special problems for the female professional is that of sexual inappropriata. As the vast majority of forensic patients, particularly in criminal justice systems, are male, the female professional is more likely to be the object of sexual fantasies and impulses. This is particularly true in that professional and nonprofessional female staff members are few in forensic settings, and thus patients are unaccustomed to some extent in dealing appropriately with women in the way. Surprisingly, none of the respondents in our informal survey reported any of the above problems, and most of their "horror stories" derived from other facts of forensic work.

Another way in which being female affects the course of one's work is in attitudes and transferences displayed by the patients. Being predominantly male in number, the patient population shares many of the same assumptions as society in general about women and their roles. This is most often manifest in difficulty in recognizing the female professional as the doctor. Just as attorneys and courts appear to have difficulty recognizing this, patients too will often address the ward female psychiatrist as Nurse or Ms. or Mrs. There is also a tendency on the part of the patients to assume that female clinicians provide more caretaking and mothering sources than they would expect of similar males. The female therapist functioning in a forensic setting is also the subject of more intense transferential relationships. Such patients often have long histories of problematic relationships with women, and frequently their victims have been women. The transference may then take on quite hostile or sexual overtones not generally seen overtly in other settings.

The therapists' own attitude and facets of the countertransference are affected by their gender as well. As many victims are indeed women or children, the female professional may more easily identify and empathize with the victim than would a male colleague. Thus, one may struggle with one's own feelings when having to discuss in a supportive and therapeutic way the circumstances of a rape or an instance of child abuse or murder. One's socialization as a woman also may create internal and personal issues around aggression and violence and how they should be handled. It may be difficult for us at times to successfully address such matters with male and female patients. Our own internal conflicts about aggression may also lead us to either unduly minimize or over-respond to indicia of dangerousness in the patients entrusted to our care.

Assets of Women in Forensic Psychiatry

Despite the fact that the female professional in forensic mental health faces a variety of problems, there are indeed assets that compensate to a significant degree for gender-related stresses. First and foremost, forensic mental health presents to the practitioner questions of great diversity and intellectual challenge. Much forensic work still addresses itself to the traditional questions of competency to stand trial or legal insanity. In recent years, mental health professionals have increasingly been called upon by the court to assist in the adjudication of many other matters such as child custody, the impact of personal injury or the psychological costs of sexual harassment. Assisting the court in answering these types of questions requires of the evaluator not only clinical skills, but also understanding of the law which may apply, carefulness of thought and capacity to communicate psychological matters effectively to the lay person. Thus, forensic psychiatry and psychology present many opportunities for complex problem-solving. The field offers many opportunities for professional growth and development. Coupled with this are the freedom and independence that this type of professional work provides. One manages one's own time and can set about collecting information to answer the proposed legal question in a way that one professionally feels is intellectually honest, productive and relevant. Almost all of the respondents to our survey commented on these two areas of job satisfaction.

In addition, functioning as a woman in forensic mental health can, in and of itself, be an asset in assessing gender-related issues such as sexual harassment or the psychological impact of rape. One's status as a woman as well as one's role as a mental health professional can assist the evaluator in framing a more thorough and helpful forensic opinion. Moreover, many attorneys feel that having testimony in such matters presented by a female professional enhances its credibility. In working with male clients, one's status as a woman functions occasionally as an asset in that it highlights the client's psychopathology in terms of his relationships with women. On other occasions, as women are socially seen as more empathetic and feeling-oriented, male patients may find it easier to be more open and to share more of their feelings when talking to a female professional.

There are also a variety of other assets and rewards in the forensic field. Expertise in forensic mental health is becoming a highly marketable skill, and the field in general appears to be expanding as mental health professionals are drawn into an ever-increasing variety of socio-legal questions. Since the demand for persons with forensic expertise is increasing, the financial compensations for this type of professional work are significant and cannot be overlooked. Other assets include occasions for travel and the opportunity for interacting with persons outside the mental health fields in interdisciplinary consultation.

In addition to the many personal assets of a career in forensic mental health, there are assets for the profession as a whole that derive from the increasing inclusion of women in its ranks. Not only are practitioners predominantly male, but so are clients sent for evaluation. Thus, it becomes easy for the profession to adhere to a variety of sex-related stereotypes. It is indeed the persistence of these stereotypes which makes for difficulties when the forensic examiner is a woman. The presence of women in the profession, therefore, enhances the growth of forensic mental health by bringing another critical point of view to social problems, psychological make-up and resolution of conflict. Additionally, increasing numbers of women in this field may well act to humanize it. Given the contentious style of the courtroom, it is easy to get drawn into a rather prosecutorial or adversarial position as a mental health professional. While women, of course, are subject to the same pressures, other aspects of their socialization may allow them to maintain more readily a helpful, nonjudgmental and understanding position.

Conclusion

This brief chapter has addressed the problems and pleasures of working in forensic mental health as a clinician. Issues of training, jobs, interaction with institutional staff, legal personnel and the judiciary have been addressed.

In conclusion, the authors suggest several coping strategies which they have found helpful in dealing with the forensic system as it exists today. The primary healthy psychological defense is a good sense of humor. In addition, it is also helpful to remember that much of what appears hostile in the courtroom is part of the adversarial "game" and not primarily personal.

Collegial support and consultation are crucial. The collegial network must include others besides female forensic mental health clinicians. Attorneys, judges and their nonforensic clinicians help to broaden perspectives. A working knowledge of the growing literature of female professionals is helpful. With these strategies in mind, the clinician can perform forensic evaluations and participate in legal decision-making with increased understanding of the problems and rewards of forensic mental health.

References

[1]Miller JB, Nadelson CC, Notman MT, and Zilbach J: Aggression in Women: A Re-examination, in Klebanow S. Changing Concepts in Psychoanalysis. New York: Gardner Press, 1981.

[2]Blum HP: "Feminine Masochism, The Ego Ideal and the Psychology of Women," in Blum HP, ed., Female Psychology. New York: Grune and Stratton, 1944.

[3]Gutheil TG and Appelbaum PS: Clinical Handbook of Forensic Psychiatry. New York: McGraw-Hill Book Company, 1982.

[4]Pollack S: The Role of Psychiatry in the Rule of Law. Psychiatric Annals 4:816-831, 1974.

[5]Benedek EP and Criss M: A Survey of Violent Incidents in a Forensic Center, Unpublished.

[6]Levy and Hartocollis: Nursing Aides and Patient Violence. American Journal of Psychiatry, 133:429-431, 1976.

20

Private Practice: Springboard or Stumbling Block for Women Leaders?

Martha Kirkpatrick, M.D.

Associate Clinical Professor,
Department of Psychiatry,
The University of California at Los Angeles (UCLA)

Diana Miller, M.D.

Private Practice, and
Assistant Clinical Professor of Psychiatry,
UCLA

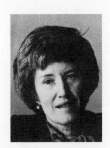 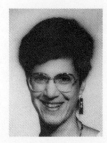

Martha Kirkpatrick, M.D.   Diana Miller, M.D.

20

Private Practice: Springboard or
Stumbling Block for Women Leaders?

The Problem

Remember when you got grades for leadership in elementary school? It was usually the goody-goody smug little girl with Shirley Temple curls or the teacher's pet who sported the A in leadership. You knew it just meant she did what she was told and did it quietly and ran errands for the teacher. Boys were rarely high in leadership qualities. Playground status was a different matter. There the rough and tumble battles for leadership were judged and rewarded by peers, and boys often wouldn't let the girls play. The girls were the audience. Life outside the home has been the big boys' playground for a long time, and A's in "leadership" which meant conformity and obedience are useless and misleading for women who venture onto that playground. Perhaps you think it's time the playground became feminized, and perhaps it will be when the socialization of women includes support for feminine individuation and feminine interest in power.

Women in private practice, like women in medicine in general, took the risk of nonconformity. They entered the playground, but their socialization instructed them to be audience rather than actor, faithful follower rather than fearless leader. Perhaps this is why the percentage of women physicians entering private practice has traditionally been lower than the percentage of male physicians. This has been true for psychiatry as well, despite the fact that the private practice of psychiatry has unique advantages for women, es-

pecially those with children. Psychiatric practice can be easily adapted to a home office, which allows for more flexibility in scheduling than a salaried position. Unlike other specialties the overhead is low, and opening an office is not predicated on assuming a large bank loan, a responsibility women often find frightening.

Leadership and power for women are ambivalently desired goals since women are taught to see them as antithetical to or destructive of the integrity of their womanhood. Our socially constructed world informs our definitions of masculine and feminine as equivalent to leader and led. Thus women are vulnerable to internal as well as external stress if they perceive themselves as leaders. For example, one of the authors (D.M.) was startled at the response of a woman physician, a president of a local county medical chapter, when asked how she had achieved this position. She replied, "It was nothing I did. They asked me, and I felt honored and obligated to serve. I enjoyed the work very much, but I would not actively seek future positions." This method of reducing interpersonal stress by denying personal instrumentality in assuming leadership clouds the picture of women in leadership. It clouds the demographic facts of women's leadership as well as deprives other women of models, mentors and a history of personal routes to power. We lack a sense of continuity with women leaders of the past and historical validation of the value of women's leadership.

In considering women's experience of leadership, one searches for a definition and/or a means of quantification. Leadership comes in many forms. The essential features appear to us to be that it occurs in a social context in which some other is led or influenced by the power, position, or capacity contained in or identified with the leader. This very broad definition does not require self-awareness or intent on the part of the leader, and says nothing about the temporal or geographic relationships between leader and led nor about the ratio of leader to led. In this sense every mother is a leader to her children, every teacher a leader to her pupils, every psychiatrist a leader to her patients, etc. While these are indeed positions of profound influence, the most profound for individual development, they do not imbue women with a sense of themselves as leaders nor prepare them for the recognition or use of their *public* power.

Public power operates in the wider community where the playground rules apply. Leadership in this public sense requires self-awareness, intent or at least willingness to acquire public power, and a belief in the appropriateness and value of one's individual efforts toward influencing a whole community. It requires a tolerance for loss as well as gain, for shifts in popularity, for disapproval, for nonconformity, for admiration and applause.

Women are more sensitive to social context and nuance seemingly from birth. They are more easily socialized. Social acceptance and support are more meaningful and more necessary to their sense of well-being. Thus it is more difficult for a woman to stand out or to stand alone, especially along from other women.

Women's organizations, so often begun in an ecstasy of sisterhood and equality but often founder and not infrequently fragment when differentiation begins and leaders emerge. The fate of women leaders is often to be "trashed" by their own constituency as being either co-opted by the male enemy or exploitative of other women because of their ambitions. They have betrayed the sisterhood. These painful possibilities lead women to shrink from the recognition of their individual power and to eschew a desire for leadership. However "woman power" is less taboo than it used to be. Histories of women of power are flooding women's book lists and women are now on the playground as players. Leadership as a state of mind, i.e., an acceptable expectation of the value and power of one's thoughts and a per-

sonal identity with leading, has been encompassed by the feminine ego boundary at last.

Women psychiatrists in private practice are nonconforming women both by virtue of becoming doctors as well as by working for themselves under their own leadership. This stretches the capacity for nonconformity and social role strain to the limit for many. We learned in our group of women psychiatrists in private practice that many felt isolated from male colleagues whom they experienced as unwelcoming and from non-professional women whom they experienced as either envious or disapproving or both.[1] They expected punishment for their nonconforming ambition, not praise and support. Ambition for public power or leadership was felt to threaten their social acceptability even further.

The Data

Little data exists on women psychiatrists in leadership positions and even less on women psychiatric private practitioners in leadership positions. We will survey the data that are available and pertinent to this topic and attempt first a profile of women psychiatrists in private practice. We will include consideration of the numbers of women psychiatrists in private practice, their income and marital status, and then their participation and leadership roles in the American Psychiatric Association (APA).

How many women psychiatrists choose private practice as their primary setting? A survey questionnaire mailed to all members of the APA in December 1982 indicated that 52.9 percent (1,352 of 2,556) of the women psychiatrist respondents and 57.6 percent (9,137 of 15,860) of the male psychiatrist respondents were working primarily in a private practice setting.[2] This percentage is similar to that of women M.D.'s in general who are in private practice.[3] The APA 1982 question-

Table 1. Age by Gender Among Active Respondents with a Primary Work Setting of Private Practice

Gender	Age					
	<30	30–39	40–49	50–59	60–69	>69
Male	240	1608	2356	1986	1157	635
(%)	(3.0)	(20.1)	(29.5)	(24.9)	(14.5)	(8.0)
Female	25	344	322	225	159	87
(%)	(2.2)	(29.6)	(27.7)	(19.4)	(13.7)	(7.5)

Note. Valid cases = 9144; invalid cases = 1345.

naire also provided information on the age distribution of women and men psychiatrists in private practice. We note in this snapshot picture of private practitioners the larger percentage of women psychiatrists in the 30-39 year age group, i.e., 29.6 percent of women psychiatrists versus 20.1 percent of male psychiatrists (see Table 1). So almost one-third of women psychiatrists in private practice in 1982 were beginning their practices in their prime childbearing years.

What are the income levels of women psychiatrists in private practice? The 1982 APA questionnaire revealed that women psychiatrists in private practice earn less than their male counterparts. Table 2 shows that nearly one-half of the male psychiatrists earn more than $100,000 while 42 percent of the women psychiatrists earn less than $60,000. Women psychiatrists in private practice share their lower incomes with women psychiatrists and women M.D.s in general. *Medica* in October 1984 reported that the median *gross* income for women psychiatrists was $65,000.[4] Self-employed women psychiatrists earned slightly more, $68,000. This can be contrasted with the figure reported in *Medical Economics* (2/7/83) of a *net* income for all psychiatrists of $70,350.[5] Women M.D.'s incomes have been analyzed by the American Medical Association (AMA). A recent report from the Socioeconomic Monitoring System of the AMA Center for Health Policy Research[6] found that women M.D.'s earn 24 percent less than male M.D.'s. This figure takes into account any income discrepancy caused by difference in number of hours worked.

Although we know that women psychiatrists in private practice are making considerably less than their male peers, the explanation for this is not

Table 2. Gross Income by Gender Among Active Respondents with a Primary Work Setting of Private Practice*

Gender	Gross Income in Quartiles				
	<$60,000	$60,000–$74,000	$75,000–$99,000	≥$100,000	Total
Male	673	838	1296	2540	5347
(%)	(12.6)	(15.7)	(24.2)	(47.5)	(100.0)
Female	311	167	133	117	728
(%)	(42.7)	(22.9)	(18.3)	(16.1)	(100.0)

Note. Valid cases = 6075; invalid cases = 4414.
*Active respondents include members who reported a current work status of active, semi-active, or temporarily inactive.

Table 3. Average Weekly Hours Worked in Psychiatry by Gender Among Active Respondents with a Primary Work Setting of Private Practice*

Gender	Average Weekly Hours Worked in Psychiatry				
	<20	20–39	40–59	>59	Total
Male	288	1147	5260	1838	8533
(%)	(3.4)	(13.4)	(61.6)	(21.5)	(99.9)
Female	85	428	605	134	1252
(%)	(6.8)	(34.2)	(48.3)	(10.7)	(100.0)

Note. Valid cases = 9785; invalid cases = 704.
*Active respondents include members who reported a current work status of active, semi-active, or temporarily inactive.

obvious. Factors such as age--younger practitioners may earn less than their more experienced colleagues--and number of hours worked must be accounted for before other influences (lower fees set by women, sexist practices, etc.) can be assessed.

As noted in Table 1 the age distribution of women and men psychiatrists in private practice is roughly comparable except for the differences noted in the 30- to 39-year-old age group and to a lesser extent, in the 50- to 59-year-old age group. One possible conclusion is that there are more younger women (30-39) earning less and fewer older women (50-59) earning more. However, if we look at men and women psychiatrists of the same age we still see income discrepancies. For example, in *Medica*'s 1984 analysis, women psychiatrists between 45 and 54 years of age have a median gross income of $63,500 compared to the male psychiatrists in the same age range, whose median net income is $91,200.[7]

Is the income discrepancy accounted for by the number of hours worked? As we can see in Table 3 women in private practice work fewer hours than men in private practice. This is a common finding.[8-16] Possibly most of the many women psychiatrists who work a 20-39 hour week are constrained to do so because of family commitments.

There are no figures available specifically for women psychiatrists in private practice, but there are data for women M.D.'s relative to family responsibilities. These data point in two directions. Women M.D.'s are more likely to marry now than they were three decades ago.[17] Sixty-seven percent of women M.D.'s have children,[18] with an average of 1.8 children. Women M.D.'s are like other highly educated women in these areas.

Census bureau findings show that the number of children is inversely related to income and educational level. The higher the income and education, the fewer births and the greater probability of plans for no children. The 1980 Census data made two predictions about women with five or more years of college: 1) they plan to have fewer children (1.7) than their non-high school completion peers (2.4), and 2) 20 percent plan no children. These predictions matched the actual data for women M.D.'s who are beyond their child-bearing years (40-44). These women averaged 1.9 children and 15.5 percent had no children. The childless figure has tripled in the last decade for women M.D.'s. So although more women doctors are marrying they may be having fewer children, and a significant number plan to have no children. Divorce in women M.D.'s has also increased although the figures are very low in women M.D.'s in their thirties, since women M.D.'s marry late. When the 55 and over age group is examined, their divorce rate (14.8 percent) is more than twice the national figure (7.3 percent).

In summary, it is not clear that the lesser number of hours worked by women doctors is explained by their family commitments. We do know from a study done by Drs. Martha Kirkpatrick and Charlotte Robertson that those women psychiatrists who do marry and have children feel a conflict between their profession and child care.[19] This area of women professionals' responses to the challenges of career and family is undergoing continual study.

Turning to look at figures that reflect women psychiatrists' positions of leadership in their specialty society, the APA, we first examine membership level. In 1984 women psychiatrists made up 17.9 percent of the APA membership (Table 4). This is an encouraging increase from 13 percent in 1979.[20] The percentage of women M.D.'s in the AMA shows a similar increase (from 18 percent in 1979 to 25 percent in 1983);[21] however, the levels of participation for both women

Table 4. Demographics of APA Membership

	Members (% of total members)	Non-members (% of total non-members)	Total (% of Total)
Female	5,395 (17.94)	2,365 (18.7)	7,760 (18.2)
Male	24,407 (81.17)	8,237 (65.0)	32,644 (76.4)
Unknown	268 (0.9)	2,061 (16.3)	2,329 (5.5)
Total	30,070	12,663	42,733

Source: Marta De Lalla, Director of Member Services, American Psychiatric Association.

and men M.D.'s are considerably lower in the AMA (47 percent in 1983)[18] than in the APA (70 percent in 1984).

Does this trend of increased membership mean increased percentages of women in leadership roles? Ten years ago the APA established a task force to examine the unexplained low participation of women in leadership roles. Many more women have participated on components and in the APA programs as a result of the task force efforts. The current picture of women in leadership reveals a woman president, the first, Carol C. Nadelson, two women on the editorial board of the Journal of the American Psychiatric Association, no women on the board of directors of the College of American Psychiatrists and women's leadership levels remaining constant for the last five years (1979-1984) (see Table 5).

At the local level change is more evident. In 1984 there were more than twice as many women presidents-elect as current women presidents in both district branches and chapters (Table 6).

Although women's struggle for equal percentage leadership in the APA is far from over, the situation is considerably better than that for women in other medical organizations. In 1979, the AMA reported there were only 51 women in elected state positions in the 40 responding states and only 114 women in elected county positions.[22] In a 1980 survey of 17 specialty societies, there

Table 5. Women Leaders in the APA

	1979	1984
Administrative Level (Professional Staff)	2 of 8 (25%)	2 of 9 (22%)
Assembly Executive Committee	1 of 23 (4%)	1 of 23 (4%)
Assembly	10 of 150 (7%)	17 of 158 (11%)
Minority Representatives	3 of 10 (30%)	3 of 12 (25%)

were only 15 positions held by women.[21] In another 1980 survey of the officers and directors of the membership organizations of medical specialties, only 3 percent were women (11 of 364).[23]

In summary, it is clear that the data available provide only a few fragments of the relevant picture. We see that slightly fewer than half of women psychiatrists are primarily engaged in private practice. They earn less than their male counterparts, which is not wholly explained by the fact that they work fewer hours. The influx of young women into the field increases the percentage of women who are just beginning practice. Probably they share characteristics of women M.D.'s in that more are marrying now than 30 years ago, they are having fewer children, and a sizable percentage plan no children. Thus it is not clear what part family responsibilities play in accounting for fewer hours worked and lower incomes or in limited participation in their professional organizations. We do know that women psychiatrists enjoy higher levels of leadership positions than women M.D.'s in general, but we have no way of knowing what percentage of this increased participation comes from the private practice group.

Commentary

Some women may choose private practice as a route to maximum freedom for individual leadership with patients and minimum expectation of public leadership. Robertson in an unpublished presentation compared the responses of male and female psychoanalysts as to the pleasures and burdens of their work and found that male analysts described the pleasure of "reconstructing" or "achieving success with disabled people" while female analysts saw themselves less as active agents and more as servicing or supporting *patients'* power and growth.[19] Nevertheless one *leads* one's own professional life in private practice. For women who enjoy that freedom yet aspire to participation in the public arena as well, no protocol or manual exists. (Machiavelli did not write a "Princess" volume to accompany "The Prince.")

Factors which are often seen as limiting or burdening in private practice include isolation, uncertainty of income, 24-hour direct responsibility for outpatient care, minimal if any support services such as secretary, research assistants, tele-phone tie line, Xerox equipment, computer service, library, etc. Collegial watering holes or collegial crossroads are few. There is no direct access to mentors, no apparent ladder to success and no direct line of ascent to power or public attention. In fact public attention which might be valuable for other specialists in private practice is burdensome to patients in psychotherapy and therefore to be avoided in psychiatry.

However, the option of a home office and the flexibility of time management are of great value to the woman practitioner especially during years involved with child rearing. Limited time for professional work during these years is usually seen as a handicap: i.e., women lose their position on the ladder, lose contacts, may lose competence and require re-entry training. These are real dangers for women in academic or salaried positions. The woman in private practice can easily maintain a part-time practice, especially with a home office, and can benefit enormously from the personal experience of child care, the intimate sharing of the non-professional woman's life, and the opportunity to participate in community affairs on a volunteer basis. There are also opportunities to learn leadership skills and make community contacts which can enhance later professional life. The availability of competent child care and a spouse who shares this responsibility can make this period in a professional woman's life a time of rich learning and expansion. Even if it is a fragmented and frazzled time, it need not be time professionally wasted. It may even be a propitious time to begin involvement with a committee, newsletter or program in a local organization. Willingness to participate, reliable attendance and serious response to issues make one a valuable member of any committee. Often becoming expert in a certain area or issue will provide a platform for further advancement. Models and mentors are invaluable. Women inside the power system can and should provide examples and practical help for younger women, but one can also find equally sincere and generous support from male mentors.

Table 6. Local Levels of the APA—Women Leaders

	Presidents	Presidents-Elect
76 District Branches	4	8
91 Chapters	3	8
Totals	7	16

Be willing to be a reporter or a moderator during annual meetings, become familiar with those who plan, assist or speak at meetings and develop contacts with others in areas of common interests. Join the clinical faculty of the local medical school and supervise or teach. Begin to write; having a writing buddy often helps. A part-time secretary and/or a computer word processing system are enormous aids. A secretary may not be a necessary part of your practice, but he/she forms the core of a support system for all other professional activities. Speak up at meetings, be brief, be relevant, but be heard. If this is hard for you, get some coaching in public speaking and practice whenever possible. Don't ignore opportunities to speak and to become familiar with organizational life in P.T.A's, clubs and political groups as well as in hospital, university, clinic and professional organizations. Become familiar with their program needs and participate in planning or speaking for programs.

These practical suggestions are meaningful only to women who feel free to be ambitious for leadership and see themselves as appropriate leaders. Inhibitions and fears are often tenacious obstacles to achieving this autonomy. Women's greatest obstacle too often is not powerlessness, but fear of power. The support of women's groups, a consciousness-raising group, a women's committee, a women's writing group, etc., often provides a medium for growth and the discovery of power. Individual therapy may also be helpful, but one experience does not take the place of the other.

Conclusion

The lack of institutional buffers between psychiatrist and patient increases the private practitioner's appreciation of both the psychological and social hardships of patients. In our minds this emphasizes the importance of women private practitioners' roles in public policy decisions and the need to pursue positions of leadership actively.

There is excitement, stimulation and satisfaction to be found on the big playground. It is not a rose garden, but it is filled with people who maintain their youth, their interest, their ability to flower by remaining on the growing edge of their profession.

References

[1] Kirkpatrick M: A report of a consciousness raising group for women psychiatrists. Journal of the American Medical Women's Association 30:206-212, 1975.

[2] Kennedy T: Survey manager: Biographical directory and professional activities survey questionnaire. American Psychiatric Association Manpower Department, December, 1982 (private communication).

[3] Heins M, Smock S, Martindale L, Stein M, Jacobs J: A profile of the woman physician. Journal of the American Medical Women's Association 32:421-427, 1977.

[4] Diamond P: What women doctors earn. Medica 2(5): 32-36, 1984.

[5] Psychiatrists' earnings: will the boom last? Mental notes, March 1983 (see White, Journal of Medical Economics, Feb. 7, 1983).

[6] Socioeconomic Monitoring System of the American Medical Association Center for Health Policy Research. Quoted in the L.A. Co. Medical Women's Association Newsletter V(3):1-8, 1984.

[7] Nelson B: The bottom line, income and practice profiles of women in four specialties who responded to our 1983 survey. Medica 2(1):33-37, 1984.

[8] Heins M, Smock S, Martindale L, Jacobs J, Stein M: Comparison of the productivity of women and men physicians. JAMA 237: 2514-2517, 1977.

[9] Dykman RA, Stalnaker JM: Survey of women physicians graduating from medical school, 1925-1940. Journal of Medical Education 32:3-38, 1957.

[10] Powers L, Parmelle D, Weisenfelder H: Practice patterns of women and men physicians. Journal of Medical Education 44:481-491, 1969.

[11] Renshaw JE, Pennell MY: Distribution of women physicians, 1969. Woman Physician 26:187-195, 1971.

[12] Pennell MY, Renshaw JE: Distribution of women physicians, 1970. Woman Physician 27:191-203, 1972.

[13] Pennell MY, Renshaw JE: Distribution of women physicians, 1971. Journal of the American Medical Women's Association 28:181-186, 1973.

14Weinstein M: Psychiatric manpower and women in psychiatry. Journal of Nervous and Mental Disease 145:364-370, 1968.

15Nadelson C, Notman M, Lowenstein P: A follow-up study of Harvard Medical School graduates, 1967-1977. Journal of the American Medical Women's Association 36:51-62, 1981.

16Yager J, Pasnau R, Lipschultz S: Journal of Psychiatric Education 3:72-85, 1979.

17Diamond P: The private lives of women doctors. Medica 2(6):40-45, 1984.

18Today's woman M.D. Medica 1(1):40-45, 1983.

19Kirkpatrick M, Robertson C: Observations of the life styles and thinking styles of women and men psychiatrists/psychoanalysts. Presented at the American Psychoanalytic Association. Western Division, Los Angeles, March 20, 1979.

20Kirkpatrick M: Psychiatry, women and the future. Special lecture presented at the American Psychiatric Association annual meeting, Chicago, 1979.

21Fletcher S: Women physicians: old times or a new era? The Pharos Winter 2:9, 1982.

22Women physicians in organized medicine. Connecticut Medicine 43 (11):729-731, 1979.

23Braslow J, Heins M: Women in medical education, a decade of change. New England Journal of Medicine 304:1129-1135, 1981.

21

Women Psychiatrists as Consultants
to Obstetrics and Gynecology

Perspective A

Miriam Rosenthal, M.D.

*Associate Professor of
Psychiatry and Reproductive Biology,
Case Western Reserve University School of Medicine
Cleveland, Ohio*

Perspective B

Elisabeth Chan Small, M.D.

*Clinical Professor of Psychiatry and
Clinical Associate Professor of Obstetrics and Gynecology,
University of Nevada School of Medicine,
Reno, Nevada; and
Co-Medical Director, Med-Stress Unit,
Sparks Family Hospital
Sparks, Nevada*

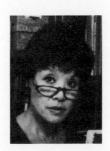 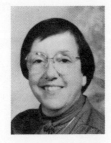

Elisabeth Chan Small, M.D.   **Miriam Rosenthal, M.D.**

21

Women Psychiatrists as Consultants to Obstetrics and Gynecology

Perspective A

Franz Reichsman defines a psychiatric liaison service as one in which the psychiatrist works and teaches psychosomatic medicine in the setting of another department. I have worked as a psychiatrist in the Department of Reproductive Biology at Case Western Reserve University School of Medicine where medical students are assigned to a pregnant woman at the very start of their studies. They follow this patient, generally referred to as "my mother" through her labor and delivery and through the first one and a half to two years of her life with her new child. It is the setting in which Kennell and Klaus looked at attachment behaviors of mothers and babies. There is also a long tradition of respect for "hard" science, the newest technical innovations, numerical data, biochemical reactions, and machinery. The department produces numerous professors, directors, and practicing clinicians. I arrived one year before the Supreme Court legalized abortion and for that year had the opportunity to talk with every woman in our hospital considering pregnancy termination. After the law changed, I remained and broadened my interests and activities considerably.

I went to a women's college, Mount Holyoke, where the department chairs, numerous distinguished scientists, the college physicians, including the psychiatrists, were women and many classmates went to medical school. In my medical school, George Washington University, however, there were three women in a class of one hundred and very few women on the faculty. By far, the best teaching was in the department of obstetrics and gynecology. The department director was innovative, a gifted teacher and an outstanding clinician who taught his staff how to talk to patients. More students chose that specialty than any other, but no women in our class did and I can't recall any women house-staff. I entered a residency in internal medicine at an academic institution and married one of the interns.

This hospital had a long tradition of women physicians since a chief benefactor had made admission of women to the Johns Hopkins University School of Medicine medical school a condition for her to give her money. There were many medical couples living and working at that hospital then, but I can recall the residency director asking me what my husband's plans were for the next years so I could make suitable arrangements.

Two years later, our first child arrived and soon after, a second. I never considered working full-time and we moved as my husband's career unfolded. I enjoyed the children and worked part-time. Many of my closest "support groups" were women physicians home with young children, trying to keep together family and career. I worked part-time in genetics in Baltimore, in enzyme chemistry in Boston, and at a rehabilitation and geriatric hospital in Cleveland. As my husband climbed the academic ladder and I longed for a chance to have some specialty training, we had another baby.

In Cleveland, at a medical wives' club meeting during my first weeks here, I met Dr. Janet Dingle, who had graduated from Reserve at the top of her class, raised a family, practiced internal medicine, and worked for Planned Parenthood. She recruited me to do office gynecology and contraceptive planning in the clinics of this organization and this was my re-entry and the turning point in my career.

Planned Parenthood clinics were held in various places throughout the inner city. The women who came to these clinics were making a strong attempt to control their reproductive lives and in that way their lives in general. They wanted to talk about more than their physical needs. This seemed to me to be the ideal time and place for interventions that could help their future mental health. The patients were women from young adolescence through menopause. We taught classes in family planning, sexuality, and informed patienthood. At one period, we had a bus fully equipped as a gynecological office that parked in churchyards with a huge sign reading, HELP IS HERE, and in small letters, Maternal Health Association. Many women climbed aboard expecting a religious message, but stayed when they found a medical message. Despite strong opposition from local doctors, these clinics flourished. My interest in the physical and mental health of women, especially the issue of reproduction, was nourished, and when all my children were in school, I did a residency in psychiatry.

Case Western Reserve's Department of Psychiatry was offering part-time residencies. I was 39 years old and had three small children, a supportive husband, and a housekeeper who offered to come five days a week. First, a few words on part-time residencies. I was always impressed by the idea that in the 1950's Bobby Brown, a famous baseball player, did a part-time residency in orthopedic surgery at Tulane and brought great prestige to his institution. What one does with the other half-time of one's residency is very significant. I can recall how irritated a residency director was when he learned I had spent some time off at a PTA meeting! I loved psychiatry and hated spending all night at the hospital two or three times a week. My family helped enormously with meals and housework and we often ate at the hospital cafeteria. My son, to this day, gets nauseated when he sees or smells hospital cafeteria

food. I was launched on a new career, in a new direction, and a question for me was how to combine my interests.

Consultation-liaison psychiatry has always been a strong part of the residency at Case Western Reserve. Headed by Dr. David Agle, residents entered with reluctance and left six months later having been very pleased with this part of their training. I chose to work in obstetrics and gynecology, needless to say. An obstetrician who had been on the faculty for many years was also doing a part-time residency in psychiatry. MacDonald House, in 1970, was a 120-bed maternity hospital which each year did over 2,000 deliveries, 1,700 surgical procedures, and had 28,000 clinic visits. The staff obstetrician-gynecologists were facing some very difficult issues because the changing roles and expectations of women often challenged their values. Abortion, sterilization, parenting problems, teenage sexuality and pregnancy, and rape were part of their daily practices. Even though they were not especially psychologically minded, many of these physicians attributed psychological causes to conditions they couldn't understand like nausea of pregnancy, dysmenorrhea, and pelvic pain (Lenane and Lenane). They were called on to help with major life decisions regarding pregnancy which they didn't always wish to do. As a resident, in addition to abortion counseling with patients, I met with staff who frequently had great resistance to terminating pregnancies, while also working with high-risk pregnancy patients. Referrals of other patients also steadily increased as our presence became a part of daily work rounds.

I finished the residency in four and a half years because I finally began doing it full-time. In 1972, I was hired by the new chief of the Department of Obstetrics and Gynecology, Dr. Brian Little. There were 15 residents doing their training in obstetrics and gynecology and a psychiatric resident who stayed for a six-month rotation. Eight to 12 medical students rotated through a core clerkship every two months. The staff also included an obstetrician-gynecologist who had finished his psychiatric training, a psychiatric nurse clinician, and three social workers. We met regularly to discuss cases and staff problems and gave weekly seminars for medical students on the woman patient, the psychology of pregnancy, abortion and contraceptive counseling, rape, menopause, and sexual history-taking. We compiled an excellent reading list and included the Nadelson-Notman books on *The Woman Patient*. We attended rounds, high risk and OB/GYN conferences, and gradually had an increasing number of patients referred by OB/GYN physicians for a variety of conditions. The variety was enormous, and the examples are endless:

A has a twin pregnancy. One twin is normal and one has Down's Syndrome. Please counsel.

'B,' said a frustrated and angry obstetrician, 'has been infertile for ten years and has had numerous procedures and tests. Now she is pregnant and wants an abortion.'

C has just learned she has a male infant on ultrasound, but she doesn't want a male child. Please talk to her because I don't do abortions for sex selection.

My special interests grew in decision-making regarding pregnancy, denial of pregnancy, infertility, and the psychological issues surrounding reproduction, from conception to the attachments of mothers and babies.

Although Horney, Benedek, Deutsch, and Rubinstein had written extensively in the 1920's and 30's about the psychosomatic aspects of obstetrics and gynecology, there was relatively little written about the liaison psychiatrist working in this setting. Some of the papers describing this work began with John Romans and Anthony Labrum at Rochester, Carol Nadelson and Malkah Notman at Beth Israel in Boston, Robert Pasnau at UCLA, Elisabeth Small at Tufts, John Astrachan at Cornell, and others.

Carol Nadelson came to Reserve to talk to our medical students and faculty in the 1970's and I began to feel a need to talk with others doing similar work. I attended my first American Psychiatric Association (APA) meeting in Miami in 1976 to give a paper on liaison psychiatry in OB/GYN and took a course given by Helen Kaplan in sexuality. There, I met Elisabeth Small, learned more of her work on the gynecology service at Tufts and how much she accomplished there. I visited her in Boston, joined her rounds and saw her teaching medical students and house staff.

I learned of The American Society of Psycho-somatic Obstetrics and Gynecology, a national organization of people interested in this area. It had begun as a subgroup of the American College of Obstetricians and Gynecologists and separated, as did most of their groups. I became quite involved. A major project Elisabeth Small and I worked on with a group from several schools was the development of a curriculum in psychosomatic OB/GYN to be included in the training requirements of the Council on Resident Education in Obstetrics and Gynecology (CREOG). A number of these suggestions have been included in the most recent edition.

Brenda Solomon, at the time chair of the APA Committee on Women, came to Cleveland, talked to the APA district branch on women, and addressed the issue of how to become active in APA. I followed her directions explicitly and was appointed to the APA Committee on Women.

Locally, the women faculty of the medical school decided to organize to look into salaries, and have workshops on getting grants, financial planning, dual careers, promotion, and tenure. The guiding organizer was a psychiatrist, Maria Bailas, and the response has been growing. We compiled a directory of women faculty outlining their interests so students can contact them if they wish.

As for liaison psychiatry in an OB/GYN setting, it is estimated that 60 percent of patients attending medical clinics have a primary psychological diagnosis, and this may be even higher in an OB/GYN clinic. Sexual problems are estimated to be very high. In ambulatory outpatient settings, there is some evidence for the cost effectiveness of brief psychotherapy in decreasing utilization of expensive medical resources and in increasing prenatal care and possibly in decreasing prematurity. The cost effectiveness of psychiatry in other settings needs research. The problems of integrating psychological care into this kind of medical setting have been considerable, but barely touched upon. The financing of liaison activities is certainly a major problem, even more so now that many insurance programs have been unwilling to include mental health benefits in their plans because of the tendency to see psychological data as "soft" and not really relevant. The time schedules of busy OB/GYN practitioners differ considerably from those of psychiatrists as do values and personality styles. There is little doubt, however, that psychiatrists have a very major place in teaching, service, and research in medical and surgical settings.

This seems to be the time of leadership by women. The American Psychiatric Association and the American College of Obstetricians and Gynecologists are led by women. Our school now has well over 40 percent women in each entering class and over half the house-staff in OB/GYN are women. The face of medicine is changing so drastically. What will this mean?

Recently, I have become active in the local academy of medicine and in the APA district branch as well as in faculty committee work. As resources become scarcer and economics more problematic, political involvement, or at least an understanding, becomes more important. Frankly, I would most love a chance to spend the next years studying the psychological aspects of pregnancy and how it affects psychological functioning. The combination of psychiatry and obstetrics is a natural!

Perspective B

The liaison psychiatrist, or a more current term, the consultant psychiatrist, treads a marginal line and often suffers the consequences of an undefined identity while working in mixed disciplines of psychiatry and a non-psychiatric medical specialty. Having been born in Peking, China, in the 1930's on German legation territory, of an American-Chinese mother and a Chinese father, I have three nationalities: American, Chinese, and German. From the beginning, the ethnic-cultural identity was a mixed experience, ending in feelings of marginality, yet with identification with several cultures. This may well have been the antecedent of the choice of a professional setting which offered a similar context.

In Chinese culture, as in many other cultures, food plays an essential role in socialization, as well as in the process of negotiation and the transaction of business. The role of eating as a means other than that of nutrition has been well understood, and the use of Chinese food for both nutrient and non-nutrient purposes seems universally applied, as attested to by the ubiquitous presence of a Chinese restaurant in some of the most remote areas of the world. (It also may reflect the sheer numbers of Chinese, but I prefer the more romantic interpretation.)

Expectations for a daughter in a Chinese family in a traditional setting would have simplified the task of feminine identification insofar as role determinants are concerned. But such was not my case. The Japanese invasion of Manchuria in 1937 forced the issue. Due to my mother's foresight of impending disaster and war and her insistence, my father left his secure position as professor of political science at Peking National University and took the last train out of Shanghai with his American-Chinese wife and two small daughters. The family returned to California, the home of my mother's forebears. My maternal great grandfather had come to California in the days of the gold rush and the building of the Transcontinental Railway. He had been a merchant, settling in the mining country of Ukiah. My grandfather was born in the mountain country, learning English on his own, as Chinese children were not allowed in schools at the turn of the century. He became publisher of the first bilingual American/ Chinese daily newspaper in the country. His daughters, not being traditional Chinese women, were all active, professional women who worked outside the home. My mother graduated with a baccalaureate degree from the University of California at Berkeley in 1929, a rare occurrence at that time for women in general. Walking on the marginal line between home and the outside world was not new with me; the role models were the women of my mother's family and her generation.

After receiving my medical degree from UCLA School of Medicine, I moved to Massachusetts where I completed a rotating internship at Newton Wellesley Hospital, an affiliate of Tufts University. More than half of the year was spent on the surgical services. Following internship, experience as assistant director of the venereal disease program in the Massachusetts Department of Public Health brought the reality of the value of a psychiatric understanding in the medical care of patients to a level of concreteness which I had never before realized.

This led me to pursue a residency in psychiatry in the 1960's in a psychoanalytically oriented program at Tufts University-New England Medical Center in Boston, where interest in the interaction of the Department of Psychiatry with other clinical departments was strongly supported by the department chairman, Paul G. Meyerson. Having an obvious interest in medical problems, I was selected to act as liaison psychiatrist to the medical service during my second year of residency, and proceeded to serve as chief resident in C/L in my last year. Familiarity with and a sense of belonging in a medical/surgical setting, as well as a true empathy for the stresses and strains of my nonpsychiatrist colleagues, were factors which preexisted the assignment and persisted.

It is my personal feeling through observations of colleagues that those who enjoy the marginal role of a liaison psychiatrist are often those who have had experience in nonpsychiatric practice. This experience gives a direct understanding and an in-depth appreciation of the needs and the clinical and management problems of a given specialty.

My psychiatric experience in a tertiary care university affiliate (New England Medical Center) allowed a variety of exposures in several specialties: research psychiatrist in gastroenterology; psychiatric consultant to the renal dialysis unit, and finally, liaison psychiatrist in obstetrics/gynecology, where I served in both a part-time and a full-time capacity in the years 1968 to 1981.

Theoretically, the inclusion of psychiatric principles into the teaching of obstetrics and gynecology is a logical step towards the complete care of women. The era of the 1960's, with the feminine revolution and the entry of greater numbers of women into medicine, focused greater attention on the social and emotional factors in the health care of women. The concept of a psychiatric component in obstetrics/gynecology in our institution was theoretically and positively received by the department chair, Dr. George W. Mitchell. He was in the forefront of progress in this area in his willingness to fund a full-time psychiatrist in a Department of Obstetrics and Gynecology.

To have achieved this end point was difficult. The initial steps to acceptance began as the usual assignment of a psychiatrist by the Department of Psychiatry to a given service. An average of three hours per week was funded to provide psychiatric consultation, usually to a conference or a group contact basis. My introduction to involvement was a slow one, beginning with the problem of several cancellations of appointments to meet the gynecology attending because of his being delayed in the operating room. It was a clear lesson to me that the surgical modus operandi often did not mesh with the typical 50 minute hour I was accustomed to in my psychiatric scheduling. Something had to change in order to communicate, and

it was me!

In private practice at the time, I was committed to the 50 minute hour for income and survival purposes, and because of the psychodynamic treatment format, but this had to change. On the afternoons I was present at the traditional consultation rounds, I scheduled no patients. I sat through the case discussions, and realized that *I* had a great deal to learn. It was evident that I had forgotten to consider the subtleties and complications of specific medical-surgical disease states and I was reminded of the complexities of surgical procedures. I was impressed that each aspect of gynecologic diagnosis and management had its special emotional component and psychologic meaning and realized that I needed to learn more about gynecology in order to be more effective psychiatrically. I needed to tread the marginal line with better balance and so asked to accompany staff on rounds to see patients directly. The gynecologist/oncologist, Dr. Douglas Marchant, was receptive and pleased, stating, "I thought you'd never ask." From a traditional three hours per week set up, subsidized by the Psychiatry Department, extension to six hours per week with half the stipend paid by Obstetrics/Gynecology followed. The development of the relationship became progressively more involved as six hours per week stretched to ten, and then to 20, until finally in 1977, to full-time, with my entire salary funded by Obstetrics/Gynecology.

The Department of Obstetrics/Gynecology at Tufts New England Medical Center includes divisions of Maternal-Fetal Medicine, Oncology, Reproductive Endocrinology, and Psychiatry. There are 14 full-time physicians including four oncologists, two endocrinologists, one neonatologist, one cytologist, one cytogeneticist, and one psychiatrist. The psychiatrist worked on the service, seeing patients along with the gynecological staff, assessing patients' emotional needs at the time of admission. Both oncological and benign disease problems were addressed with particular emphasis on the problems of gynecological cancer. The emotional needs of the staff were also recognized, particularly the stresses of dealing with death and dying, the difficult patient, and problems of compliance. The need for pre-operative and post-operative emotional management was recognized as a gynecologic issue in surgical situations such as exploratory laparotomy, tubal ligation, mastectomy, hysterectomy, ileostomy, vulvectomy, vaginoplasty, and pelvic exenteration. Sexual dysfunction as a result of surgical or medical intervention required special attention. Management of pain and analgesic therapy and problems of disease and its effect on family members were also a part of the overall care. Clinical problems which include psychologic factors such as trophoblastic gestational disease, hyperemesis gravidarum, anorexia/bulimia, infertility, artificial insemination, sterilization decisions, abortion and contraception, and toxic psychosis were also seen as gynecologic management problems and not left to the psychiatrist alone. No formal consultation was required for a visit from the psychiatrist, since she was part of the team and, thus, there was no stigma attached to the consultation. The information, both gynecologic and psychologic, is thus intermingled, resulting in an immediate and total approach to the patient.

It was easier to convince senior staff of the relevance of psychiatric factors than it was house-staff. Although the duties of all of the full-time physicians included teaching, the psychiatrist's role was initially not fully considered seriously until house-staff seminars were scheduled after the operating schedule was completed for the day, and Chinese food was brought in for dinner. "I don't want to be bothered, I just want to cut," was the typical attitude of the neophyte resident. By the time the residents had arrived at the senior level, most of them had a different perspective as they anticipated their forthcoming responsibilities in practice. They also had an association of psychiatric learning with a feeding experience, linking mental and physical nurturance.

Teaching students and residents around the clock, on the wards, in lectures and seminars, in collaboration with the obstetrics/gynecology department also integrates the information for the trainee. For example, the concept of hysterectomy includes not only the pathology and treatment, but automatically includes the emotional aspects of loss of reproductive capacity and the meaning of such loss for the woman. Being available to house-staff and nursing staff to mediate conflicts, to counsel, or to refer for therapy should such need occur also facilitates a more smoothly functioning service. The availability of emotional support for house-staff also demonstrates to the young physician the value of paying attention to human needs and reinforces the importance of empathy.

Of course, I did not arrive at consultation/liaison (C/L) without a great deal of influence from the experience and writing of others. Those who stand out include Franz Alexander, Flanders Dunbar, George Engel, Thomas Hackett, F. Patrick McKegney, James Strain, and Robert Pasnau. A.J. Lipowski affected me most in devising a full-time commitment, having read his classic papers and meeting him from time to time to discuss practical issues involved in such an endeavor. Malkah Notman and Carol Nadelson are Boston colleagues and neighbors, who share interests in the care of women and are collaborative and supportive. Miriam Rosenthal, whose work situation is similar to mine, is a close colleague and collaborator in many research and teaching projects. At a time when there were few psychiatric consultants in obstetrics/gynecology, we found comfort in one another, if only to share "war stories" and methods of survival.

The Asian philosophy of the dynamic harmony between opposites, the Yin and the Yang (male and female principles), has logically set a background for my career as a liaison psychiatrist. There is much personal gratification in walking the marginal line between psychiatry and obstetrics/gynecology which allows utilizing training in both medicine and psychiatry and exercising training and knowledge in the bridge between mind and body.

Bibliography

Alexander F: Psychosomatic Medicine: Its Principles and Applications. New York, Norton & Co., 1956.

Engel G: Is psychiatry failing in its responsibilities to medicine? Am J Psychiatry 128:1561, 1972.

Hackett TP: The psychiatrist: In the mainstream or on the banks of medicine? Am J Psychiatry 134:432, 1977.

Lipowski ZJ: Consultation-liaison psychiatry: An overview. Am J Psychiatry 131:623, 1974.

Lipowski ZJ: Psychiatric consultation: Concepts and controversies. Am J Psychiatry 134:523, 1977.

Lipowski ZJ: Psychosomatic medicine in the Seventies: An overview. Am J Psychiatry 134:233, 1977.

McKegney FP, Weiner S: A consultation-liaison psychiatry clinical clerkship. Psychosom Med

38:45, 1976.

Pasnau RO: Psychiatry and obstetrics-gynecology: Report of a five-year experience in psychiatry liaison. In Seminars in Psychiatry. Edited by RO Pasnau. New York, Grune and Stratton, 1975, pp. 135-147.

Small EC, Mitchell GW: Practical aspects of full-time liaison psychiatry in gynecology. J Reprod Med 22:151-155, 1979.

Strain JJ, Grossman S: Psychological Care of the Mentally Ill: A Primer in Liaison Psychiatry. Englewood Cliffs, NJ, Appleton-Century-Crofts, 1975.

22

Feminine Leadership in Community Mental Health

Raquel E. Cohen, M.D., M.P.H.

*Professor,
Department of Psychiatry,
University of Miami Medical School; and
Director, Program Development,
World Health Organization Center,
Miami, Florida*

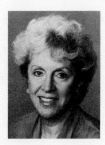

Raquel E. Cohen, M.D., M.P.H.

22

Feminine Leadership in Community Mental Health

Hispanic women's leadership in mental health during the last twenty years is best understood in comparison to the changing career paths and the leadership opportunities of all working women in the United States. The following chapter will analyze these leadership opportunities within the following contexts: 1) role issues, 2) experiences within the historical framework of the 1960's, 3) barriers to leadership, 4) opportunities for leadership, and 5) a personal case history.

Role Issues

The sociological definition of "role" is the way in which a woman behaves according to the rule governing her performance, and this rule varies widely according to the cultural, internalized guidelines assigned to her feminine functioning. This academic definition needs to be complemented by the very specific characteristics of Hispanic cultural and subcultural groupings within the United States. Women who are natives of Hispanic countries and who have become acculturated to the United States have very different role characteristics than women whose parents emigrated to the United States and who were themselves born in the United States. Also, the many nationalities that have Hispanic roots, the Cubans, Mexicans, Latin Americans, and Spaniards, transfer a rich cultural heritage and weave it into the experiences that they have had in this country. Although no single pattern of a feminine Hispanic role characteristic emerges, some important traits appear with some consistency in Hispanic women. These traits, some strong and some with lesser influence, include passivity, acceptance of masculine superiority, strong values for the maternal role, and primary care of children and households. In addition, sincere religious beliefs and ethical ideas of morality are essential to the rearing of young women within Hispanic households.

How do these basic ego ideals relate to leadership? A review of the various definitions of "leader" indicates the concepts of director, head, supremacy, mastership. These concepts contradict many of the feminine characteristics embedded in the Hispanic tradition.

Leadership is associated with words like superiority, initiative, domination, directing, influencing, governing, and dominating. These are not words that describe the traits that Hispanic parents promote in their daughters. Leadership roles and behavior are not programmed for the Hispanic woman. By contrast, her psychic personality and emotional responses are modulated early in her development by the subtle cues of approval within her environment where she interacts in an intimate and emotional manner. Each parent conveys approval, encouragement, and support or critical/shaping responses when she manifests some dominant or leadership behavior. The young Hispanic woman begins to rely strongly on these shaping signals and, although incorporating them into her repertoire of infantile social guidelines, she needs them even in adulthood to set her course.

It is important to hypothesize that there are other existing conditions that must be recognized in order to identify Hispanic women as some of the professional leaders who have recently emerged in the United States. Some findings in psychological research suggest that personal, individualistic characteristics of parents/mentors in interactions with historical, social, and political events can influence an individual's latent psycho-emotional characteristics and lead to leadership. Once these personality characteristics emerge in the Hispanic woman, leadership can result in self-satisfaction and increased self-esteem. This initial awareness of success and ability allows Hispanic women to review the barriers imposed by the formative Hispanic roles and consider the alternative Anglo environment, where support for feminine leadership is stronger and more consistent than within the Hispanic family. If circumstances are appropriate, young women move up professional career ladders and arrive at levels of latent or actual leadership. An interesting hypothesis might be proposed to answer the issue of whether women develop leadership positions if they are educated in all women's schools, or in co-educational institutions. A large percentage of Hispanic women attend private female schools which serve as basic supportive environments for the development of leadership qualities. The potential for competitive abilities to emerge in multicultural and co-educational institutions should be recognized.

Changes in the 1960's

Many historical and political programs that emerged in the 1960's supported potential leadership for women and minorities including Hispanic women. In communities, women emerged as identified leaders with powerful skills and abilities. This climate also supported their entry into academic careers and the pursuit of intellectual skills and professional gains. As the Hispanic woman emerged in leadership positions, her own inner identity potential was reinforced.

Barriers to Leadership

Her inner conflicts between traditional values and unique opportunities appearing in her social world for independence, assertiveness, and competition became a source of difficulty for the Hispanic

woman. Surrounded by strong messages from American culture about "feminine self-actualization," the Hispanic woman feels pressured to find her way of life in terms of what is important to her individually and her self-realization. She has to battle the same fears and conflicts as her Anglo peers, conflicts between the domestic ideals of motherhood and home versus the sense of realizing her human potential as a female. Issues of language, familiarity of interactions with men, and comfort with power and influence appear in many career paths. When a Hispanic woman takes command, participates with the group that controls the rules, and/or influences men, she appears to become hesitant and ambivalent before she finally can process the difficulties stemming from her own heritage.

Opportunities for Leadership

In the mental health field, the Hispanic professional has increased opportunities for leadership in areas with a large Hispanic population. Many of the skills and characteristics of the Hispanic female are sources of ability and competence in the mental health field. Supporting, responding empathetically and sympathetically, and using patience and sensitivity in order to cope with emotional problems of patients are natural qualities of many Hispanic women. To these basic qualities, she can add responsibility and can accept opportunities that offered the possibility of proving her competence and latent potential for leadership. These emerging qualities in the Hispanic woman have been accepted in a variable way by Hispanic and Anglo males. Examples range from programs that had difficulty in accepting a Hispanic female as director to others where her leadership was appreciated and served to unite various factions from different levels of the mental health field. Mental health center programs that were based on community support and that expressed the values of the community represented a historical opportunity for women to emerge and to develop skills that might not have been possible within other bureaucratic systems. As these programs have diminished in the 1980's, the Hispanic women who originally had an opportunity to acquire leadership skills are now beginning to transfer their expertise into the many financial systems that are delivering mental health services within the private sector.

Other programs in emerging mental health programs that helped to promote leadership in the Hispanic woman were the Head Start programs, deinstitutionalization and community-based programs for chronic mental patients, and the geriatric subspecialty. Where we still see few Hispanics is in the academic leadership ranks and as heads of research clinical teams.

Case History

As a Hispanic, senior psychiatrist in the United States, I can offer my career path as a case history. As in all case histories, the individual factors can be considered as a probability of a sample only until more confirmatory data are accumulated. My career path exemplifies some of the opportunities, challenges, and barriers that minority, foreign women have encountered during the last thirty years in psychiatry. European women in this field have excelled. Hispanic women, on the other hand, are rarely found in any top-level academic or administrative posts.

I want to highlight the concept that the small, kaleidoscopic fragments of my personal, psychological, and parental heritage, as well as cultural guidelines for behavior and chance opportunities all combined to interact with the historical events in my professional pathway.

As I write this retrospective sequence of my professional activities, there is a symbolic recognition that I am currently working in Miami, Florida. This was the destination of the first plane ride that I took from Lima, Peru, in my quest to further my education in the United States, where I came to obtain a graduate degree in public health. My goal was based on strong, life-long experiences with the children in my community who were doomed to malnourished growth and defective development because of poverty. After acquiring skills in nutritional, maternal, and child programs, I hoped to return to my country and join professionals who were active in trying to solve these problems. I was advised to apply to one of the graduate schools in Boston, Massachusetts. Aided by a group of professional women, I was admitted to the Harvard School of Public Health.

This year of study at Harvard was interwoven with the events affecting academia during the terminal era of World War II. Two independent issues influenced my plan of returning to my country with a masters degree in public health. My teachers advised me that I needed more education, including an M.D. degree, if I wanted to exert any leadership in my country. Coincidentally, the admissions committee of Harvard Medical School was getting ready to break the tradition of "only men need apply." With the support of mentors and teachers, and the reluctant acceptance of my parents, I completed all my documentation, lived through the interviews, and was one of the women accepted to the first class which included women medical students.

As I reflect on the years of learning and training to become a doctor, I can select the following group of experiences that may be considered kernels for early formation of leadership: 1) the available *role models* of male medical leaders, 2) the environment of intellectual stimulation and vision toward the frontiers of modern medicine, and 3) the internalized identity of being part of an institution that was recognized as a leader in world medicine.

Years later, as I became part of other faculty in various departments of psychiatry, and self-awareness allowed me to examine the interfaces between institutional patterns and individuals, I became aware of the troublesome interactions between institutional racism, minority discrimination, and feministic strivings. My awareness developed against the backdrop of national ideologic forces, governmental policies, and ethical commitments of medical schools striving to offer balance between candidates with excellent academic records versus unskilled students with good potential needing further educational training. In the setting of these debates, women physicians emerged as natural candidates to take the banner for their "sisters." Senior faculty members were recruited to be both "sole" members on all types of committees and to constitute a minority of women's power groups.

This setting of historical events began to shape both my skills and my sense of leadership identity in the United States. Beyond the walls of Harvard, other events began to identify me as a Hispanic professional. Programs like the War on Poverty, Head Start, and community mental health programs heralded an increasing sensitivity to psychosocial factors in health and illness. As these programs began to extend themselves into the community, professionals came face to face with the special needs of pluralistic populations. Joining my public health prevention philosophy and my interest in Hispanics, minority issues, and discriminatory practices toward women, the opportunity to participate in this historical phase of American history became accessible to me because of my specialty and psychosocial expertise, my identity as a physician, my ethnic and cultural upbringing as a Peruvian, and my legitimization as a "minority professional." These opportunities allowed me to break from the traditional patterns that governed so many of my young adult years in spite of the travels across the American continent, in spite of receiving an excellent medical education and in spite of my developing role as a wife and mother of three children. It was in the exercise of participating events and episodes where the opportunities begged for leadership, where mistakes could be made and not noticed by admired male colleagues, where small increments of satisfaction were accumulated as problems were solved, as programs emerged, and as opportunities for Hispanics and minorities increased.

Today, I can reflect on these events that constituted the early efforts of what today are well-established, almost institutionalized Hispanic programs in the field of mental health. I have to acknowledge that chance events allowed me to learn my first lessons in leadership. Leadership behavior, once established, can be applied in different settings. My medical expertise with a specialty in psychiatry continued to evolve as I developed the first community mental health program in the northeast section of Boston. Again, these efforts were exercised against the national patterns of service delivery developed by legislation supporting new patterns of care in the Kennedy era.

After five years of daily practice in the community, I returned to academia as a staff person with the Laboratory of Community Psychiatry at Harvard Medical School. As Associate Director of the Laboratory, I participated with Dr. Gerald Caplan in his pioneer efforts and teachings. He represented the many men who offered role model behavior, methods of thinking, and approaches to solutions that I have emulated during my professional growth. The argument for male and female role models is presented, because the lack of women leaders as a reason for a lack of female role models and as an explanation for the meager number of women leaders is insufficient. I believe that, although a woman model is helpful for

women to develop leadership, this does not explain satisfactorily the lack of women in the top levels of our profession. Other barriers besides lack of female mentors exist and reinforce in a circular manner the difficulties of rising to the top. Skill and knowledge have to be ingredients of accumulated experiences. Parallel local and national opportunities to participate as a leader of programs, committees, and workshops within my specialty exist. For example, I developed a special interest in assisting victims of natural disasters both in this country and in Latin America. These efforts led to establishing relations with the Pan American Health Organization and writing a practical book on procedures for treating victims of post traumatic reactions. This method of participating, observing, organizing the material into patterns, and trying to extract some simple principles useful in the practice of psychiatry has characterized all my publications. In addition, this interest in conceptualizing phenomenology was fueled both by innate interest and by the practical ethos of academia to publish for the progression upward into professorship rank. The development of a specialized academic area of expertise assisted me in progressive fashion to develop leadership in assistance programs for disaster victims. These specialized areas of knowledge paralleled other academic activities generic to the training and clinical mental health areas of my job.

Having concluded a successful training program of a large number of leaders in community mental health, the Laboratory of Community Mental Health at Harvard came to closure, and subsequently the staff members engaged in other activities. I was asked to participate in the design of an emerging program for child abuse which was part of the historic national effort to address this severe problem. This center, located in Boston, was to serve as a support program for all the New England states in training and service of their state and public programs. This opportunity gave me the perspective of examining interstate public services with the accompanying multiprofessional groups that come together to control, attend, and legally punish the perpetrators of abused children and to examine the contributions of the mental health profession regarding these issues. This job required public speaking, management skills, conceptualization of program design, and the ability to condense many systems related to the specific problems that emerge from the field of child abuse. This increased administrative ability and experience led to my candidacy and ultimate selection as superintendent of a large mental health center in Boston. Again, the interlocking of historic opportunities and increased development of abilities and skills exemplified the potential for a Hispanic woman to emerge as a leader.

Following four years of these activities, the desire for further research and academic opportunities was explored and a year's leave of absence was requested and granted by the academic institution where I held a professorship. Another historical event coincided with these plans and I was asked to participate with the Office of Refugee Resettlement in working with the refugees coming from Cuba in what has become known as the "Mariel boatlift." This led to a year's activities in the refugee camps involved with acculturation and adaptation of Cuban adolescents who had come to the United States of America without parents.

This experience led to increased knowledge within the field of crisis and stress responses.

Then in the city of Miami I had the an opportunity to become director of training in child psychiatry and clinical director of the ambulatory care system for children and adolescents. This was another example of good timing of historical events and of a leadership opportunity because this job required basic knowledge about Hispanic culture, language, and mental health in addition to leadership skills.

It becomes evident that the total configuration of personality factors, knowledge, expertise, and opportunity arising through political and/or historical events needs to be combined in order to analyze feminine leadership.

An interesting question to explore is whether these environmental factors have greater influence in the opportunities for leadership for women than for men. Women appear to react with complex sensitivity to outside events and may be potentially ready, if the right configuration of forces come together, to support qualities of management, assertiveness and strong belief in the pursuit of meaningful behavior.

23

The Woman Psychiatrist
in Public Administration

Mildred Mitchell-Bateman, M.D.

Professor of Psychiatry,
Marshall University School of Medicine,
Huntington, West Virginia

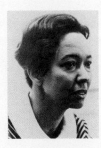

Mildred Mitchell-Bateman, M.D.

23

The Woman Psychiatrist
in Public Administration

In recent years more women have been appointed as the "top" administrative officers of governmental service units. The areas of responsibility have included public utility commissions and agencies dealing with welfare, the environment, employment security and health. Women have been elected as mayors, county commissioners, state treasurers, secretaries of state and governors. This increasing visibility of women as leaders in government parallels a similar increase in business and some levels of education. In this paper, I will present some observations and ideas on women in public administration based on my experience as a state mental hospital superintendent and director of a state department of mental health covering a span of nearly 20 years.

This period of service began at a point in time when public mental hospitals were bursting at the seams in all states. Nationally, forces were being mobilized towards the "Bold New Approach" which was forerunner to the era of the community mental health program development. The role of the director/commissioner of state mental health departments had to become that of a juggler to maintain and improve support for patients in hospitals, while trying to obtain new funding and resources for the rapidly increasing need for services in the community. Add the task of challenging traditions of care delivery, of changing philosophies about where the primary locus of treatment should be, patronage systems of employing staffs with civil service systems, of revising commitment laws that are unconstitu-

tional and then appoint a woman psychiatrist as director for a real interesting time!

Several questions might be asked at this point. Can the outcome of a particular program be directly influenced either positively or negatively by the gender of the administrator? Has the socialization of women as physicians and/or as psychiatrists inhibited their interests in or selection for administration? I do not attempt to address these questions here. As noted by Talbott and Bachrach, there is a real gap in the representation of psychiatry in administration and in public mental health programs. They encourage a continued effort to look at issues that might enhance tapping the potentials of women psychiatrists to fill this gap.

It is quite possible that one of the major deterrents to actively seeking careers in psychiatric administration by men and women is the perception that one must be able to absorb huge quantities of abuse. This is in many respects quite true, but with understanding of the nature of public mental systems and their intricate interrelationships, the administrator can be creative and successful in seeing some goals achieved and progress made towards others. While programmatic outcome should be a significant measure of the effectiveness of leadership, the judgment of success or failure is in the "eye of the beholder." In other words, the definition of "outcome" may vary extensively. Thus, such a direct one-to-one relationship between the nature of the leadership and the outcome is often not the sole measure by which an administrator is judged as a "good one," or a "poor one," as effective or ineffective.

In the public arena there are many constituencies of any given program and each one has its own agenda. Each one forms some opinion about the management of the agency, as well as the quality of the outcome as compared with that constituency's expectation. Some of the constituencies are as follows:

1. The appointing authority--a mayor, a governor, or a board of directors.
2. The legislative arm is prominent in the case of state level positions, but comparable relationships may exist with county commissioners.
3. The recipients of services, their collaterals and their advocates form the largest constituency. Yet the needs of this consumer constituency often become compromised as the administrator attempts to balance service demands with available resources and/or the demands of other constituencies.
4. There is a constituency which is composed of the peer professional community. Many professionals in the private sector or in other agencies have a sense of responsibility and concern for their colleagues in the public agency and for its program delivery. Members of this group can be advocates or adversaries.
5. Finally, there are the constituencies that are internal to the organization, especially the professional and supportive staff of the agency. The well-being of this group can directly impact on the effectiveness of programs. However there are times when the aspirations and needs of members of this constituency may seriously impede service delivery.

This description of constituencies is applicable for any leader of either sex. The list is not complete or refined into the numerous subgroupings that are responsible. For example, as a state mental health director, I found it important to develop communication networks with county clerks, sheriffs, juvenile and intermediate court judges, prosecuting attorneys and county commissioners throughout the state. This was accomplished through meeting with their respective state organizations and finding key persons in each group for ongoing involvement in our planning. Without the resultant mutual understanding of each group's needs, and the support system that

formed, we would have had a much longer siege in getting legislative changes in commitment laws and in the redirection of certain tax revenues towards local mental health services.

It would be interesting and useful if the interactions with constituencies could be examined on the basis of the gender of the administrator. It would be important to try to assess to what extent preconceived expectations of the woman administrator enter these relationships. She needs to be aware of the likely existence of these stereotyped expectations. Awareness, however, can become a stumbling block if one overreacts. I did just that on one occasion when we were having a particularly difficult time with budget appropriation.

One of the senate finance committee members had targeted me for personal attack. I had refused to intervene on behalf of an employee who was seeking an inappropriate merit raise. While speaking with the senate president prior to my budget hearing, he indicated I might expect challenges from the other senator. Then he said, "You're too much of a lady. Bang the desk!" Finance presentation time came. It flowed without interruption and the floor was opened for questions. As predicted, the disgruntled senator immediately took the floor. However, rather than challenging the budget or even the program, he began personal attacks that were so inappropriate that not a single reporter took notes. When it became apparent that the chairman was not going to curtail this harangue, I decided this was a good desk banging time. I interrupted the senator in loud but not shrill tones and stated that I would not use this budget hearing time for replying to personal accusations, none of which were true, incidentally. For that he could see me later. This time was needed for consideration of the mental health budget and any discussion the committee members wished to have about the programs for which support was being requested. There was a seemingly long silence and then another senator said, "The doctor has a point. These are not matters for this committee, but she is highly educated and we are plain folk, most of us. She didn't have to cut down our colleague with such big words." Curiously some of the observers laughed because they thought this senator was being purposely facetious. He wasn't. He was serious and the committee members were still uneasy. Nevertheless, the laughter broke the tension. Somebody posed a pertinent question and we were back on track.

Inside, I didn't feel very good about my table banging effort, although my staff was delighted. I knew that the real issue in the first senator's attack was my rejection of his untenable request, translated into a personal rebuff by a woman. The issue with the second senator was not "big words," but a woman "putting down a man," worse yet in the presence of his colleagues.

I believe "awareness" of the preconceived notions about women enable the woman administrator to be less surprised and not thrown into a defensive or counter-offensive mode of reaction which may lead to predictable "female" behavior. Sometimes the expected behavior is so firm in a person's mind that it is attributed to the woman anyway. That same senate president mentioned earlier was a panelist at a seminar for mental health volunteers on how to effectively work for passage of legislation. At the end of his presentation, the senator said, "Anytime your director of mental health is up there, I get ready to vote the way you want. I just hate to see her cry." There was laughter again, but fortunately not much because most of the people in that audience belonged to a constituency with which we had diligently worked and they knew differently. But the senator had very neatly discounted the quality of my presentations and follow-through with the legislature.

I have spoken and written about this next item before, but I feel it should be mentioned again in the context of this chapter. Women administrators who are psychiatrists have a triple threat in working with many of the constituent groups listed earlier. In some public policy circles, there is the attitude that physicians generally make poor administrators. This belief is especially prevalent in legislative and executive branches of government, but not infrequently physicians treat their administrator-colleagues as second class members of the profession. In the constituency of professionals, medical and non-medical, many hold this view that psychiatrists make poor administrators. The net result of these feelings, plus a persistent shortage of psychiatrists willing to enter public administration is that most directors and commissioners of state mental health programs are now non-physicians. A similar trend is present in community mental health centers and public mental hospitals. As a result, in many programs the physician leader is the clinical director or chief medical officer. Hopefully, the administrator/

physician team is compatible in terms of trust, respect and mutuality of goals. When this is not the case, and double or even contradictory messages go out into the system, the entire service delivery is compromised and valuable support from constituencies can be lost. If one of the members of this team is a woman psychiatrist, we are in the triple threat situation. There is an even greater risk because of the propensity to rationalize many conflicts on a sexual basis. When this happens we may lose sight of the fact that such partnerships can and do fail when no gender differences are involved.

Ideological differences may be the real problem, sex notwithstanding. The woman administrator who fails to keep in focus all the possible ramifications of management conflict may succumb to the feeling that her difficulties are related to her being female. This will prohibit, or delay getting at other factors, e.g. communication styles. It could be that she is having to espouse fiscally or even administratively sound policy that is unpopular or poorly understood. On the other side of the coin, one or more of our constituencies may hesitate to accept the particular changes in any circumstances but may confuse this with uneasiness with the soundness of program decisions coming from a woman.

A legislator who was especially supportive of mental health came to see me about six months after my appointment as head of mental health. "Well," he said, "the boys out there say you do pretty good, but they have one complaint. You're more interested in getting docs and nurses than fixing-up the barns." This one remark captures the essence of the subtle philosophical differences that lay the seeds for splitting clinical and program matters from business and fiscal matters at state and local levels in the mental health system. As I worked with this development and as I have observed its evolution, it seems clear that in today's climate the triple threat still remains in many organizations for the woman who is a physician with a specialty in psychiatry. In addition this triple threat has taken on a new dimension in light of broadening roles for all mental health professionals. Hopefully, a sufficient amount of maturity has developed in all the constituencies to support the premise that the most important consideration in selecting the administrator or the administrative team are--given the mandate, mission and goals of the particular agency; given the current stage of development, short-range objectives as well as long range--who has not only the appropriate knowledge base, but the vision and the creativity to integrate the resources to maximize the outcome in services. This approach would mean eliminating the closed shop, short-term approach policy which may recruit a woman so long as she is not a psychiatrist.

In the opening paragraph, it was indicated that there are increasing numbers of women in public administrative positions. However, this is not as true in state level mental health programs. The movement of women psychiatrists from primarily clinical management positions to broader administrative responsibilities in the organizational structure seems to be moving at a slower rate. I feel it is contingent upon those who are concerned about the quality of mental health programs to address the deficiency in psychiatric services. Further, efforts to improve the representation of psychiatry in the policymaking and administrative structure of public mental health systems are under way, but they need more intensive support and greater visibility. Vigilance against a closed shop approach

is imperative. Women psychiatrists do represent an untapped resource for infusing public mental health administration with the added insights of the clinician/psychiatrist to policy formulation, resolution of organizational conflict and creative use of all resources for the desired outcomes in providing services.

Finally, the public mental health arena still encompasses a vast grouping of unserved and underserved persons with seriously handicapping mental disorders. The psychiatrist has a unique opportunity to see his/her input ameliorate the illness of single individuals or of hundreds of individuals, but to accomplish this the psychiatrist must be there.

The enormity of the task of encouraging psychiatrists, especially women psychiatrists, to enter public mental health administration calls to mind the words of John F. Kennedy: "All this will not be finished in the first one hundred days. Nor will it be finished in the first one thousand days, nor in the life of this Administration, nor even perhaps in our lifetime on this planet. But let us begin."

24

Women Psychiatrists
and Public Administrators

Mary Jane England, M.D.

Assistant Dean and Director,
Mid-Career Masters in Public Administration Program,
John F. Kennedy School of Government,
Harvard University,
Cambridge, Massachusetts

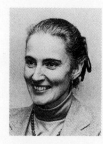

Mary Jane England, M.D.

24

Women Psychiatrists
and Public Administrators

I grew up in Brighton, Massachusetts, a working-class neighborhood in Boston, and attended medical school at Boston University. In 1962, at the end of my sophomore year, I married and we moved to Brookline, a Boston suburb. I spent 1966 in San Francisco at Mt. Zion Hospital where my husband took a residency in internal medicine and I trained in adult psychiatry. Then we returned to Brighton to live in my family home while we completed our respective residencies in cardiology and child psychiatry.

It's been an important part of my life that I live in a working-class neighborhood and that, as an adult, I am living in the same neighborhood I grew up in. My neighbors and my community are very supportive and proud of me as a woman professional and of my family. No one has ever said to my kids, "Your mom should be home instead of out working."

I was educated by the Sisters of St. Joseph for sixteen years, finishing at Regis College, and my children were educated at least in part by them, too. I knew many of the women who taught my children, because we had gone to school together or they had been my teachers.

The theme of my life and my career as a doctor, a psychiatrist, and a public administrator has been empowerment, helping others to get power over their lives. The sixties and seventies were periods of social change around the issues of civil rights, women's rights, the rights of the poor and the disadvantaged, or, as the sixties' chant put it, "Power to the People." I have spent much of my career responding to these issues, especially in community health services, mental health, and desegregation.

Again, it was my family, my school, and my community which empowered me and gave me the confidence and the trust to do the job. It was their support which allowed me to develop the commitment to what Catholics call "service" and the Puritans describe as a "calling." You might say I took my own background, being a Catholic and growing up in a working-class neighborhood, and used it to shape a career of service. I thought about becoming a doctor fairly early in my life, I guess when I was in high school, maybe even earlier. My mother was a nurse, a health professional, and eventually an administrator, and there is no question that she was an important role model for me. She was ahead of her time in feeling that women should be accomplished. She was definitely not the traditional housebound housewife.

Mother had an important job running the respiratory unit at Massachusetts General Hospital, and friends of mine who were in training there often came to her for advice and support. She was a role model for many other women besides me. She was personally strong, and she also had strength for others. I think my friends liked her because her advice was sound and she wasn't rigid.

Early in her professional life, Mother was interested in becoming an obstetrical nurse and at one point thought of going to Appalachia. Instead, she went to the Florence Crittenden Home for unwed mothers in Brighton. In the thirties older women as well as younger ones came there, because it was a place to hide. My mother talked a great deal about the horrors of childbirth. She thought the doctors overmedicated women, and she believed that with more education, women could help deliver their own babies. She eventually ran the Crittenden Home, moving, as I would myself, from practitioner to administrator.

My parents married in 1937; my mother was 30, my father 40. Father didn't feel he could marry until his brothers and sisters were able to support themselves without him. Many people were dependent on him during the Depression and that's why he became a policeman. He viewed his job as a public service and a helping profession.

My father always felt that I could do whatever I wanted to do, that there was no limit to my ability and he was unambivalent in his encouragement. A supportive, encouraging father is extremely important in a woman's success. A study done at Simmons College of 250 women[1] shows that the clear, unambivalent support of their fathers is a common element in the backgrounds of successful women managers. Obviously it helps in becoming a confident woman that you don't get a mixed message from the important man in your life when you're growing up.

After my parents, the Sisters of St. Joseph were the second greatest influence on my life. They are a teaching community whose mission is to educate young people. They are also a very progressive order. The Sisters were themselves women who came from working-class Irish or Italian families whose religious community supported them in the development of professional careers.

People often ask me if the Sisters taught me to sew. The Sisters of St. Joseph were real feminists. They didn't teach needlepoint. They emphasized the classic liberal arts education: literature, Latin, mathematics, and science. But they also recognized a need for elocution, dramatics, and debating and that kind of training has been very useful to me in my career. The Sisters of St. Joseph believe that women have a real responsibility to produce, not just reproductively, but intellectually. Professionally they gave me a clear message.

One of the reasons I went to medical school was to help women and children. At first I wanted to be an obstetrician because women were discrimi-

nated against by male physicians. It particularly bothered me that women had no control over childbearing and that the men took women's bodies away from them.

In the sixties, with the new emphasis on women's civil rights, it became an issue that women should be able to participate more in their own pregnancy and delivery. Our Bodies, Ourselves,[2] with its emphasis on women controlling their bodies and their destinies, came out in the early seventies. Until fairly recently, no men, not even doctors, were allowed in the delivery room when their wives delivered. The Lamaze method and natural childbirth date from the late fifties. When I was in medical school and pregnant with my first child, I had to go to Harvard to find a doctor, Clement Yahia, who was familiar with the Lamaze method.

While the issue of childbearing and women's control over that process continued to be an important concern to me, when I began to spend more time on hospital wards as a medical student, I realized that the issues women were grappling with had more complex societal and psychological origins. I saw so many depressed women, women overwhelmed by poverty and by being single parents. They would come in to say "I'm pregnant," and then they would talk about their hopelessness.

They had terrible anxiety, many were phobic and never left home. They would keep one child home in order not to be alone and to have an excuse to stay home themselves. When I was at the Brighton Neighborhood Health Center, my treatment plan would be to get these women to come to my office, and then I would gradually increase their independence. I was especially concerned about adolescent girls. Adolescence is a time of painful vulnerability for all women, but especially for lower income women. They may be physically mature, but they are unprepared for life. The data show that if they become pregnant in their teenage years, they are likely never to complete their high school education and then they have no option but to get on welfare.

In fact, until 1971, pregnant public school students were not allowed to remain in the classroom. I testified in the first federal case that secured a pregnant woman's right to stay in class, Ordway V. Hargraves. We went to court to put to rest the myths that 1) pregnant women might be jostled in class and suffer undue stress and strain, and 2) that they were contagious, i.e., if one girl in the class became pregnant, the others were bound to follow suit. I entered the case as an expert witness and testified as a psychiatrist that it was not harmful either physically or emotionally for a pregnant woman to be in a classroom.

My interest in psychiatry was stimulated in medical school by an awareness of women's problems, how their feelings were being devalued, how their view of their own powerlessness held them back. The choice of psychiatry was reinforced by some of the women who became my role models in medical school.

There aren't many women role models in medical school to begin with. Women do not attain positions of importance in academic medicine partly because we don't publish much, as a Harvard Dean once remarked to me. "And," he added, "you don't publish because you have so little uninterrupted time to yourselves." That may partly be because our style of managing, being available, being accessible, doesn't leave us much time, an issue I'll discuss later.

A quick look at the history of women in medicine may clarify why there are so few role models. Women doctors in America have had a curious history. It begins in the mid-1800's, with the founding of the Woman's Medical College of Pennsylvania, the first regular medical school for women in the world. Women began entering the medical profession in increasing numbers in the second half of the nineteenth century, and then after the turn of the century, for the next sixty years, there was a dramatic reduction in the number of female admissions. The numbers increased during World War I, when the number of male admissions dropped and women doctors took over in hospitals and acquired new status. Then the men came home and women were edged out. They weren't needed. During World War II, women acquired military status, but after the war, both the prestige of women M.D.'s and the number of women in medical school again diminished, the latter dropping to around 5 percent. Harvard did not take its first woman student until 1948, because, as many women doctors will recall, one of the Harvard Medical School Faculty insisted that women had smaller brains than men. The same thing is often said of Blacks.

In the sixties, only 8 percent of medical students were women, and both numbers and percentages did not really increase until the early seventies. Today the percentage of female medical students is closer to 30 percent.

Particularly because there are so few women in medicine, women who distinguished themselves in psychiatry when I was in medical school stood out. For a variety of reasons, women were able to move ahead in child psychiatry. And I was lucky enough to meet some of the more outstanding ones in Boston. When I was in medical school at Boston University, the women students would gather together in the Gregory Room, named for the Gregory who founded the first women's medical college in Boston. At the turn of the century, it went co-ed and became the Boston University School of Medicine. Down the hall from that room was the office of Eleanor Pavenstedt, a renowned child psychiatrist.

Dr. Pavenstedt was a very handsome woman, admired and respected by the faculty at the medical school for her work with poor people and children. One of the highlights of our social life were the women-only dinner parties at Dr. Pavenstedt's home in Cambridge.

Dr. Eveoleen Rexford was another important role model and influence. Dr. Rexford was Professor and Director of Child Psychiatry at the Boston University Medical School. I had specifically come back from California to work with Dr. Rexford in child and adolescent psychiatry.

She was by any standards an extraordinary woman, interested in and good at administration, as well as an excellent psychiatrist. She cared a great deal about minority issues and poverty and I had a unique and very practical child training experience with her. My training was not only in the traditional, intensive one-on-one psychotherapeutic model. I also worked in settlement houses, organized mothers in housing projects, and saw patients at the Roxbury Court Clinic.

I learned a great deal about the judicial system in my psychiatric residency, particularly how it affected the lives of disadvantaged people. That's a concept which the middle class often has trouble understanding, since we have little immediate experience with it. Nobody knocks on our doors and looks under our beds. The judicial system is not a big part of our daily lives. Among the poor, however, the district court is part of the family. In Roxbury we were often seen as helpers.

I greatly admired Dr. Rexford for her outspoken support of community mental health and her clear statement of women's competency. She was personally very supportive to me as a wife and mother, as well as a professional child psychiatrist.

Dr. Suzanne van Amerongen, a child analyst who was one of my supervisors, was another important role model. Dr. van Amerongen was from the Dutch royal family and fought in the Resistance. She was a marvelous clinician, sensitive, caring, able to clarify adolescent issues for both men and women. I learned a great deal from her, as I did from Dr. Beverly Dudek, another woman physician who has continued to be a close personal friend.

It's been asked whether a man can be a role model for a woman. The answer is, emphatically, "Yes." Fortunately for Massachusetts, in 1973, Governor Francis Sargent invited William Goldman, M.D., whom I had met in California in 1966, to become Commissioner for Mental Health and Retardation. Bill became an important role model and influence in my development as a public administrator.

By 1973, I had three children, and was living in Brighton in the home I was born and brought up in. The seventies was the era of community mental health and deinstitutionalization. I was very involved with schools and community agencies, and had put programs in some very diverse places, for example, day care agencies in church basements. I personally started a mental health center clinic in a local convent and developed a neighborhood health center in a low-income housing development. I believe I was able to do these things because I was part of my neighborhood, and that along with my expertise in psychiatry allowed me to develop trusting relationships with local school personnel and community groups.

The issue of the day was neighborhood-based community programs. We were intent on putting services close to or in the neighborhood instead of in large institutions. The idea, indeed the point of deinstitutionalization, was to bring services to the people, instead of putting people in institutions. I had become increasingly concerned that government was not providing sufficient services for children, particularly in the school system, and for children with special needs, so I became involved in writing legislation which ensured education for all handicapped children. The bill, Chapter 766 as it was called, was the forerunner of the national special educational legislation, P.L. 94-142. As the time approached to implement

Chapter 766, I worried that the Massachusetts Department of Mental Health was not sufficiently prepared to implement the bill. I formed a delegation to approach Dr. Goldman and ask him what he was doing to help children. That evening he called me at home and suggested that since I had so much to say about how government ought to be run, especially for kids and adolescents, perhaps I'd like to come and work for him and do it.

It didn't take me very long to decide to go to work for Bill. The year I spent with him became a benchmark in my career. Bill was a psychiatrist who understood the world of psychiatry and an administrator who recognized the resemblances among large institutions like hospitals, medical schools, and state bureaucracies. He was the first person I had met and worked with who combined the qualities of leadership, and the ability to clarify a mission, with the commitment to citizen boards and an understanding of the bureaucratic systems which impact on health care. Bill recognized the need for involving managers and administrators in order to implement change successfully. He realized that you could not just work with clinicians and hope to implement such a major agenda. He had already brought many civil servants in the department around to his way of thinking and, when I came to work for him, he told me to spend time with the administrators, the budget people, the personnel people, and the institutional management people in the agency.

Bill felt it was important to involve community boards as a way of preparing neighborhoods for the location of group homes and other essential services in their community. He traveled tirelessly across the state to communicate the mission and get support. The roadblock to neighborhood health services was usually the reluctance to have certain services on their block. Most people think it's fine in theory to have group homes for the mentally retarded, for adolescents, for recovering alcoholics and addicts next door--as long as it's someone else's next door.

Another lesson I learned from Bill was that budget drives policy. He pointed out that if I wanted to make major shifts in policy I had to understand the budgeting process. That's when he assigned me to Joseph Finnegan. I worked closely with Joe, who was then Assistant Commissioner of Administration. I shared my clinical knowledge with him, he shared his knowledge of budgeting, personnel, and administration, and we both came out stronger.

My experience with Joe and especially with Bill Goldman shows that women can have male role models, that what's important is the sharing of common goals and missions, as well as mutual respect. The issue of sexism and limitations imposed because of your sex cannot be an issue or it will seriously interfere with your ability to learn successfully or to teach others.

Working for Bill and working with public sector employees helped me clarify my management style. There's very little written about the differences between the way men and women manage. One of the few references I've come across is *Management Men and Women: Closed and Open Doors.*[3] The description is not only literal, but symbolic. Women managers are usually more accessible emotionally as well as physically to employees and staff.

I mentioned that at Mental Health, Bill urged me to make the rounds of the Mental Health Department and talk to everyone. At Mental Health I took pride in knowing the senior staff at all the institutions. I met with them personally and I left myself open to questions about union, management, and policy issues. I can call the Department of Mental Health today, and although I haven't been there since 1979, a clerk will say to me, "Oh, Dr. England, how are you?" They knew me and what I was doing!

Later, when I became Commissioner of the Department of Social Services (DSS), which was divided into six regions and then further into forty catchment areas, I made it a point to travel the state and visit local offices whenever possible.

Personal presence is very important in public administration, and particularly in the public sector. It counts especially with young people. They're not paid very much, compared to what they could earn elsewhere, so you must help motivate them, and be willing to work with their youth, their idealism, and their enthusiasm. For them, that is often compensation.

The personal presence of the top administrator not only provides access and strength but clarity about the goal of the agency. At both Mental Health and DSS, I wouldn't necessarily talk a lot myself, but I would open a meeting with a discussion of goals. At Mental Health, the goals were moving clients from institutions to community settings. At DSS they were getting children back

home. That's what I mean by presence reinforcing clarity. Everyone was clear on where I was coming from, because they heard it from me. They couldn't say, "Geez, what did she say?"

An important part of the manager's job is communication, and accessibility is another aspect of that. I always felt comfortable with more information rather than less, and my habit of walking around the agency often led to picking up information. Walking around helps a manager pick up climate as well as information. Otherwise you don't really know what's happening to the little people in the agency.

Micromanagement, i.e., redirection and overdirecting your subordinates, is a possible drawback of accessibility. The other potential dangers of accessibility for the manager are too much time spent responding to others, and information overload, while the danger for subordinates is dependency. I think a good manager can avoid these.

The Department of Mental Health prepared me for the responsibilities I would have as Commissioner of the Department of Social Services. In 1975, when Michael Dukakis became Governor of Massachusetts, Bill went back to California. That same year, Dukakis appointed me Associate Commissioner of the Department of Mental Health. I was the first woman associate commissioner in the state, and it was the biggest job I'd ever held. I was responsible for directing a $400,000,000 budget, 20,000 employees, nine state hospitals, and six state schools. That was where I got my real management training, with my feet to the fire, so to speak. The commissioner who succeeded Bill was more interested in policy and left the management pretty much to me. After that, I wanted to run my own shop and set my own policy.

In 1978, partly due to a series of scandals involving child abuse, the Massachusetts Legislature pressed for legislation to create a new social service agency. Both the legislation, which I helped to write, and the administration of the agency were great challenges. The thrust of the new legislation was to separate Social Services from the Department of Public Welfare (DPW) which had an unprofessional workforce and was protected by the unions. My objective as a psychiatrist and community health professional was to create an agency for children and families that would deliver needed services with dignity while providing every child with a home.

In deciding how to deal with DPW's workforce, we had three choices. We could follow the example of the private sector when it needs new people and a new direction, i.e., Reduction in Force as it is called, or RIF. Simply put, RIF means fire the old guys and gals. Or we could follow the usual pattern of public service agencies in such circumstances, which is to take the workers from the old agency and move them over to the new one. That's referred to as "grandfathering." Or we could take the middle course and find a way to broker the change. We chose the last.

Our goal was to provide a home for every child and to do that we needed a well-trained, sophisticated workforce. We insisted that every supervisor at DSS must have a master's degree in a clinical field, social work, psychology, etc. Many supervisors in the old DPW would not qualify. Essentially, we created a career ladder with the worker salary level just below supervisor's level which matched the old DPW supervisor salary. That allowed the DPW supervisors to come into DSS at the worker salary level just below supervisor's level which matched the old DPW supervisor salary. If they did want to get a master's degree, both educational leave and tuition reimbursement were available. That way, social workers who wanted to go back to school (at the department's expense) could be upgraded. If not, at least they could retain their salary. I thought that was a decent compromise.

We also went from 5 percent minority staff to 20 percent, allowing us to build an agency that more reflected our clients, so people couldn't say that DSS was the same old people doing the same old work, because it wasn't.

We had a tough time fighting a union bill for grandfathering, but we had the personal support of Speaker of the House, Thomas McGee, and Chairman of Ways and Means, John Finnegan, who is currently the State Auditor. The bottom line was that they, too, wanted good programs for the kids. And the deal was that no one lost a job. Many people stayed with the old agency in income maintenance, but at least they had security.

I'm very much opposed to following the private sector's RIF model in government. People who go to work in the public sector know they won't have a large salary. But they do expect security if they do their job and I think government owes them that. They can be retrained for new direc-

tions. Undoubtedly, security can lead to bad habits; when it does, I think that's often the fault of the manager.

In the human services area in particular, salaries are just above the poverty line, particularly for institutional workers. We have a responsibility, if we're shifting the goals of the agency, to retrain the workers and the superintendent as well.

In essence that's my program at Harvard's Kennedy School of Government, i.e., retraining mid-career professionals. We take people who have a minimum of five years in the public sector and put them through a nine-month program which introduces them to new skills. It's a program for practitioners who can choose to learn to do what they're doing better, or how to move into new areas.

It's a critical function of leadership to be able to work with people already there on how to assume new roles. That includes women coming back into the workforce. It also raises the question of women in leadership roles. It's interesting that *In Pursuit of Excellence*[4] decided that a critical attribute of leadership was intuition, a quality which has, in large measure been recognized as special to women, and therefore devalued.

It's also interesting that the fastest growing area for women managers is the public sector. In the public sector, women assume CEO positions earlier and take on more responsibility earlier than they do in private industry.

Also, the public sector is risky, at the senior levels of management, and women are more inclined to take risks. A manager is lucky to last four years in administration. On the average, Commissioners of Mental Health last one and a half years, Commissioners of Social Services, two and a half years. In his second term, Nixon asked for the resignation of everyone in his cabinet, just in case. What's more, many men won't work for the salaries public sector jobs pay, so there are particular opportunities for women there.

I think there are also going to be more opportunities for women doctors to move into administration as we become overpopulated with doctors, and as doctors become increasingly concerned with non-doctors making decisions about how medicine should be practiced. Today the question of who pays influences medical practice tremendously. Doctors who don't want to be browbeaten by fiscal types will start returning to health administration and public policy. And they will undoubtedly be looking for retraining either in business or in public administration and many of them will be women.

The reality is that women will go into public administration in order to manage. This is a logical move for women physicians who already tend more than men not to be in solo practice and, of course, tend to work for less money.

I'm often asked, especially when I talk about women doctors becoming administrators, should women go to medical school. Emphatically, yes. An M.D. after your name means respect. I've often felt that being an M.D. gave me an advantage with men in terms of status, though not necessarily with other physicians. By and large, when someone meets a woman doctor, they know she has had to be smart, dedicated, and hard-working to get through the training. She's not someone you're going to send out for coffee. She's also not necessarily someone you're going to take out for a drink. Of course, as a psychiatrist, I have a further exotic distinction in that I am presumed to read minds.

After being asked if women should go to medical school, I'm then often asked how a woman doctor should deal with a family, if she chooses to have one.

I'd say it's very trite but true that the husband a woman M.D. picks had better be a hard-working professional because women M.D.'s will work long hard hours and a straight 9 to 5 person will resent his partner's not being readily available. My husband is more of a traditional doctor than I am. He's intensely involved in his work and with his patients, and he also writes and lectures in cardiology.

I'd also say a woman doctor should marry a competent guy who is not threatened by her, nor is so narcissistic that he needs a woman to be in adoration at his feet. I must say that most of the senior women I know in medicine who are married are married to doctors.

As for children, I had my first child while I was in medical school and my second and third during residency. I took two weeks out for each, but I have never believed that because I did it one way, so should everyone else. I think one thing women doctors must do is help other women doctors get maternity leave. We're working through the American Medical Women's Association, of which I am president-elect, to establish a maternity leave policy for residents. The American

Medical Women's Association is an important asset to women M.D.'s. I have personally felt my involvement with them to be enriching and they are a warm and supportive group. The networks developed through the Association have proved to be very helpful. The doctors I have met there share the same values, and perhaps more important, they are caring colleagues who have become close friends.

As to how the kids feel about my working, someone once asked my daughter, Alexandra, what she thought about not having her mother at home when she was a kid, and Alexandra answered, "Well, I don't think if she had been home, I would have survived my adolescence."

We had, and have, a lot of family routines. We set aside lots of time for the kids. We have Sunday dinner at our house no matter what. Bob may go out to buy Chinese food for Sunday dinner, but we have it together at home.

I guess I'm ending where I started, in terms of the strength I've derived from my environment, my home and my community, and the strength and service I've always tried to return. That's my mission, my calling, as I see it.

In terms of what government service means, I remember Hubert Humphrey saying that a government is judged by how well it takes care of its poorest, its most disadvantaged. That's always been my idea of what government should be.

Additionally, I like to remember Senator John F. Kennedy's speech to the Massachusetts legislature when he said:

When at some future date, the high court of history sits in judgment on each one of us,....we will be measured by the answers to four questions: Were we truly people of courage, courage to stand up not only to our enemies, but to our associates; were we truly people of judgment, of the future as well as the past, of our own mistakes as well as those of others with enough wisdom to know what we did not know, and enough candor to admit it; were we truly people of integrity, who never ran out on the principles we believed or the people who believed in them; and were we truly men and women of dedication, devoted solely to serving the public good. Courage, judgment, integrity, dedication, these are the historic qualities of the leader.

References

[1]Hennig M, Jardimann A: The Managerial Woman, Anchor Press, Doubleday, New York, 1977.

[2]The Boston Women's Health Book Collective, Our Bodies, Ourselves, New England Free Press, Boston, 1971.

[3]Josefowitz N: Management Men and Women: Closed and Open Doors in Harvard Business Review, Sept-Oct, 1980.

[4]Orlick T: In Pursuit of Excellence, Human Kinetics, Champaign, Illinois, 1981.

25

_____

Current Concepts
of Sexual Disorders

_____

Helen Singer Kaplan, M.D., Ph.D.

_Clinical Professor of Psychiatry; and
Founder and Director, Human Sexuality Program,
New York Hospital-Cornell Medical Center
New York, New York_

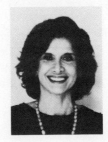

Helen Singer Kaplan, M.D., Ph.D.

25

_____

Current Concepts
of Sexual Disorders

_____

I first became interested in sexual disorders in the early sixties when the field was still in the dark ages. At that time very little accurate information about sexual physiology was available, and there were many misconceptions about the nature and causes of sexual disorders. Not surprisingly, treatment was so ineffective that persons with what we now consider simple problems were often doomed to a life of sexual disability.

But it turned out that we were on the brink of the so-called "sexual revolution" which would in two brief decades transform the field into a legitimate branch of medical science, with a technology so advanced that today sexual disorders are among the most readily treated human ailments. I was most fortunate to be part of these remarkable developments.

In 1964, under the auspices of an NIMH grant for career teachers in psychiatry, which allowed me to follow my special interests, I organized a psychosomatic service with the department of obstetrics and gynecology at Metropolitan Hospital in New York City. Our catchment area included four and a half million of New York City's poorest inhabitants. Many were on welfare; unemployment and illegitimacy were rampant; fathers were often absent; housing was inadequate; and drug traffic, violent crime and prostitution were prevalent in the streets, creating danger and tension in the neighborhoods. Sexual problems were not in my mind as I prepared to deal with (at that time) illegal and botched abortions, pelvic infections, teenage pregnancy, sterility, menstrual

disorders, dyspareunia, menopausal problems and sexually transmitted diseases. We did see our share of those, of course, but in addition, despite the overwhelming stresses experienced by these women, many asked us for help for their sexual difficulties.

I was at that time in psychoanalytic training, where it was a dictum that sexual disorders are always the product of profound and unconscious neurotic processes which derive from early childhood, and that such patients could only be cured by lengthy, reconstructive psychoanalytic therapy.

But apart from the fact that this was unfeasible in view of the large patient load and limited facilities of a city hospital, it seemed to me that our patients were, for the most part, not really appropriate candidates for psychoanalytic treatment. Apart from unconscious sexual conflicts, many of these women were consciously aware of their sexual anxieties, which often had simpler and cultural roots. Typically they were struggling with serious and real stresses in their daily lives. Many were trying to cope with abusive or absent or irresponsible partners, or partners who were as misinformed about sex as they were themselves.

My graduate work at Columbia University had been in learning theory and my doctoral thesis on fear extinction was biologically oriented. My clinical interest was on psychosomatic medicine. It was this confluence of theoretical influences which predisposed me to take a physiological and behavioral approach to the sexual complaints of the women in our clinic. Thus I began by giving our patients simple direct instructions meant to maximize both the physical and the mental aspects of their sexual experiences. These "homework assignments" were supplemented during the clinic visits by sex education and by psychodynamically oriented counseling designed to encourage sexual pleasure and to confront these women with their inhibitions, guilt and distortions about sex and men. Also, I quickly learned that if the assignments were to succeed, it was necessary to enlist the partner's cooperation, and this became an important issue in the counseling sessions.

To my surprise and immense pleasure many of the women responded favorably and, in just a few sessions, began to experience orgasm and more sexual enjoyment and even, in some cases, better relationships with their partners.

During the sixties interest in sexuality was still considered somewhat peculiar, and I remember that my work with sexual disorders was the subject of one of the faculty roasting skits presented by the psychiatric residents at our annual Christmas party at New York Medical College in 1967. But soon thereafter, in 1970, Masters and Johnson published their monumental book, *Human Sexual Inadequacy*,[1] and suddenly sex became a legitimate scientific concern. This great work supported my own observations that, contrary to long-held views, psychosexual symptoms often result from consciously perceived "minor" anxieties and that marital problems and cultural forces are frequently involved. And the most striking finding of all was that the majority of patients with sexual symptoms can be cured with brief, intensive, active, behaviorally oriented, couples-focused treatment. The extensive clinical experience that has been accumulated over the last twenty years has, in essence, supported these claims, which at the time astounded the medical establishment.

I was no longer alone. The publication of *Human Sexual Inadequacy* had made the study of sex respectable, and had blazed a trail which made it much less of an effort to pursue my own work in this area.

But, not surprisingly, the initial reaction of the psychiatric establishment to Masters and Johnson's findings was skeptical. For this reason, in 1975, I invited them to present their work at an APA symposium where it was discussed from biological, behavioral, psychoanalytic and marital per-

spectives by leading authorities in the field. (I chaired the symposium which included Dr. Robert Michels, who represented psychoanalysis; Dr. John Brady, behavior therapy; Dr. Clifford C. Sager, marital therapy; and Dr. C. Raul Schiavi, who discussed sex therapy from a biological perspective.)

In 1970, it was my good fortune that the medical students at Cornell Medical College in New York City petitioned the Dean of Students for a course on human sexuality. Dr. Richard Kohl, Medical Director of Paine Whitney at that time, and Dr. Robert Lahmon, Chairman of the Department of Psychiatry, invited me to join the faculty in order to develop and head a new human sexuality program whose tasks would include the teaching of human sexuality to medical students and psychiatric residents. At the same time I organized the post-graduate training program which has taught our integrated approach to the evaluation and treatment of sexual disorders to physicians and mental health professionals for the past fifteen years. Everyone who is on our staff today and who works with me in our private practice group is a graduate of this program and many of our trainees have gone on to other communities and other countries to open their own sex therapy centers.

Also, in 1970, I founded a sexual problem clinic for men and women within the outpatient department at Paine Whitney. This was the first such specialty clinic in a medical school and teaching hospital setting. In addition to providing a much needed service to the community, the clinic has also been a rich source of teaching and research material.

Our patients at Paine Whitney represent a highly diverse economic and cultural group and have taught us a great deal. First, it rapidly became apparent that men have essentially the same kinds of sexual anxieties and vulnerabilities and respond to the same kind of therapy as women do. That was really not much of a surprise to me; however, it was startling to observe that sexual disorders cut through wide cultural and economic differences. I had expected to see different kinds of problems among the wealthier patients at New York Hospital. But it seems that the rich and the poor, black and white and Hispanic, Christians, Jews, Moslems and Hindus all have similar sexual conflicts, similar fears of intimacy, similar struggles with their spouses, and all respond to the same treatment procedures if these are dispensed with empathy and sensitivity to cultural differences.

I am frequently asked if I encountered obstacles to my work, and the answer to that is that to a large extent the opposite has been true. The overwhelming majority of my students, colleagues, and administrators have been incredibly helpful, despite the prevailing social matrix of negative attitudes about sexuality and about women. (These antisexual attitudes are perhaps best illustrated by the following: in 1971 a letter to me from the New York State Department of Mental Health, which objected to compensation for the treatment of sexual disorders, contained the following: "It is our objective to treat illness and we are not in the business of enhancing human life.")

I am especially grateful to Dr. Robert Michels, who has chaired the Department of Psychiatry at the New York Hospital-Cornell Medical Center since 1974, and to Dr. Arnold Cooper, who is the director of training, for their personal support and encouragement. Together with other colleagues, they have created a stimulating and facilitative academic ambiance without which my work could not have continued.

Some Contributions

Of the many fascinating issues I have been concerned with, two are perhaps of special interest: 1) the "triphasic concept" of the human sexual response which has spawned a new system of classifying sexual disorders; and 2) the "new sex therapy" which is a brief treatment method for sexual disorders that integrates behavioral and psychodynamic concepts and techniques.

The Triphasic Concept

Until the publication of *DSM-III* in 1980, all the various sexual dysfunctions of males, including erectile disorders, premature ejaculation, retarded ejaculation, sexual avoidance and ISD, had been officially classified as "impotence," while all psychosexual disorders of females were labeled "frigidity." And, since all sexual disorders were viewed as variations of a single pathological entity, each was treated in the same manner. The clinicians' approach and not the nature of the disorder determined the type of treatment that

was prescribed. Thus, for example, behaviorists treated all psychosexual syndromes with systematic desensitization of sexual anxiety; psychoanalysts analyzed the unconscious conflicts of all their sexually disabled patients; and marital therapists attempted to improve the couples' general relationship without considering the specific nature of their sexual complaint. Even Masters and Johnson originally used the same sex therapy protocol for all sexual dysfunctions.

Historical Perspective

This lack of nosologic precision came about because the physiology of the sexual responses of males and females was not clearly understood and had always erroneously been regarded as a single physiological event. Masters and Johnson's meticulous pioneering studies of the human sexual response of men and women greatly advanced our knowledge about sexual physiology. These investigators observed 14,000 sex acts over a ten-year period under the same strict laboratory conditions which had been used to study and illuminate all biologic phenomena with the exception of the sexual response. In their publication, *The Human Sexual Response*,[2] in 1966 they gave us at last an accurate description of male and female sexual physiology. Masters and Johnson described four stages of the "sexual response cycle": excitement, plateau, orgasm and resolution. The value of Masters and Johnson's observations cannot be overestimated. Their four-stage scheme is extremely useful for descriptive purposes and gave us a standard vocabulary which facilitated communication in the field.

However, Masters and Johnson's four-stage system was still based on the old monistic model which regarded the sexual response as a single "cycle." The fundamental and important facts that desire, excitement and orgasm are neurophysiologically and anatomically discrete responses, and that disorders of desire, excitement and orgasm are separate syndromes is not accounted for in this scheme.

In order to organize and make sense out of the clinical diversity of the psychosexual disorders I felt that a different system based on the true triphasic biological infrastructure of the sexual response was needed.

It was apparent to me early on that orgasm and excitement phase disorders are clinically and

pathologically distinct syndromes which respond
to different treatment strategies (Kaplan, 1974,
1977). Actually the distinction between orgasm
phase and excitement phase disorders was first
discovered for males. Although he did not specifically articulate this concept, ejaculatory and
erectile disorders were clearly differentiated by a
urologist named James Semans who in 1956 cured
eight patients with "ejaculatory impotence" (PE)
using the stop-start method.[3] Semans thus demonstrated that premature ejaculation is different
from impotence in that this syndrome responds to
a specific treatment intervention: interrupted
stimulation. Later Masters and Johnson used their
"squeeze" variant of this method with equally
good results. I have postulated that the essential
therapeutic ingredient of both methods is that interrupted stimulation focuses the patient's attention on and heightens his awareness of the erotic
sensations premonitory to orgasm. This experience
creates the conditions whereby sensory-sensory
integration can take place, which is required for
the acquisition of voluntary control over all reflexes.[4] On the other hand, impotence responds to
different therapeutic techniques. The "sensate
focus" and "nondemand" methods developed by
Masters and Johnson diminish the patient's performance fears. This approach is excellent for
treating erectile disorders, but does not cure PE.

I made a similar distinction between the orgasm
and excitement phases and also between orgasm
and excitement disorders of females.[5] Many
women with inhibited orgasm have a normal sex
drive and enjoy a normal excitement phase in that
they lubricate and feel pleasurable erotic sensations. Anorgastic women get "stuck" only at the
point of climax. Patients with this diagnosis respond to a combination of clitoral stimulation and
relaxation together with distraction from self-
observation by fantasy. By contrast, women who
can climax, but suffer from inhibited excitement
are more likely to improve with sensate focus
exercises and nondemanding coitus.

Later the study of treatment failures in sex
therapy led me to recognize that sexual desire is a
third and separate phase.[6] One had come to expect
such a high rate of cures with the orgasm and excitement phase dysfunctions that any treatment
failures warranted a hard look. It turned out that
a significant proportion of our treatment failures
for what had appeared to be retarded ejaculation,
impotence and anorgasmia could in fact be traced

to our failure to recognize that the essential pathology in these cases was really the inhibition of
sexual desire. The erectile and orgasm dysfunctions of these patients were a secondary consequence of their trying to make love despite their
lack of interest.

Harold Lief, founder and head of the Family
Council of Philadelphia, independently recognized
and described desire phase inhibition, and he also
realized that we were dealing with a related but
distinct clinical syndrome with its own set of
causes and its own pattern or response to treatment.[7]

The analysis of the current sexual experiences
of patients with inhibited sexual desire (ISD) led
me to hypothesize that, in many cases, the immediate cause of ISD is the suppression of erotic
imagery and also a self-destructive tendency to
put themselves into a negative emotional state.
Such patients inhibit their sexual feelings by
focusing their minds on critical thoughts about the
partner or on self-deprecating images or on
stressful extraneous matters while making love. I
have called these self-induced negative mental
states "anti-fantasies." The psychosexual and
family histories of these patients suggest that on a
deeper level ISD is often associated with more
serious intrapsychic and marital problems than the
genital phase dysfunctions are. For this reason the
treatment of ISD tends to be stormier and
lengthier, often requiring a greater emphasis on
the psychodynamic aspects of therapy. While some
psychodynamic exploration is often necessary in
the treatment of the genital phase dysfunctions, it
is not unusual to cure impotent and anorgastic
patients primarily with behavioral methods.[6]

The Three Phases and Their Syndromes

According to the triphasic concept, the human
sexual response of males and females is composed
of three related but neurophysiologically and
anatomically distinct responses: desire, excitement
and orgasm. On a physiological level, orgasm in
both genders consists of the reflex contraction of
certain genital muscles. Male orgasm is composed
of two subphases: emission and ejaculation. Emission is the reflex contraction of the smooth
muscles of the internal male reproductive organs,
and squeezes the seminal fluid into the posterior
urethra. A split second later, 0.8 per second clonic
contractions of the striated muscles at the base of

the penis propel the semen through the urethra. Pleasurable orgastic sensations are experienced only during the ejaculatory phase of the male orgasm.

Female orgasm is analogous to the second or ejaculatory phase of the male orgasm and is also characterized by pleasurable, 0.8 per second clonic contractions of analogous striated muscles. In the female these muscles surround the vaginal introitus.

The essential physiologic feature of the excitement phase in males and females is the reflex vasodilitation of the sexual organs which prepares them for their reproductive functions. In the male, congestion of the penile blood vessels occurs within the confined space limited by Buck's fascia and produces erection. A more diffuse vasodilation congests the tissues surrounding the vagina and labia during the female excitement phase. This produces vaginal lubrication as well as the characteristic redness and swelling first described by Masters and Johnson.

Both the orgasm and excitement reflexes are mediated by neural centers located in the spinal cord. These are connected with higher erotic inhibitory and facilitory regions in the brain. But different and discrete spinal reflex centers and nerves and different higher cerebral centers serve the orgasm and excitement reflexes.

The third phase of the human sexual response is appetitive. Like other drive states, such as hunger and thirst, the neurophysiologic mechanism subserving the sex drive involves activation of certain pathways and centers of the brain. The "sex circuits" are located in limbic, hypothalamic, and cerebral areas and, in males as well as females, require testosterone to function normally. Evidence suggests that the sexual and the pleasure centers of the brain are closely related.

The separate and discrete anatomy of the reflex arcs and neural connections of the three phases holds the key to the new classification of sexual disorders and constitutes the biological mechanism which makes the selective inhibition of each sexual phase possible.

The triphasic model and the classification system to which it has given rise is not a mere academic exercise but has important implications for the medical as well as the psychiatric aspects of the clinical management of sexual disorders.

Organic Sexual Disorders

The importance of disease states and medication in the etiology of sexual disorders is just now being recognized. In my book on the evaluation of sexual disorders I emphasized the usefulness of the triphasic concept for the medical management of sexual disorders. Since each phase of the sexual response involves different anatomic structures, different disease states and medications are implicated in disorders of orgasm, excitement and desire in men and women. Thus, impaired desire in men as well as women may be associated with testosterone deficiency, prolactin secreting tumors of the pituitary, depression and beta blocking medication. But impotence is more likely to be caused by diabetes, penile circulatory deficiencies and antihypertensive drugs, which all must be ruled out when evaluating men with erection difficulties. On the other hand, deficient vaginal lubrication (excitement phase disorder of females) is not caused by any of these, but is frequently the result of estrogen deficiency. Still different medical causes are associated with orgasm and ejaculatory disorders. Although in their primary form orgasm phase syndromes are most often psychogenic even when the symptoms are not situational, delayed or absent orgasm may be associated with MAO inhibitors, advanced diabetes and spinal cord lesions. Secondary PE on the other hand may constitute the first sign of organic impotence.[8]

The Psychosexual Disorders

The major impact of the triphasic system has been on the psychological aspects of treatment. More specifically, if a person is intensely conflicted about sex, she or he is likely to become totally asexual. However, in the usual course of events only one of the phases is inhibited while the others are spared. Thus anorgastic women often feel desire and lubricate; impotent men frequently have a strong sex drive and many can ejaculate with a flaccid penis; premature ejaculators function well apart from their rapid climax; and patients with sexual anorexia or ISD may continue to function genitally, albeit with little pleasure.

The triphasic concept has given rise to a new classification system which describes diagnostic criteria for eight separate syndromes. (This system has been adopted by the American Psychiatric Association in *DSM-III*, by the American Psychological Association, and by the World Health Association.) Six represent the selective inhibition of desire, excitement or orgasm, while two types of disorders are not phase specific. 1) *Inhibited female orgasm* (anorgasmia) and 2) *Inhibited male orgasm* (retarded ejaculation) are both characterized by delayed or absent orgasm. The essential clinical feature of 3) *premature ejaculation* is the lack of adequate voluntary control over the ejaculatory reflex which causes the man to climax too rapidly for adequate lovemaking. 4) *Inhibited excitement of males* or *impotence* is characterized by the inability to attain or maintain an erection, while the essential feature of the analogous disorder, 5) *inhibited female excitement*, is a lack of erotic sensation and inadequate vaginal lubrication during sexual excitement. 6) *Inhibited sexual desire* has similar clinical manifestations in males and females. This syndrome is characterized by a loss of sexual appetite which may be partner specific or result in a total loss of libido (sexual anorexia). The two remaining sexual syndromes described in *DSM-III* are not associated with a specific phase. They include 7) *psychogenic dyspareunia of males and females*, and 8) *vaginismus*, a disorder associated with painful genital muscle spasms in females. Functional ejaculatory pain in males logically belongs in this category as well.

Finally, *sexual phobias* are specifically omitted from psychosexual disorders in this category. Although sexually phobic patients are not really dysfunctional in the sense that their sexual reflexes are intact, dysfunctions and phobias share similar clinical and psychopathological features. More specifically, both types of disorders are caused by sexual anxieties, both result in the couples' sexual disability, and both respond to similar sex therapy methods. There is one important exception, however. In my clinical experience approximately 30 percent of patients with a phobic avoidance of sex have an associated panic disorder, while the proportion of patients with other sexual complaints who also have panic disorder is considerably lower. This observation is of clinical significance because most patients with panic disorder fail to respond to sex therapy unless antipanic medication is administered to protect them from experiencing panic attacks during the treatment process. This type of medication has no place in the treatment of "simple" sexual phobias or sexual dysfunctions that are not associated with panic disorder.[9,10]

Etiology

The detailed analysis of the current sexual experiences of patients with different psychosexual dysfunctions led me to hypothesize that the currently operating causes or *immediate defenses* against sex are *highly specific* for the different syndromes.[6,8] Because of this specificity each dysfunction is amenable to different and specific behavioral interventions and for this reason I and others as well have developed specific behavioral protocols to treat the various dysfunctions.[11] Thus, for example, the immediate cause of vaginismus is an involuntary conditioned spasm of the vaginal muscles. The behavioral aspects of the treatment for this syndrome consist of gradual and systemic dilatation of the tight muscles that close off the introitus. The behavioral aspects of the treatment of the phobic avoidance of sex are quite different and entail general in-vivo desensitization methods that gradually expose the phobic patient to the irrationally feared and previously avoided sexual situation, which is the immediate cause operative in that disorder.

In sharp contrast I have found *no* evidence that the content and origins of the *deeper causes* which often play a role in sexual disorders are specific for the various sexual dysfunctions. Identical sexual conflicts of cultural and neurotic origins, and identical kinds of destructive struggles with love objects appear in the family and sexual histories of patients with all the different types of sexual disorders. But there is considerable diversity in the *intensity* of the underlying neurotic processes and marital difficulties. In general, with some exceptions, patients with impaired orgasm and excitement and also vaginismic patients tend to have relatively milder intrapsychic conflicts and relationship problems compared to patients with ISD. Thus patients who are *mildly* conflicted about sexual pleasure, because of unresolved oedipal problems or because of guilt about sex induced by a strictly traditional and/or devoutly religious upbringing, are likely to develop anorgasmia or impotence or PE. But *intense* conflicts with the same contents and of the same origins are more apt to result in ISD.

Because of the lack of specificity of the deeper causes, the psychodynamic aspects of treatment of the various dysfunctions do not address specific dynamic issues but vary considerably in scope and complexity with each case.

The New Sex Therapy

The success of Masters and Johnson's brief behavioral sex therapy methods prompted some critics to claim that psychoanalysis had thereby been invalidated and should now be discarded. But it makes no sense to abandon our rich psychodynamic heritage merely because behavioral techniques are more effective for curing certain sexual symptoms. Clearly, psychodynamic therapies also have their share of cures and both methods have a coherent conceptual base. It seemed to me that it would be more logical to identify the best and most useful elements of both systems, and to attempt to establish criteria for the appropriate use of each.

But at first glance the behavioral and psychodynamic approaches to sexual disorders seemed hopelessly contradictory and diametrically opposed.

According to behaviorists sexual disorders are learned responses which are acquired according to the laws of *conditioning* by the temporal association of sexual experiences with fear or pain. Although extremely disadvantageous to the patient, the symptom is maintained because it is *reinforced* by the avoidance or the reduction of anxiety. Thus, according to learning theory, impotence is caused by a learned fear response and is maintained by a self-perpetuating cycle of anticipatory anxiety and sexual failure. In order to cure the patient it is necessary to extinguish his sexual anxiety and to modify the performance pressures which are reinforcing the symptom.

On these assumptions behavior therapists had initially attempted to cure sexual dysfunctions by means of "systematic desensitization" which had shown promise for the treatment of phobias. These techniques were designated to extinguish the patient's sexual anxiety by pairing gradually more intensive mental images of the feared situation with body relaxation, which was sometimes augmented with short-acting barbiturates. Logical though this seemed, this approach was largely unsuccessful. But Masters and Johnson were extremely successful with an "in-vivo" desensitization approach which they used within a systems context. Based on their belief that per-

formance fears and inadequate communications between the couple play a major role in sexual disorders, Masters and Johnson prescribed gentle, nondemanding, progressively more stimulating sexual interactions between the symptomatic patient and his partner. This exposes the patient to constructive sexual experiences which he had previously avoided because of the anticipation of failure. Masters and Johnson's "exercises" diminish performance anxiety by creating a relaxed, reassuring and intimate ambiance in the ongoing sexual relationship. Some of the original Masters and Johnson exercises (sensate focus and nondemanding sexual interactions and training in communication skills) are so effective that they still constitute the backbone of the behavioral aspects of modern sexual therapy.

Psychodynamic theory, on the other hand, holds that psychosexual dysfunctions are caused by complex intrapsychic neurotic processes which are relatively independent of the patient's current reality. Most often these center around unresolved oedipal and in some cases pre-oedipal conflicts. These complexes operate on an unconscious level and originate in early childhood. Pathologic interactions with family members give rise to traumatic sexual conflicts which are repressed and lie dormant, only to create serious sexual conflicts and symptoms later in adult life. For such neurotic patients sex is not a natural, pleasurable experience, which under appropriate circumstances is neither dangerous nor immoral. To these unfortunate individuals sex has become symbolically and unconsciously an incestuous, competitive, dangerous, and sinful act and, not surprisingly, the sexual experience becomes fraught with anxiety. The pathway to cure, according to the psychodynamic view, can lie only in insight into, and resolution of, the patient's unconscious sexual conflicts. While psychodynamic therapies are considered by many clinicians to be the treatment of choice for personality disorders and neurotic behavior, the cure rate for sexual symptoms has been disappointing.[12]

Behaviorists and psychoanalysts have each maintained that their own system is correct and irreconcilable with the other. But the apparent dichotomy between the behavioral and psychodynamic approaches is false. The two theories do not contradict each other but merely describe human behavior on different levels. They occupy different conceptual niches that do not offer competing explanations. Each deals with different, but equally valid, phenomena and each intervenes on different and equally valid psychopathological levels which are appropriate in different clinical contexts. Thus, the success of one should not cast doubt on the validity of the other.

My clinical experience with sexually dysfunctional couples led me to the view that both approaches are correct in some respects and wrong in others. On the one hand, there is little doubt that psychoanalysts have correctly identified the importance of neurotic distortions about sex, love and pleasure that derive from childhood experience, and the bitter marital struggles that result from parental transferences in the etiology of many psychosexual difficulties. But equally striking is the crucial role which demanding partners, performance anxiety and negative self-judgments play in most cases of psychosexual disorders, which supports the behavioral position.

And both approaches also have significant limitations. The concept of unconscious mental processes is anathema to behaviorists who dismiss this notion as unscientific and "unprovable." For this reason, behavioral approaches lack the capability to handle the resistances which arise from unconscious sexual conflicts and neurotic problems in the couple's relationship. How do you deal with a couple's destructive parental transferences to each other if you deny the existence of unconscious neurotic processes? Can you "systematically desensitize" a patient's unconscious oedipal distortions if you maintain that there is no such thing as intrapsychic material and deal only with consciously perceived current reality? It is because of this "blind spot" to psychodynamics that behaviorally oriented techniques fail to help patients with more profoundly rooted sexual problems.

On the other hand, psychodynamically oriented therapists are equally biased in the opposite direction and tend to dismiss learning theory concepts of psychopathology and behavioral methods that attempt to modify symptoms directly as patently simplistic and naive. While psychodynamically oriented approaches do have the capability to deal with unconscious sexual conflicts they neglect the immediate and currently operating defenses against sex, which are critical in or to producing and maintaining the sexual symptom.

This omission arises out of two erroneous assumptions: 1) that sexual symptoms always have deep neurotic roots, and 2) that the symptom should automatically disappear when the underlying conflict from which it originally arose is eliminated. But sexual symptoms are not always associated with deeper conflicts about sex, and even when they are, often acquire a life of their own which is maintained and reinforced by the contingencies created by the patient's current sexual experience and may then persist indefinitely after the original conflict has been resolved. Thus for example, long after a woman has attained insight into, and has given up her hopeless wish for her father, she may still not be able to have an orgasm, because her obsessive pattern of self-observation and performance anxiety has become habitual. Sexual symptoms which persist in successfully analyzed patients who have derived benefits in other respects often respond with little resistance to a brief course of behaviorally oriented sex therapy, because the deeper sexual conflicts which originally gave rise to the symptom have already been resolved.

An Integrated View

Although the integrated treatment of sexual and also other types of disorders has recently gained wide acceptance, some critics still regard eclectic approaches as creating a confusing "mish-mash" from a research point of view.[13] But on a clinical level no confusion arises when behavioral and psychodynamic modes are combined within a coherent, rational system, such as described in the *New Sex Therapy*.

I have found that a hierarchical model of psychopathology with views that causes of sexual disorders as operating in layers provides a useful theoretical structure for conducting integrated treatment in an orderly manner (Kaplan, 1974, 1979, 1983). According to this metaphor, all sexual symptoms are ultimately caused by currently operating behavioral antecedents in the form of performance anxiety, obsessive self-observation (spectatoring) and negative thoughts and images (antifantasies). These destructive mental processes create anxiety and tension in the patient's current sexual situations and produce symptoms by interfering with the sexual reflexes on a physiologic basis. This is the dual common pathway by which symptoms are produced and constitutes the most superficial or immediate causal layer.

On a deeper level, neurotic sexual conflicts, guilt and shame about sexual pleasure from early anti-sexual messages, and destructive relationship struggles are regarded as the deeper psychodynamic infrastructure that in many cases lies "beneath" the immediate causes and the sexual symptom.

These remote or psychodynamic causes give rise to the immediate currently operating causes described above, and may mobilize anxiety and resistances to the rapid improvement of the sexual symptoms during the treatment process.

Integrated Treatment

The new sex therapy uses an amalgam of structured sexual interactions which the patient or couple conduct in the privacy of their home, together with active, psychodynamically oriented psychotherapeutic interventions in the therapist's office. As long as this basic model is maintained, sex therapy appears to be equally effective when conducted by a team or a solo therapist, daily for two weeks as originally devised by Masters and Johnson, or on a once a week basis over a longer period of time.

The behavioral interventions are used to modify the immediate, currently operating causes of the sexual symptom. If treatment succeeds in modifying the immediate behavioral obstacles to sexual functioning, the patient will be cured no matter what other intrapsychic and/or relationship problems exist. Conversely if the immediate causes persist, so will the sexual symptom, no matter how valid the patient's insights, and no matter how harmonious the couple's relationship is in other respects.

The main objective of the psychodynamic aspects of therapy is to resolve or bypass resistances to the rapid modification of sexual symptoms which are beyond the capability of the behavioral interventions.

The skillful and sensitive handling of resistances is the true art of psychosexual therapy and the key to successful treatment in many cases. This requires that the therapist work from an in-depth understanding of the psychodynamics of each partner and also of unconscious forces in their relationship. In the sessions, along with encouragement and support of pleasure and sexuality, the therapist also confronts both spouses with their unconscious resistances and with the destructive distortions from the past which both bring to the marriage. The dual steering mechan-

isms of empathic support and active confrontation are used to control the therapeutic process and to ensure that it proceeds at an optimal pace.

When resistances are too powerful to be bypassed, the unconscious material which fuels those must be dealt with. Toward this end the interpretation of dreams and fantasies is often useful. Transference toward the therapist is interpreted only when this constitutes a resistance to treatment, but transferential distortions between the partners often present obstacles to sexual improvement and must therefore be dealt with explicitly in many cases. As a general rule, in brief psychodynamic therapy, an attempt is made to keep interpretations of unconscious material on an ego-syntonic level in order to avoid mobilizing undue resistances. Thus, for example, confronting a patient with his unconscious sexually self-sabotaging behavior is usually more effective than suggesting that he wants to make love to his mother.

The process as well as the outcome of psychosexual therapy produces rapid significant changes in the couple's system, and on that account may be threatening to both spouses. The therapist's skill in conjoint treatment, his ability to tune into the covert dynamics of a couple's relationship, and his effectiveness in enlisting the unambivalent cooperation of the nonsymptomatic partner holds the key to the success or failure of many cases.

Sex therapy lends itself particularly well to the combined and integrated use of behavioral and psychodynamic approaches. When conducted according to an orderly hierarchy there is no dichotomy or confusion between the two methods. On the contrary, behavioral and psychodynamic techniques complement each other, compensating for each other's shortcomings, and when combined in a flexible, creative manner create an exciting synergy. The behavioral assignments, apart from serving the purpose of desensitization, also confront the couple with emotionally charged erotic and intimate experiences which they had previously avoided because these were too threatening. Thus defenses are removed and crises are created. In this manner the behavioral aspect of the therapeutic process often taps into highly sensitive latent material which then becomes accessible to the patient's conscious awareness and available for psychodynamic exploration during the therapy session. On the other hand, in depth understanding of the couple's psychodynamics, their vulnerabilities, their insecurities, their un-conscious transferences and the distortions which derive from the past will equip the therapist with the insights needed for devising astute behavioral assignments that fit the patient's individual psychological requirements, and whose therapeutic impact can extend far beyond mere mechanical desensitization and education in sexual techniques.

References

[1]Masters W, Johnson V: Human Sexual Inade-quacy. Little-Brown, 1970.

[2]Masters W, Johnson V: The Human Sexual Re-sponse. Little-Brown, 1966.

[3]Semans J: Premature ejaculation: a new approach. South Med J 49:353-358, 1956.

[4]Kaplan HS: The New Sex Therapy. Brunner/Mazel, 1974.

[5]Kaplan HS: A new classification of female sex-ual dysfunctions. Journal of Sex and Marital Therapy 1:124-138, 1974.

[6]Kaplan HS: Disorders of Sexual Desire. Brunner/Mazel, 1979.

[7]Lief H: What's new in sex research? Inhibited sexual desire. Medical Aspects of Human Sexuality 2:94-95, 1977.

[8]Kaplan HS: The Evaluation of Sexual Disorders: Psychological and Medical Aspects. Brunner/Mazel, 1983.

[9]Kaplan HS, Fyer A, Novick A: The treatment of sexual phobias. Journal of Sex and Marital Therapy, Vol. 8, No. 1, 1982.

[10]Kaplan HS, Klein DF: Sex Therapy and Medication in the Treatment of Sexual Phobias. Brunner/Mazel (in press).

[11]Barbach L: For Yourself: The Fulfillment of Female Sexuality. Signet, 1975.

[12]O'Connor JR, Stern LO: Results of treatment in functional sexual disorders. NY State J Med 72:1927-1934, 1971.

[13]Eysenck JH, Beach R: Counterconditioning and related methods in behavior therapy, in Handbook of Psychotherapy and Behavioral Change: An Empirical Analysis. Edited by Bergin AE, Garfield LD. John Wiley, 1971.

26

A National Survey of Women Physicians in Administrative Roles

---

Leah J. Dickstein, M.D.

*Associate Dean for Student Affairs
and Associate Professor,
Department of Psychiatry and Behavioral Sciences,
University of Louisville School of Medicine,
Louisville, Kentucky*

Judith J. Stephenson, S.M.

*Instructor,
Department of Psychiatry and Behavioral Sciences,
University of Louisville School of Medicine,
Louisville, Kentucky*

The senior author expresses gratitude to Judith J. Stephenson, S.M., for assistance in questionnaire design and for all of the statistical analyses.

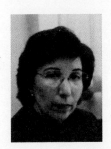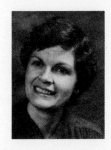

Leah J. Dickstein, M.D.   Judith J. Stephenson, S.M.

26

A National Survey of Women Physicians in Administrative Roles

Women have been entering medicine relatively unopposed for over a decade, but it is not yet time for them to relax and assume that barriers to advancement have disappeared. Women physicians remain underrepresented and underused in medical administration. Previous studies of women physician-administrators have dealt only with those in academic positions.[1-10] This study of 778 women physician-administrators presents data on an extended sample of medical administrators in academic and other positions.

Studies of women in academic medicine uniformly show that they cluster in lower-level positions and that their advancement is slower than men's. According to Scadron, "Women have been moving at a glacial pace in penetrating the upper echelons of medical school administration," and "Women have been clustered in low, characteristically untenured faculty positions, largely in traditionally 'nurturant' specialties and primarily in administrative posts dealing exclusively with student and minority affairs."[5] Braslow and Heins concurred: "What has not occurred to any notable degree, however, and is disconcerting to all women in academic medicine--both students and faculty--is a meaningful increase in the number of women at the senior professorial ranks, in the number of women occupying departmental chairs, or in the percentage of women in administrative positions in academic medicine."[1] Wallis, Gilder, and Thaler compared women's and men's promotion rates and found "that women physicians are promoted more slowly than men at all levels of

the academic ladder and that an increase in the representation of women in colleges does not ensure equalization of promotion rates."[9]

The commonly cited reason, apart from sexism, for women's poor showing in leadership positions is that women choose not to be leaders: that they lack interest and skill in leadership and that they choose to devote their time to their families rather than concentrating their attention on professional advancement. Talbott and Bachrach compared men and women psychiatrist-administrators and found that men liked wielding power, making decisions and managing more than women did.[11] Women do not have a history of wielding power at work, and their socialization and education actually inhibit leadership, whose most important quality, according to Rendel, is "self-confidence and a will to lead, to stand out."[12] In this study, women physician-administrators reported that they do enjoy power and decision-making and that specific training in leadership would be helpful.

Method

A 39-item questionnaire was mailed in 1984 to 1233 women physician-administrators in internal medicine, pathology, pediatrics, psychiatry, and public health, the specialties that traditionally have attracted the most women. The mailing list was compiled by a private listing agency recommended by the AMA (American Medical Association) and augmented by national specialty societies, state health departments, VA (Veterans Administration) hospitals, medical schools, and the Association of American Medical Colleges. The 778 valid questionnaires, a return rate of 63 percent, supply the data for this study. Cross-tabulation determined significant differences in the sample age and specialty.

Demographics

Most (84 percent) of the physicians were Caucasian, 8 percent Asian, 5 percent Black, the remainder other. Only 1 percent were under 30 years old; 21 percent were between 30 and 40, 29 percent between 40 and 50, 29 percent between 50 and 60, and 21 percent over 60. In birth order, 13 percent were only children, 44 percent oldest, 43 percent other. By specialty, 26 percent were in pediatrics, 23 percent in psychiatry, 19 percent in internal medicine, 14 percent in public health, 9 percent in pathology, 8 percent in pediatrics and public health and 1 percent in other combinations of the five specialties.

Role Models

Lack of role models is frequently cited as a handicap for women professionals. Questions about parents, education, and mentors provided information about role models. Forty-four percent of fathers and 18 percent of mothers worked in administrative positions. Of mothers who did not work outside the home, 34 percent were leaders in volunteer organizations. A large proportion of the physicians therefore had family role models for administrative work.

Data suggesting that women who attend women's colleges find it easier to be independent led us to ask about this point: 28 percent of the physicians attended women's undergraduate schools, and 8 percent had male mentors and 20 percent had female mentors. Sixty-seven percent of the physicians who had mentors said that the mentors helped them gain their administrative roles.

Family and Family Support

Of the physicians, 17 percent were single, 68 percent married, 12 percent separated or divorced, and 7 percent widowed. As might be expected, single physicians tended to be younger (40 and under), and divorced and widowed physicians tended to be older (divorced 45-plus, widowed 50-plus).

Thirty-two percent had no biologic children, 11 percent had one child, 25 percent two children, 19 percent three children, and 14 percent more than three children. Of the 13 percent who had stepchildren, adopted children, or foster children, 5 percent had one, 4 percent two, 2 percent three, and 1 percent more than three. Seventy-four percent had no children living with them, 11 percent had children under six years old, 15 percent had children 6-12 years old, and 20 percent had children 12-18 years old. Nine percent of the physicians had an older person living with them.

In response to a question about wage-earning status, 62 percent described their current families as dual-career families, 11 percent were the sole supporter, and 9 percent were the only professionals in their immediate families.

Table 1. Route to Administration

	Percent Yes	Percent of Responses*
Immediately after training	28% (210)	8%
After years in practice	39% (293)	11%
First on a part-time basis	27% (206)	8%
Immediately full-time	39% (297)	11%
To accommodate family needs	21% (159)	6%
Desire to be in administration	21% (159)	6%
Through teaching	28% (213)	8%
By accident	21% (160)	6%
Through interest in organizational systems	26% (196)	8%
Always was a leader	36% (269)	10%
Enjoy the challenge	61% (462)	18%

*Multiple responses: average 3.5 answers per person.

Table 2. Advantages of Administrative Roles for Women

	Percent Yes	Percent of Responses*
None	7% (53)	2%
Better work schedule	43% (330)	12%
Being a role model for other women	62% (470)	17%
Being assigned typical women's roles	2% (16)	1%
Better financial remuneration	25% (189)	7%
Changing health policies	49% (374)	14%
Prestige	45% (339)	12%
Creative opportunities	64% (483)	18%
Working with other than private patients	25% (188)	7%
Easier lifestyle with family responsibilities	32% (243)	9%
Other	6% (47)	2%

*Multiple responses: average 3.6 answers per person.

In response to a question about family attitudes toward their professional roles, 87 percent reported that they had the emotional support of their families of origin, and 93 percent reported that they had the emotional support of their current families.

Career

Of all the physicians, 74 percent held academic positions: 16 percent were professors, 15 percent associate professors, and 14 percent assistant professors. Only 4 percent were instructors, and a total of 19 percent held clinical positions. Thirteen percent worked for educational institutions, 19 percent for hospitals, 7 percent for the federal government, 13 percent for state governments, and 9 percent for local governments. Eleven percent combined work for hospitals with work for educational institutions, and the remainder held other combined affiliations. Twenty-six percent of the physicians had held only one administrative position, and the remainder held two or more.

Twenty-eight percent began working in administration immediately after training, 39 percent after years in practice. Twenty-seven percent

began administrative work first on a part-time basis; 39 percent began full time. Only 21 percent said that they chose an administrative position because they wished for it, 26 percent selected an administrative role out of their interest in organizational systems; 21 percent characterized their appointments as "by accident" (see Table 1).

Questions about sexism revealed that 46 percent never experienced difficulties because of being female; 27 percent experienced a little difficulty, 19 percent some difficulty, and only 7 percent a lot of difficulty. Thirty percent reported having competed with equally competent men, 7 percent with equally competent women, 42 percent with less competent men. Sixty-eight percent reported gender bias on the part of employers or promoters. Predictably, a small number of physicians reported no difficulty because of being female but also reported gender bias on the part of an employer.

Asked whether they experienced sexism from other women who don't think women belong in administration, 26 percent said yes. Thirty-eight percent reported that male peers related to them as mothers, expecting support and nurture. Only 37 percent felt misperceived or misunderstood

Table 3. Disadvantages of Administrative Roles for Women

	Percent Yes	Percent of Responses*
None	37% (271)	29%
Lack of networks	33% (239)	25%
More rigid schedule	13% (98)	10%
Discomfort with being assertive	27% (198)	21%
Other	19% (137)	15%

*Multiple responses: average 1.3 answers per person.

because of their administrative style or because they are women, and 60 percent found it difficult to say "no" because of wanting to please others.

In response to questions about formal training in administration, 68 percent agreed that formal training in the use of power would have helped them, 65 percent that training in decision-making would have helped, 44 percent that training in working as a minority would have helped, and 75 percent that training in styles of leadership would have helped. Only 38 percent said that they had found networking among women useful.

Seventy-seven percent reported that they use a traditionally male administrative style, i.e. relying on individual decisions, and 87 percent reported using the traditionally female cooperative or joint approach. (Obviously, many physicians use both, and a common written response was "I use what works.")

Asked whether they wanted to advance further in administration, 36 percent said yes, 59 percent no, 5 percent not sure. Twelve percent voiced regret about having chosen the administrative path, but 87 percent felt no regret.

The large majority of physicians reported that they obtain satisfaction from administrative work: 93 percent from decision-making, 92 percent from leadership, 86 percent from managing, and 85 percent from serving as role models.

Two questions with multiple responses asked about advantages and disadvantages of administrative roles for women. Very few women saw no advantages in administrative work, and only a very few reported being pleased with their traditionally feminine role (see Table 2). An analysis of these multiple responses showed an average of 3.6 answers per person, with the most common answers being: better work schedule (12 percent), prestige (12 percent), changing health policies (14 percent), being a role model for other women (17 percent), and creative opportunities (18 percent).

Thirty-seven percent reported no disadvantages in holding an administrative position, 33 percent agreed that the lack of networks and role models for women is a disadvantage, 13 percent complained of the more rigid schedule, and 27 percent felt discomfort in being assertive and feared being called aggressive. Analysis of these multiple responses showed 1.3 answers per person, the most common response (29 percent of the answers) was that there are no disadvantages in administrative work for women (see Table 3).

Discussion

Most of the administrators were 40 to 60 years old, which could be expected, for studies show that women advance slowly in medical administration. Although the mailing list was as comprehensive as possible, perhaps some younger physicians beginning careers in administration were inadvertently left out. It is a common finding, and also predictable, that more than half of the physicians were only or oldest children.

Almost half, though not the majority, of physicians' mothers and fathers had experience as administrators and leaders, and two-thirds of the administrators reported having had mentors. Families and teachers provide important role models for administrative work. Furthermore, almost 90 percent of the administrators had the support of their families of origin and of their current families.

An interesting finding that appears to contradict earlier studies is that the physicians in academic positions (over two-thirds of the total number held at least partial academic appointments) were evenly spread across professorial levels. Probably what accounts for this discrepancy is that all these physicians are administrators; perhaps what should be surprising is that so many hold positions of power without high academic rank.

It is common for successful women to deny that they have ever experienced sexism. Almost half of these administrators reported never having experienced difficulty because of being female, and only 7 percent reported having experienced a lot of difficulty. Probably these numbers are influenced by the administrators' determination not to see sexism. Often people who report no sexism in general, remember specific instances--unequal pay, for example. Additional comments on questionnaires suggested that such was the case for at least some of these administrators.

Questions about the usefulness of formal training revealed that even these very successful administrators wished they had had or could have training in using power, decision-making and working as a minority, and in styles of leadership. An interesting point is that only 38 percent have found networking useful. These findings point to the need to educate women physicians in organizational systems and survival techniques so their numbers in administration will increase.

The questionnaire received enthusiastic response; many of the administrators are lone women in their organizations and were eager to relate their experiences. The most important finding of the study is that women feel competent to wield power, that they like forming health policy, that they enjoy being role models--that they view administrative careers as offering a creative and satisfying opportunity to help patients and health providers.

References

[1] Braslow JB, Heins M: Women in medical education: a decade of change. N Engl J Med, May 7, 1981, pp. 1129-1134.

[2] Farrell K, Witte MH, Holguin M, et al: Women physicians in medical academia: a national statistical survey. JAMA 241:2808-2812, 1979.

[3] Harris AS: The second sex in academe. AAUP Bulletin, Fall 1970, pp. 283-295.

[4] Robinowitz CB, Nadelson CC, Notman, MT: Women in academic psychiatry: politics and progress. Am J Psychiatry 138:1357-1361, 1981.

[5] Scadron A: AMWA's experiment in planned change: a report on the "women in medical academia" project. JAMWA 35:299-301, 1980.

[6] Scadron A, Witte MH, Axelrod M, et al: Attitudes toward women physicians in medical academia. JAMA 247:2803-2807, 1982.

[7] Scully AL: From the halls of academia. JAMWA 37:265, 1982.

[8] Wallis LA: Academic promotions: a plan of action. JAMWA 37:180, 1982.

[9] Wallis LA, Gilder H, Thaler H: Advancement of men and women in medical academia. JAMA 246:2350-2353, 1981.

[10] Witte MH: Death in an untenured position. JAMA 246:2356-2357, 1981.

[11] Talbott JA, Bachrach LL: Administrative psychiatry: what sort of job is this for a woman? In Administration in Mental Health, Vol. 12, no. 4, Summer 1985, pp. 253-263.

[12] Rendel: Changing Roles of Women in Industrial Societies. Bellagio Conference, 1976, Rockefeller Foundation, 1977.

27
___

Women Administrators:
New Hope and New Dilemmas

___

Jean Baker Miller, M.D.

Clinical Professor of Psychiatry,
Boston University School of Medicine; and
Scholar-in-Residence,
Stone Center for Developmental Services and Studies,
Wellesley College,
Wellesley, Massachusetts

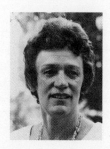

Jean Baker Miller, M.D.
Photograph by Bernard Cole

27

Women Administrators:
New Hope and New Dilemmas

Until recently, most administrators have been men. Therefore, men have provided the models of what an administrator should be. As women become administrators, they inevitably confront the task of deciding explicitly or implicitly, whether they will strive to emulate the only models so far available. If taken up explicitly, this decision offers the opportunity for reexamination of the assumptions underlying the commonly accepted models. It also opens the possibility for new kinds of problems.

Today, most people work within large organizations where they may be ground down and diminished, or helped to enlarge and grow. Most of us would agree that we are very short on the latter. Since these problems are not solved in countries with other socioeconomic systems, e.g. socialist countries, or those with fuller welfare states, changes in the larger socioeconomic system have not provided answers.

In our workplaces there are two major categories of questions. One concerns the provision of decent economic standards and basic working conditions. These essential needs are not yet met for everyone. The second concerns the creation of a structure of relationships which fosters the development of the people within the institution.

It is fair to say that in our history, those people who have concentrated on finding ways to foster the growth of other people have been women.[1-3] Women have long practice in the complex, emotionally and cognitively integrated activity of helping other people to develop.[4-6]

Women have provided growth-fostering relationships for many people, children, husbands and other women and men in the home and in the workplace. Equally important, women have carried out this kind of activity within an "institutional" context. That is, women have concentrated on trying to make the "institution" of the family "work" for all of its members.

Despite obstacles and difficulties, women have tried to learn how other people feel and what their needs are. Struggling to understand these many varied feelings, they have often mediated skillfully among family members. (That women alone cannot solve optimally all the issues in the family or at work is another, larger topic, which involves the question of the whole structure of families and of our society.)

A closely connected aspect of this emphasis on relationships is that most women do not feel their deepest pleasure in "winning out" over others. Indeed, most women feel pain if their own enhancement results in another person's pain.[7] There are women who appear otherwise. However, this stance is usually reactive, a defensive way of acting, arising out of perceived or real threats from others. Many women who act this way are left feeling distressed because no matter how "tough" they may appear on the surface, they often feel alone and isolated and pained at the image of themselves as destructive. Women, however, do not want to be hurt themselves. Most women want the kinds of connections with others that allow them to hear and understand the perceptions and desires of others, and in which the other person is able to hear their perceptions and desires. Emerging out of this psychological experience, most women feel a greater sense of well-being, self-worth and effectiveness if they feel their actions arise from a context of relationship and, in turn, lead on to a greater sense of connection with others, as opposed to a sense of distance or so-called "independence." This is to say that women feel better and more worthwhile if we feel that our activities have come out of the interchange and workings of a relationship.[6,7]

Men need these kinds of relationships, too, but at this point in history most men have been led to feel that each is more worthy and effective if he believes that he, personally, is a strong, highly developed individual, that he "is his own man."[8] Men have not been raised to feel that it is their *primary responsibility* to foster the growth of others; and their own development has not focused on preparing them for building relationships which benefit others as well as themselves. Instead, men have been encouraged to concentrate on developing and advancing themselves. Indeed, they are pressured to do so. It follows that men have learned to seek their own advancement, status and power, usually including *power over* others. This is a very different form of activity and a very different way of being in the world.[1,2]

Thus, women have a realistic history of practice which leads them to enter large institutions with a very different approach and different set of values. These may be close to precisely the values and the approach which our institutions lack and *need most* at this time.

While women have these motivations and values they have been affected by countervailing forces, as well. Thus, building a structure of relationships which are truly mutually enhancing is not easy on any level, either in personal or public settings. But it could be at least a stated goal to be put forward.

How can we do this? Perhaps consideration of a few concrete examples can serve as a starting point. In these examples, I will disguise the facts, but try to preserve the essence of the events. In an institution in which I worked in the past, a beginning resident, a gifted person who already had some clinical experience, expressed a great desire to be in a third-year seminar on group therapy. I had to tell him that his first-year supervisors believed he did not have enough ex-

perience for it. He was disappointed and angry. I said two or three more times that I was sorry, but it was just a question of experience and he would acquire that in time.

During the months that followed, this resident appeared to be at the center of considerable difficulty on the service. He seemed to be the person who was always filling fewer clinical hours than he should. This put an extra burden on other staff, especially at certain rushed periods. I'm not sure that this extra strain resulted in poorer service to the patients, but it is likely that this occurred. All of this was time-consuming and psychologically negative for the other residents and for staff members.

This resident also played a major role in aggravating, nonproductively, the other trainees' various complaints. While many of the complaints were valid, the modes of dealing with them were not. The disgruntlement of the trainees led to more difficult and time-consuming interactions with their supervisors. In addition, some of the staff were sucked into a vortex of opposition to the leadership of the service.

This resident also violated rules by taking on the kind of patients that he was not supposed to take, and for whom he was not sufficiently trained. Some of these patients proceeded to manifest serious difficulties.

As a result of these incidents a large part of the staff's time and energy was consumed in activities which were less than optimal. They consisted of trying to pick up the pieces of bad situations and to deal with negative dynamics which had been set in motion within the work group.

While my interaction with one resident was obviously not the whole cause of these problems, let us discuss it as if it were, for the purposes of illustration. (It is also not a question of an individual's character or psychodynamics, but of a way of working for a whole staff.) The entire situation could have been handled in another manner. I think I could have paid more attention to the disappointment of the resident and to my own emotions which make it difficult to disappoint anybody and also to be the recipient of anger. One possibility would have been to have had an early meeting with the residents, or with the residents and relevant staff, to discuss matters of this sort. The resident could have been encouraged to express his anger, disappointment and hurt. I think he might have said that he felt that the decision was a put-down and a devaluation of him, which I believe was the most significant feeling involved. This is a feeling many people experience in institutions, often for valid reasons. The other trainees might have been able to talk about the ways in which they were feeling similarly. He might have felt heard and understood by others. This support would have helped to allay his need to muster "support" in the more negative fashion he employed.

Equally important, I think I could have expressed to the residents, directly, some of my feelings--e.g., that it is hard for me to disappoint people and to experience their anger, but also that there are appropriate groupings for people of different levels of experience and that this does not necessarily imply devaluation of anyone. Staff and trainees would probably have seen this as valid and felt less devalued. They may have been more able to see me as an ordinary person with hang-ups, and less as a "villain."

I would probably have suggested to the trainees, as a group, that there were some routes open to them to bring about more of what they wanted. For example, if enough were interested in a topic, they could form their own discussion group. We could then provide an experienced person to meet with them after they had worked on formulating their own central questions. In fact, I had suggested this to the resident. He had not been able to hear it or to act upon it. An even better possibility is that out of these kinds of exchanges the trainees might have generated their own ideas for activities which could offer more satisfaction for them. Although there are always constraints, some of their desires could have been met.

In some institutions this use of time probably would have been seen as inefficient or even "silly." As the events demonstrated, it probably would have been much more efficient and would have saved much of the large amount of time that was used later in much less productive ways. It is also very possible that holding this series of discussions could have been perceived as a manifestation of indecisiveness and of being and encouraging others to be "too emotional," some of the very common ways in which women, especially women administrators, risk being labeled. On the contrary, I think it would have drawn on the already existing bases of strengths which are present in women and which can be tapped in men.

If we all had had a greater opportunity to express emotions, particularly those that are more difficult to express such as feeling hurt or put down, I believe that the subsequent actions by all parties could have proceeded in a way in which intellect and emotions were integrated more positively. As it happened, emotions were expressed in nonproductive actions. Clearly, emotions don't go away. This is a prevalent illusion within institutions.

I'm certain that my initial approach to this situation was a reflection of my background in the institutions in which I have worked and was trained. Nobody thought much about the feelings of a first-year resident. A decision would have been made at the top (even possibly a good decision) and transmitted accordingly. I would certainly never have thought of such actions as telling the director how hurt I felt and, least of all, how angry I was.

Another example may illustrate a similar set of forces which led to a different result. It concerned a major snafu about a call for an emergency consultation on a weekend. The first person on call could not be located by telephone. The second person made an estimate of the situation and said that in his judgment it did not require an emergency consultation. The people calling grew more upset and dissatisfied and tried to reach the third person on the list. She could not be found. They then phoned the fourth person who said that he was in the middle of a social event and shouldn't be required to come because he was fourth on the list. He told them to try again to find the other three people before bothering him again.

I need not go into further detail about how such a situation can escalate. If the identified patient was not sufficiently disturbed initially, by the time the people around grew more and more upset, he as well as others may well have needed attention. It was also part of our stated working approach that we view problems in a "social context," meaning that we recognize that in many instances it's not a single individual who is in need of help, but rather that it is our obligation to attend to the complex of people involved in any situation.

In this situation a number of people might have been called on the carpet, with good justification. Instead, the administrator chose to see it as a manifestation of misunderstandings and negative emotional forces within the staff. She held a number of meetings, seemingly very time consuming, at which staff and trainees were encouraged to express all of their various complaints and opinions about the emergency procedures. These discussions led on to consideration of other topics as well. Out of them came a review of the principles and procedures for dealing with emergencies and other matters. The staff felt involved in all of these decisions; most understood and agreed with the rationales. In the following several years there has been no recurrence of this kind of problem. In fact, emergencies have been used in a most productive way. Discussions about them have led to fruitful preventive activities, i.e., staff members have developed ideas for influencing some of the factors contributing to some of the most common types of emergencies in that setting.

Here, too, all of the meetings and expressions of emotions could have been seen as manifestations of indecisiveness by the leadership, of encouraging people to be emotional, and especially as inefficient. Instead, I'm certain that if measurements had been made they would have shown a decrease in actual time and money costs. Most important, the new programs benefitted the people served.

The characterization of indecisiveness is inaccurate. Decisions were made. They were made by a different process. The common image of decisiveness need not be the only or the best guide to decision making. As mentioned above, the characterization of anything or anyone as "too emotional" is also incorrect. It is more accurate to say that the existence of emotions was recognized and an attempt was made to provide pathways to deal with them in a productive fashion.

These examples suggest one feature which is relevant for all institutions: no one knows *the right way* to do things. Further, because institutions are composed of people, they are *alive* and therefore always in motion, in a state of change. At this time, an optimal path may be to search for an improved *process* for working together. Such a process should enable those "at the bottom" to bring forward their experience, and those "at the top" to accept the proposition that they are never and can never be "right." While those at the top have certain kinds of information they are out of touch with other kinds of information—precisely the information about a large part of

what's really happening where it is happening. Maxwell Jones[9] made this point about mental health service institutions, but it seems true about all institutions. By working to develop better processes for relational development within institutions we will be encouraging simultaneously the growth of people at all levels.

These remarks obviously assume a hierarchal institution. Many women today (and women and men past and present) have criticized hierarchal institutions. In recent years, many women's organizations have conducted courageous struggles to create more collective organizations.[10] Some have evolved very valuable models which can serve as guides for professionals and others. One example which is now available in written form is the collection of handbooks and manuals written by the North Vancouver Island Women's Self-Help Network.[11] There is not yet a generally agreed upon model for large organizations, and there are many unsolved issues. However, these women's ideas and experiences provide, I believe, the most creative guides currently available for further work.

Closely related to the question of hierarchies is another overriding and unsolved topic: power—both the drive by those in power to keep things the way they are and simultaneously to seek greater power. This drive clearly is not the same as seeking the good functioning of the institution and the development of everyone in it.

In many situations within institutions the participants are deflected from dealing with the real matter at hand. They are playing in another "game" which is geared to protecting themselves, and/or advancing themselves, in a situation in which the major determinant will be power. In general each participant seeks to obscure doubts or possible deficiencies lest these be used to diminish him/her. This tendency obscures reality because we all have doubts and deficiencies along with our abilities and potential. In general, this tendency leads to a debate around a topic which is never the real one, instead of a dialogue on the real issue.

Here women confront a major problem. There are a great many women who are not motivated to engage in this kind of power seeking. It is also true that some women are. Others have come to believe that it is absolutely necessary to do so because that "is how the world is." However, the new and creative possibility is that those women who do not value that form of activity can continue to come together to try to find and to define their preferences. We do not know how to do this well yet. But some women do it better than others. We can all learn from them.

We have all been affected by "the way the world is" and have incorporated many non-constructive ways of acting. On the other hand, most of us have other motivations as well. Thus, most of us live with a great deal of conflict. We might start with a recognition of this conflict and of the painful ways in which each of us experiences it.[12] A fuller recognition and expression of the various components of our conflict may release the new and creative possibilities which also are present in us.

In summary, I've tried to suggest only a few examples of the many ways in which women administrators' desires and actions can be misperceived and misunderstood. There are many others. The very characteristics which may be misunderstood and mislabeled can be the characteristics which women can redefine accurately as very valuable bases for leading into new forms of functioning within institutions. These new ways of working reflect the values which women, in general, tend to have. These values arise from a grounding in the kinds of activities that women actually have already practiced in life. In general, we might say that they rest on the belief that it is in the interactions between people that all people develop; that the best ideas and ways of functioning can emerge from mutually enhancing relationships between people rather than from the enhancement and advancement of any one individual.

It is difficult to find the institutional forms by which to put these goals into practice. It is harder, still, to think in terms of creating major changes in institutions so that they become places which enhance people rather than places in which the few gain power and prestige at the expense of the many. However, what are institutions if not places which should benefit everyone who works in them and everyone who is supposed to be served by them?

Women do have the right to say that institutions should function for us in ways that work for us. Women enter the institutional scene with a different background. The danger is that in the face of formidable and powerful institutions women will fail to recognize and value the truly valuable parts of this background. Instead, we might try to articulate explicitly our particular values and goals.

References

[1] Miller JB: Toward a New Psychology of Women. Boston, Beacon Press, 1976.

[2] Miller JB: The development of women's sense of self, in Work in Progress, Number 12. Wellesley, Stone Center Working Papers Series, 1984.

[3] McIntosh M: Feeling like a fraud, in Work in Progress, Number 12. Wellesley, Stone Center Working Papers Series, 1984.

[4] Jordan J, Surrey J, Kaplan A: Women and empathy, in Work in Progress, Number 2. Wellesley, Stone Center Working Papers Series, 1982.

[5] Jordan J: Empathy and self boundaries, in Work in Progress, Number 16. Wellesley, Stone Center Working Papers Series, 1984.

[6] Surrey J: The self-in-relation: A theory of women's development, in Work in Progress, Number 13. Wellesley, Stone Center Working Papers Series, 1984.

[7] Gilligan C: In a Different Voice. Cambridge, Mass, Harvard University Press, 1982.

[8] Levinson D: The Seasons of a Man's Life. New York, Knopf, 1978.

[9] Jones M: Beyond the Therapeutic Community. New Haven, Yale University Press, 1968.

[10] Riger S: Vehicles for empowerment: The case of feminist movement organizations, in Studies in Empowerment: Steps Toward Understanding and Action. Edited by Rappaport J, Swift C, Herr R. New York, Haworth Press, 1984.

[11] The Women's Self-Help Network: Working Together for Change: Women's Self-Help Handbook, Vols I & II. Campbell River, British Columbia, Ptarmigan Press, 1984.

[12] Stiver I: Work inhibitions in women, in Work in Progress, Number 3. Wellesley, Stone Center Working Papers Series, 1982.

28

Women Leaders in Medicine:
Some Notes on Transference and Countertransference

Malkah T. Notman, M.D.

Clinical Professor of Psychiatry,
Director of the Women's Resource Center,
Tufts University School of Medicine
and the New England Medical Center; and
Training and Supervising Psychoanalyst,
Boston Psychoanalytic Institute,
Boston, Massachusetts

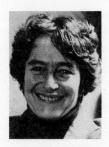

Malkah T. Notman, M.D.

28

Women Leaders in Medicine:
Some Notes on Transference and Countertransference

Leaders acquire their authority for a variety of reasons. They can attain their position because of their own efforts, be chosen by some other authority, or be elected. Someone can spontaneously rise to leadership in response to a particular occasion; a position of leadership can also be inherited, even in an academic situation in which one individual is groomed for a position and is expected by all to succeed to it. There are thus many routes to leadership, and the authority and leadership itself can be quite varied, with patterns which are shifting or constant, strong or weak, divided or unified. It might appear that leaders in an academic or professional field are more rationally chosen than in the arena of pure politics. And, in fact, the basis of leadership can be the real knowledge and skill of the leader. This form of authority was termed "rational authority" by Eric Fromm.

No matter in what manner the leader arrived at a position, maintaining it involves a balance of power between the leader and the led, in which this power is given to the leader, at least where force is not involved. This is true even where it seems that personal qualities of the leader appear to be most contributory, such as when the real expertise, assertiveness, willingness to take positions, to stick one's neck out and take risks as well, the personal qualities such as charm and charisma are important. Freedom from ambivalence, indecision and doubt has often made the difference between an effective leader who can present material as compared to someone who may have very creative and new ideas, but is hesitant in conveying them. For example, it has been thought that in the early work between Freud and Breuer, the difference between Breuer's tendency to doubt and Freud's boldness helped determine which of them pursued the ideas developed from the early cases, since work with their original patients was done collaboratively. Breuer backed down when some difficulties with a patient caused him to develop self-doubts.

Those aspects of leadership which require assertiveness or willingness to take risks in a way which leaves one vulnerable to attack or challenge have not been congruent with traditional feminine qualities. Those women who attain such positions either must be prepared for some internal conflict or need to develop adaptive strategies to cope with these. This conflict for women may be more open and acknowledged in the political arena and masked and rationalized in medicine. Questions about the competence of a leader may be raised regarding a woman leader when the actual concern is with qualities that appear disquieting or "unfeminine," and what is really of concern is that she is "aggressive" or "abrasive."

In medicine, as in other fields, the basis of leadership depends not only on realistic contributions, but on the same balance of political talent and style, innovative qualities, and expertise. Sometimes the particular combinations of historical circumstances, individual talents and resources are the critical determinants in mobilizing a potential leader into a position of active leadership. The availability of women at a time when the positions for women in leadership have become somewhat more available has been important. Characteristics that are effective and needed at an early phase, however, may be different than those in a later phase, when women are more established and accepted.

In all situations, the response to a particular individual is determined not only by personal qualities but by social class, gender and other group characteristics. One has only to think of issues raised in people's minds by the emergence of a leader who may be a tough, black individual or a young person dressed in off-beat, nonconservative clothes or a soft-spoken, slim blonde woman to realize that group characteristics are extremely influential in determining individuals' responses to this leader. Sometimes these are recognized, but often they are not and appear instead to be questions about real qualifications or subtle processes of discounting. For example, women's contributions in a discussion may be ignored or minimized or their wish to speak may be passed over.[1]

Sometimes reactions to an individual's group characteristics are based on what are thought to be realistic qualities, such as concern about the educational preparation of someone who is seen as having a lower-class background or the suspiciousness and distance with which someone from an upper-class position may be regarded if problems concern the urban poor. Women have also been concerned that men cannot adequately understand or represent their interests, and certainly men have worried about women's understanding them as well. However, the symbolic aspects are often as important as the real ones, and stereotypes about groups influence how an individual is perceived.

Individuals also bring into each of those situations the potential for distortion based on their own previous experience. An important concept for understanding these reactions is the concept of transference and countertransference. Transference refers to those feelings, expectations and reactions which are part of an individual's responses to situations in the present but arise from his/her past experience. For example, reactions to authority are strongly influenced by one's own authority experiences, starting with one's own parents. Countertransference reflects a similar process and is a technical term used to refer to a particular form of transference, namely

that of a therapist or physician to a patient. It refers to the physician's attitudes to the patient which are interactions by determinants of his/her experiences from previous early relationships which may not be recognized. For example, someone with a history of relationships with parents who were dominant, controlling and critical is likely to approach a new professor with anxiety and the expectation of being criticized. That individual will also have perceptions which lead him or her to feel criticized even if comments are not intended that way. These transference reactions are present in all human interactions to a greater or lesser degree. They are often unconscious and form part of the unconscious, less rational aspect of human responses. There is always a mixture of conscious and unconscious, rational and irrational factors in a relationship, particularly in a relationship of leadership. Even if the process of arriving at the position is fairly rational, such as the selection of "the best possible candidate" to chair a temporary committee, transference responses and other unconscious and irrational elements are inevitably brought into the situation by the participants, and operate to some extent and need to be adjusted by experience with reality. Understanding these factors can shed light on apparently contradictory responses.

Of course, the leader is subject to irrationalities as well. The leader may have omnipotent fantasies of being able to accomplish anything and everything; he or she may expect to be able to solve all kinds of problems alone. The leader may feel the need to be independent, not to consult anyone because of some concern that this would indicate weakness. (This style tends to be less characteristic of women.) He or she can feel helpless in the face of what seem to be overwhelming problems, without taking the opportunity to assess them thoroughly. Women traditionally looked for consensus and worked towards compromise, with concern about alienating and losing people or making enemies. The problem of taking risks and making enemies can interfere with effective leadership. An extension of this is the idea that the solutions arrived at or the positions taken on one's own are likely to be ineffective, and taking a position is possible only by consulting with others and receiving what amount to guarantees of acceptance and support.

The unconscious responses which affect the reaction to a leader include not only those deriving from past relationship to any authority, they also reflect expectations and wishes to receive help, to be guided, taught, informed, supported and gratified. These also represent the desire for the leader to be like a helpful parent. There can also be an anticipation that the leader will be a disappointing parent, reflecting experiences with a withholding, competitive or critical parental figure in one's past.

The presence of a leader who represents someone with whom one can identify, such as a woman leader in a situation which was predominantly male, may arouse fantasies of having some "special" access. These represent realistic expectations that such a person would indeed be able to understand one's needs and wishes and help fulfill them. These fantasies also arouse wishes and expectations from earlier life, such as the feeling that at last the good mother is there and will "make things right."

When Franklin D. Roosevelt died, very widespread reactions of mourning and depression were connected with the fatherly aspect of his leadership and the wartime crisis which had just been weathered. People felt they had lost the father who had protected them, and they felt vulnerable. John Kennedy aroused different kinds of expectations, and responses to him were also strongly affected by some of the magical promise which he offered to some people during his presidency, symbolized by the Camelot legend.

Transference responses that are felt towards a woman leader are complex. As with all leaders, one can consider these as generally positive or negative, although certainly they are not entirely one or the other. If the leader is able to accomplish more because of these reactions, to mobilize effective participation, respect, trust and create an aura of strength, understanding, resourcefulness or power, which facilitate the common task, some of the transference aspects can be considered particularly "positive." Positive usually means respectful, affectionate, supportive; and negative refers to the obvious distrust, dislike and resentment. Sometimes the leader, no matter what the merits of actual policies, seems to be able to do no right, possibly because he or she is seen as a representative of a disliked group or is mistrusted without being given the opportunity to demonstrate what he or she can actually do. Negative transference responses affecting a leader can arise from exaggerated and impossible expec-

tations and wishes, which can create distortions in assessing reality. This is particularly true if the leader is someone on whom one pins unrealistic hopes which then lead to disappointments. It can also be true when resources are limited and competed for. Those who are disappointed can also re-experience the competition and losses they felt as siblings. When women are leaders, identification of the leader as a woman can play the critical role in raising hopes and expectations. Realistic limitations on their realization or the actual role the leader must assume and the multiple functions she must serve can lead to limitations and intense disappointment if one had special expectations.

The following vignette illustrates one such experience. As the elected president of any group, there are commitments to that constituency as well as to maintaining one's integrity and consistent personal viewpoints. Some years ago, I was elected one of the few women presidents of a state psychiatric society. A bill which was being considered by the legislature at that time had been in process for a number of years. The bill proposed reimbursement for psychiatric services by non-medical professionals. The society membership had been polled in the previous administration and had voted against the bill, in collaboration with the medical society who had taken a very strong position in this regard. This stimulated many complex political considerations including relationships with the other disciplines involved and the medical society. It tapped into emotionally charged issues of hierarchy and status. As we know, women in the fields of health and mental health have tended to not be the physicians and not achieve positions of highest power, but to occupy ancillary positions.

As president of the society, I believed that there was no alternative but to register the vote of the membership. A letter had been written to the legislature opposing this bill, and I signed it. Actually the letter was a revision of one that had been written by the former president and sent the previous year. It had been received by the legislature the year before without very much reaction or comment. A reporter from the local newspaper heard about this issue and tried unsuccessfully to reach me. She then wrote a story for the paper, focusing on this issue, including the letter and highlighting some phrases which could be interpreted as demeaning and critical to the non-medical practitioners. The reaction was immediate and extremely strong. I received many letters from all over the state from women who insisted that I had betrayed them. Although not members of the medical society, they had felt allied with me as a woman who had been visible and active in the field of women's health. They had also interpreted this interest as representing an alliance which would lead to political support as well. There was considerable distress at the position I had taken which was a "guild position" from a medical group. This reaction and the sense of betrayal lasted for several years, even in the face of my statements that I had not made a statement of individual philosophy, nor was this position different from the position the society had taken the year before. It was perceived as a lack of support for women rather than a reflection of a medical position.

This situation had an unexpected political impact, in that the groups were stimulated to lobby on their own and not expect support to come from another field. They did succeed in having the bill passed. Several years afterwards at a social gathering, I was introduced to someone by one person who had been quite prominent in that campaign. Both were administrators of fairly high rank. The first woman remarked that she remembered my name from the legislative issue, and she remembered me as having been on "the right side" and favorable to her position. I corrected her. But she was, at that time, disposed to a positive response to me and had the perspective of a leader and an administrator in her own field. She said, "As an administrator, I understand the position you had to take."

Both the intensity of the response and the personal sense of betrayal can be understood by paying attention to the expectation that a good mother, even in "an alien camp," would be able to set things right, to protect the women and their position. This was understood as support of the bill even though this went contrary to the stated wishes of the psychiatric and medical group. In addition, this support was thought to be of particular consequence, as it was their own efforts that were certainly important in the eventual success of their interests.

The countertransference issues also became strong. I noticed in myself an expectation that my "true self" would be recognized even though I had taken an antagonistic position. How could

anyone think I was "the enemy?" I found myself feeling some anger at being "misunderstood" and my efforts to promote peace and strengthen the alliance of the women not acknowledged. To be the "enemy" against women revived old concerns about maintaining harmony with the important women in one's life, particularly mother.

To shift to another aspect of the transference aspect in leadership, many women share, even in the 1980's, the devalued concept of being a woman. They still have deep-seated feelings and therefore suspicion that a woman may not have "the right stuff" to offer guidance in the high places that men frequent. There is also some concern about competing, particularly with other women. There have been few models and not much guidance in ways of managing aggression and competition with women colleagues. Coping with these conflicts is crucial in order to be an effective leader, but most women sense discomfort with these feelings. They bring with them residual aspects of their socialization towards a more "feminine" style rather than an openly aggressive one. They can also recall childhood experiences of feeling that open aggression and competition with others, particularly mothers, is dangerous and destructive. There have not been comfortable and acceptable channels for women's development of the direct expression of aggression except in athletics and achievement.

There is at least one study describing the reluctance of women in a particular system to choose other women as role models.[2] These women do not appear to feel that female role models would be helpful. They shy away from the stresses of managing potentially competitive relationships with people to whom one might need also to turn for professional recommendations and support.

There is some question about whether the expectations of a woman leader have more of the qualities of what one might expect of a maternal figure, such as nurturance, compassion, warmth, facilitation and support. Although it is legitimate to expect some of these from any leader, it is obviously not always possible. There are some suggestions that consequent disappointments may engender bitterness and an intense feeling of desertion and abandonment, rather than a more realistic acknowledgment of a situation which has not gone favorably.

Men respond to a woman leader with a different set of transference expectations. Although a "role model" may not be so explicitly involved, transference aspects also reflect men's experiences and expectations. If the woman leader acts in an aggressive or competitive manner, men may find themselves feeling that this seems inappropriate.

Men's reactions to women leaders contain transference aspects of their concepts of women in general and derive from their own personal experiences with the women who were present in their own lives. These include the conventional stereotypes about women. Even with the social changes of the last years which have resulted in many more women entering the professional world and becoming leaders, there has not been an eradication of attitudes about what constitutes appropriate "feminine" behavior. Even men who have elected a woman to leadership or support her in that position may find some conflict, often unconscious, between the qualities they would support in a man leader and those which they find disturbing in a woman. Among the latter are "bossiness" or behavior which is interpreted as "excessive" ambition or "excessive" aggressiveness or "pushiness." Some of the classic social maneuvers which have been reported by writers of the last 20 years or so still do take place. For example, women who participate in a group discussion which may consist of very high level people report that their contributions are attributed to the man next to them or to the one who may have preceded them. Even a woman chair who is leading a particular meeting may find that her remarks or comments are attributed to others. This may seem hard to understand unless one approaches it from the point of view of the irrational aspects of people's responses. Ignoring or misattributing women's remarks is not necessarily deliberate rudeness or lack of respect for that individual. There is a discontinuity or a dissonance set up by the combination of an assertive leader and conventional expectations of what is "appropriate" for a woman. These may be combined with depreciating or critical attitudes which may not be conscious but which may result in devaluation of the woman's contribution. These attitudes may be less likely to be expressed in behavior if the situation is a clinical interaction, but can re-emerge in a meeting or discussion.

Another form in which attitude toward a woman leader can be strongly influenced by transference factors is the sexualization of responses. Although the relationship is not in itself a sexual one, one can bring to it sexualized feelings from past relationships. This can be particularly important when a man has not had much experience with women in authority who are peers or near-peers. A man, for example, can attempt to turn a professional relationship in a direction with which he is more familiar if it is with a woman who is closer to his age and who does not readily evoke a maternal transference reaction.

The sexualization may be an attempt to establish familiar ground but also to shift the power balance. Traditionally, the male/female sexual interaction has involved the man as the more powerful figure. On one occasion at a farewell celebration for a woman leaving for a better job, one of her co-workers commented on her attractiveness as part of the public farewell speech.

As women leaders become more visible and prominent, responses to them are likely to become less exceptional. However, the potential for transference reactions influencing not only the responses to a leader but the perceptions of the effectiveness of a leader are extremely important to keep in mind. These judgments may appear to be based on objective interactions, but may at the same time contain elements of the sense of fit between one's conscious and unconscious internalized expectations of women and one's actual experiences, all of which color the assessment.

One other aspect of this dynamic pattern is that a woman may evoke less competitiveness in men, at least initially, since the interaction does not evoke the familiar male patterns of games and struggles for status. She can perhaps be listened to with some more openness, if the other aspects do not interfere.

As more women leaders in medicine emerge and social expectations change, there will be different varieties of expression of some of these underlying and enduring dynamic realities. It will be interesting to see what forms they take and how they can be utilized for effective leadership.

References

[1]Sandler B and Hall R: The Classroom Climate: A Chilly One for Women? Project on the Status and Education of Women of the Association of American Colleges, 1982.
[2]Brown S-L, Klein R: Competition Among Women in Medicine, American Psychiatric Meeting, Dallas, May 21, 1985.

29

A Conversation with
Paula Clayton, M.D.

Leah J. Dickstein, M.D.

*Associate Dean for Student Affairs
and Associate Professor,
Department of Psychiatry and Behavioral Sciences,
University of Louisville School of Medicine,
Louisville, Kentucky*

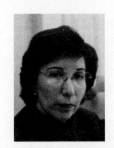 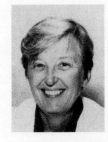

Leah J. Dickstein, M.D.   **Paula Clayton, M.D.**

29

A Conversation with
Paula Clayton, M.D.

Paula J. Clayton, M.D., has been professor and head of the Department of Psychiatry at the University of Minnesota Medical School, Minneapolis, since 1980. Prior to that, she was on the faculty in psychiatry at Washington University School of Medicine, St. Louis, where she earned her M.D. in 1960.

Interview: November 30, 1984

As an undergraduate I was a botany major, taking a major that was fun and consistent with premed. There were no doctors in my family, but my mother was a very energetic, hard-working woman, a former teacher. She stopped teaching when she got married, but she was a suffragette, so there was a family tradition of being independent and committed. My mother was very much in favor of my going into medicine and so I had a lot of support. She had this enormous amount of energy and did not need much sleep.

My father was an interesting guy who was much less energetic than mother and I have two sisters, and we all work full time and always have. One is a teacher, and the other was a teacher but became an editor of a university magazine. My father wanted us all to have college educations as he and my mother had had, but I don't think he thought beyond that. Marriage probably was what he had in mind. He did not encourage me and he was not happy with the idea that I was going to medical school. He humored me through college but was surprised when I applied to enter medical

school. By the time I graduated, however, he was quite proud and pleased with my career. He supported me financially at all times. My father, an accountant, was an executive in a clothing firm.

I didn't plan to be an administrator and in fact, it never occurred to me. When I was a medical student, I didn't know I wanted to go into psychiatry; when I decided to go into psychiatry, I didn't know I wanted to do research. And when I was running a large research project and an inpatient unit, it didn't occur to me that that was administration. Perhaps I decided to become an administrator because I thought that was what I was trained to do. If you stay around a place long enough, you assume more and more responsibilities and naturally work your way up to being a candidate for chairperson. And Dr. Guze, my chairman at Washington University, consciously trains faculty members for chairs by talking freely about problems, positions, promotions, political issues and so forth. You need mentors in all aspects of academic life--research, teaching, and administration.

Washington University is a medical school where the students are held in high regard. A lot of time is spent with them, and they are taught to be very rigorous, critical and curious in their thinking. We were required to do research projects as first year students. So I imagine the groundwork for my interest in research was probably laid in medical school. I chose psychiatry because I liked what the psychiatry faculty were teaching at Washington University. In that department every resident was required to do research. I thought that was fine and I enjoyed it, though I didn't think of myself as ever wanting to write. I certainly had no idea that I could write or give speeches, although my mother did both, something I learned after her death.

The way I started doing research was good. There were always ongoing projects in the department. At one point Dr. Winokur asked me to follow up a few manic patients. They all had psychotic symptoms and he wanted to know what their subsequent courses were. The resultant paper was written mostly by others and I wrote only the clinical histories which I found easy to do. It was a good paper. Later, I did my own project on bereavement, stimulated by Dr. Winokur, ostensibly to differentiate a reactive depression from an endogenous one and I started a big project with Dr. Winokur (The One Grand Study). Dr. Eli Robins, who was the chairman at that time, was a rigorous teacher. He had ideas about everything; titles on papers and slides, how many lines should be on a slide, what tables should look like in a paper, how to collect and analyze data, in fact, exactly how to write a paper which was "short and to the point," and he read them all! When you presented at professor's rounds, he would correct your English. He wanted everything to be perfect and clear with no abuse or misuse of ideas. I had a group of very conscientious mentors, Dr. Eli Robins, Dr. Sam Guze, Dr. George Winokur and Dr. Lee Robins.

Being a woman was as much an advantage as a disadvantage. It never mattered as a resident or faculty member except that as a woman I was on "the lunch brigade." I probably met more notable people than most young faculty members. I'm sure some speaking engagements, symposium participations, memberships in associations and elected offices, as well as chairmanship opportunities, were because I'm a woman. Growing up in a city with a significant black population like St. Louis, it would be hard to think of yourself, a white woman, as an underdog or disadvantaged.

At my interviews for possible department head, they did ask about my husband though not about my family. Although they probably were more concerned about that because I'm a woman, most committees find out if a man's wife works and if she's enthusiastic or neutral or opposed to moving. There are lots of things that aren't asked on a first visit. At the first visit I'm never sure who's

selling whom. The schools are trying to put on a good show and certainly the candidate is too. There were always women faculty members and/or women chairs on the committees, as well as other women such as nurses, social workers, students, lay people and practitioners. I wasn't concerned about whether there were other women on the faculty; I was more concerned with whether this was a job I could enjoy. Psychiatry has always been my major interest, so I was trying to assess psychiatry in those places.

When I moved, my husband was a practicing attorney, and he had to start over. He did that, but there probably was some resentment. And one child was openly resentful; in fact, for a year he was angry. The other two were in college and so it was easier for them.

I don't know what I expected this job as department head to be, but I would say that I underestimated the amount of time it would take to do it. What happens is that my research suffers. I don't have time to do my research, and I miss it. So I would say that the job is different than I expected, and I don't find it as pleasurable as I thought.

For the most part, I imagine other chairmen appreciate having a woman. I think women are different than men in that they are a little bit more direct. My impression is we don't do as well at compromise. I think there is an "old boys' network" that is consistent with the personalities of men. I find that women are often less willing to give in when they should. They don't sit down and talk and work things out as easily. My peers here might say that I am a little less compromising, which is true. Partly, however, I do it because I think that they don't always see the other side of issues. In the long run, I sort of vote the way they do, but I may bring up alternatives just to get them to think about them. We women may be less compromising but we also are less arrogant. One of my male mentors once said to me, "I'm amazed at how selfish and petty faculty members can be." Even with that warning, I'm still amazed at some of the problems and issues that surface in this department, particularly from males. On the other hand, maybe successful women are more like men. I've never thought of myself as having a Type A personality. I can usually wait in long lines without feeling stressed. But there are certain things I like to get done, so I must have some of the Type A traits.

I've met women who have been chairs in bio-chemistry and pediatrics. As a pregnant medical student I presented a Department of Medicine Grand Rounds to Dr. Sheila Sherlock, a world renowned professor of medicine from England. A basic science chairperson has his or her own set of problems that are entirely different from those of a clinical chair. And psychiatry is different from other clinical fields, so I haven't gone over problems with other chairwomen.

The faculty members are very supportive in Minnesota, both the men and the women, but the women are extremely supportive, which I guess I'm a little surprised at because I'm not as supportive as I should be to them. I really feel that women faculty members have to be promoted on the same grounds as men, and so I cannot support men's or women's promotions when they don't have what I think of as the right criteria.

Minnesota has always had many women in medicine and this has not been by accident. They really do worry about women's rights. They've always had a number of women both in medical school and in residency programs. I try to interview all prospective residents so they know how I think. We probably get more women applicants because of me, but not many. Residents come more because of the training we offer or because they want to be or stay in Minnesota.

I make time to teach the residents and each of the undergraduate medical student classes. Some women students come to talk if they're interested in psychiatry. An occasional woman comes because of psychiatric problems. We have a woman associate dean, and she is particularly interested in the women students.

I do some mentoring. I think it has to be started in the residency program, and I haven't had that many residents who've been interested in research. I started an affective disorders clinic, and I was hoping I could interest residents in doing research. So I've done mentoring in a clinical sense, but not in a research sense. I try to read papers that people ask me to read, but I do not read every paper the department produces. I am not as conscientious as my mentors. Our department consists of about 70 psychiatrists, psychologists, basic researchers, and residents.

The ideal goal as an administrator is to be creative and to develop something that wasn't there before. It may be creative to make psychiatry more visible and acceptable and available.

Developing people into the roles of researchers or administrators is another creative process. I hope some of my newer professors go on to be chairs. Serving as a department chair is slower work--you have to be patient because it takes longer than in clinical research to see the results.

As a woman you have to decide priorities because you are asked to be a representative more frequently than men. In the mid-seventies before I took this job, two events made me suddenly realize that I was prioritizing. In one instance someone offered me $2000.00 to write an interactive computer learning program on depression. I went home that weekend and tried to write these questions and found that I had no interest in it. On Monday I told them I wouldn't do it. I was glad that money couldn't seduce me into spending time on something I didn't enjoy. Then the second instance occurred when I was asked to run for president of an important psychiatric organization. I decided that I didn't want to get into that kind of administration, so I said, "No." It was quite enlightening for me to understand that I really knew what I got pleasure from, and I set my goals in that direction. You have to do that if you are going to enjoy your husband and your family.

I am convinced that research is one of the best backgrounds for administration. In order to make decisions you need to gather general information and specific data. If you're very well-trained to do that in research, without meaning to, you apply the same techniques to administrative decisions. Plus, research teaches you to interpret data and to admit what you don't know. As always, knowledge is power.

I would encourage women to do two things: First, to do research and to collect their own data. That is extremely important because you cannot expect others to do your work for you. Second, women must write those papers. These are the building blocks for an academic career.

Residents and young faculty women ask me about being department chair, but even more they ask me how to become a researcher. They are much more interested in that question. If I go to a university to give grand rounds, they may have a meeting of women faculty, and we discuss their concerns related to appointments and tenure.

I think advancing was possible for me because of the medical school I attended and the department I stayed in. They had had other women who had worked hard in research, so I wasn't a trailblazer. When I finished my residency I had three children, so I chose to work one-quarter time and I was home many hours. The department allowed me to do only research and teaching over the next eight years. I gradually worked my way to full time. The department of psychiatry I came from allowed young faculty members lots of time for research and required senior faculty to teach, to be responsible for patient care, and to administrate.

I like to work and I discovered that back in St. Louis. I came home one Saturday and my husband, who likes to garden, was out there cultivating his beautiful flowers and I said, "You know, I really like to work." That has to be part of it--I really enjoy learning.

30
——

Women and Leadership in
Departments of Psychiatry

————————

Carol C. Nadelson, M.D.

President, American Psychiatric Association;
Professor and Vice-Chairman, Associate Psychiatrist-in-Chief,
and Director, Training and Education,
Department of Psychiatry,
New England Medical Center,
Boston, Massachusetts

Patti J. Tighe, M.D.

Associate Professor and Director of Education,
Department of Psychiatry,
University of Chicago School of Medicine,
Chicago, Illinois

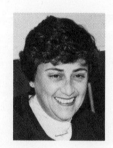 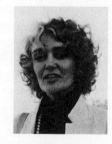

Carol C. Nadelson, M.D.   Patti J. Tighe, M.D.

30

Women and Leadership in Departments of Psychiatry

History

We can look back with pride at the gains women in medicine have made in the last few decades. Twenty-five years ago women were 5.7 percent of medical students, now they constitute more than 32 percent.[1] There has also been an increase in women faculty at all levels. There are women chairing academic departments and women are entering fields of medicine they had not previously entered. But, lest we become sanguine about our achievements, we must look carefully at our history and at current trends and indicators. Women also made great strides forward in the past, but, unfortunately, each time they have fallen back. We must wonder if our direction will be different this time.

In 1900, 24 percent of the medical students and 18 percent of the physicians in Boston were women, and the Medical College of Pennsylvania had women deans prior to its name change when it became coeducational in 1969.[2] Between 1910 and 1960 the percentage of women physicians in the United States, however, remained a stable, low 4-6 percent.[3]

As we pursue this history of women in medicine, we find a pattern of decreased participation of women with each step toward greater academic organization and formalization. Even in the 5th century A.D. women who had been leaders in public health and hospital administration were forbidden by the Council of Trent to continue in these roles. By the end of the 15th century, when

medicine became established academically in various European centers, women were increasingly excluded from formal involvement and were specifically limited to functioning as midwives. This reflected a wider societal trend and it occurred in the context of the ideology of misogyny as encapsulated in the Malleus Maleficarum (A.D. 1486). The "spiritual and mental" inferiority of women was interpreted to mean that the only roles for which they were suited were traditional caretaking ones, or those that involved the care of women and their reproductive functioning.

In early colonial United States, where there were few formally trained physicians, and no medical schools, the healing role of women was critical to survival. However, when the first American medical school was founded in 1765, it excluded women. In the 19th century, since women were barred from "regular" medical training, many were trained in homeopathic or eclectic traditions and set up practices without diplomas. In 1847, when Elizabeth Blackwell became the first woman to be admitted to and graduate from a "regular" medical school in the United States, the New York State Medical Association promptly censured the school.

By 1850, three all-female "irregular" medical colleges had been founded in the United States, but these were designed to be separatist institutions to "protect female delicacy." When Harriet K. Hunt, who had established herself in an "irregular" practice in Boston, applied for admission to Harvard Medical School in that year,

she was admitted, as were several black men.
However, she was denied her seat when the all-
male class threatened to leave if women and
blacks were admitted. It was not until almost 100
years later, in 1946, that Harvard Medical School
first admitted women.

In the United States medical societies continued
to refuse admission to women and hospitals
denied them appointments. In general, those
women who were graduated were from middle- or
upper-class backgrounds and often had fathers or
husbands in medicine so that they entered medicine to join their families in practice. The patients
of the first generation of women physicians were
largely poor women and children.

The resistance to women in medicine was consonant with prevailing views about women. An
1848 textbook on obstetrics said, "She (woman)
has a head almost too small for the intellect but
just big enough for love." In 1905, Dr. F. W.
VanDyke, President of the Oregon State Medical
Society, noted that "hard study killed sexual
desire in women, took away their beauty, brought
on hysteria, neurasthenia, dyspepsia, astigmatism
and dysmenorrhea." "Educated women," he
added, "could not bear children with ease because
study arrests the development of the pelvis at the
same time it increased the size of the child's brain
and therefore its head. This causes extensive suffering in childbirth."

Despite these views, by 1900 over 50 percent of
the class at Boston University and over 40 percent
at Tufts were women. Some medical schools at the
end of the 19th century had commitments to
admit women because they were persuaded to do
so by a variety of means. Johns Hopkins, for
example, was opened after it received a sizable
endowment from a few wealthy women on the
condition that women would be admitted on the
same terms as men. Interestingly, despite this history, Johns Hopkins has never had a woman department chair.

The situation changed for women in medicine
rapidly after the Flexner Report of 1910.
Medicine increasingly became an established
academic discipline with high standards for training and practice. As a result, a number of medical
schools were closed. Among these were the ones
that had admitted women, the less prestigious and
less wealthy schools. The number of women entering medicine began to decrease rapidly.

Flexner's explanation for this pattern stated:

"Medical education is now open to women on
practically the same terms as men. If all
institutions do not receive women, so many do,
that no woman desiring an education in medicine
is under any disability in finding the school to
which she may gain admittance. . . . Now that
women are freely admitted to the medical profession, it is clear that they show a decreasing
inclination to enter it."

This view could hardly explain recent data indicating that between 1970 and 1975, when overt
efforts were made to attract and admit women,
the number of women entering medical school
more than doubled very rapidly. Whether we look
to the misogyny of 15th century Europe or the
"learned" views of the 19th century, explanations
indicate that the belief in women's inadequacy for
leadership or intellectual pursuits has been pervasive and it clearly affects the perceptions and
behaviors of both men and women.

The percentage of women physicians remained
stable and low between 1910 and 1960 (4-6
percent). As the numbers have increased, however, some aspects have not changed substantially.
The number of women on medical school faculties
remains low, particularly as one ascends the
academic ladder, and women continue to take
longer to reach higher ranks. By 1981, 16.2 percent of medical school faculties were women of
whom approximately half were women physicians,
and women comprised 5.3 percent of professors,
13.0 percent of associate professors and 19.8 percent of assistant professors. Although the numbers
of women in medical school nearly tripled between 1968 and 1978, there was a gain of only 1.9
percent in the proportion of the female faculty.[4]

Women are proportionally underrepresented in
administrative and other leadership positions, and
few women serve on specialty boards or are
department chairs. Until four years ago, there
were no women deans (and currently there are
none), and at the present time there are no
women members of the Association of Academic
Health Centers of the American Association of
Medical Colleges. In 1978, 33 women chaired
academic departments out of approximately 2,400
positions and by 1980, 56 chairs were occupied by
women. Women occupy approximately 2 percent
of the total number of academic chairs. In pediatrics more women hold chairs than in any other
specialty, but only 7 percent of pediatric departments are headed by women, although 28 percent

of pediatric faculty are women. Today, 65 chairs of medical school departments are women; of these, 50 are full chairmen and 15 are acting or interim chairmen.[5]

If we look at other fields, we find parallels to medicine. In the last decade, the proportion of women in college and university administration declined both in women's institutions that have become coeducational and in women's colleges that have remained single-sex institutions. While approximately 26 percent of all college professors are women, women represent only 10 percent of full professors. The salary differential between women and men faculty is increasing, not decreasing.[6]

Higher female enrollments also have been reported for other traditionally male dominated professions such as architecture, engineering, the sciences and law. What is evident, however, is that in all of these areas, despite these increased numbers, there is a wide gap between the proportions of men and women in professional training and those who have attained positions of prominence and responsibility in their fields.

Less than 10 percent of judges are women. They also represent only 12 percent of local elected officials, 5 percent of the U.S. Congress and 2 percent of the Senate. While there are now 400 women, according to 1984 figures, on major corporate boards, there are 16,000 men. In spite of the dramatic influx of women into the corporate world, the women in middle management represent 5 percent and in top management 1 percent.

From one perspective, this disproportionate underrepresentation of women in positions of leadership is to be expected as the increased numbers of women only recently entering these fields have not yet had the opportunity to attain these positions. At the same time, however, we must understand our historical lessons if real change is to occur. In the past, when women have had a significant influence on health fields, external factors have often been influential, including wars, physician shortages and major cultural reorganization. Attitudinal changes have followed. The changes brought about by expedience or pragmatics, however, invariably reverted to previous patterns of gender role differentiation when circumstances changed.

When, for example, in the Soviet Union, midwives proved themselves to be effective as doctors in the Russo-Turkish War of 1870, the influx of women into medical schools began. After the 1917 revolution, when the prestige of medicine was reduced, women were admitted to medical school in even greater numbers. It is important to note that recently, as medicine has attained a slightly more prestigious position in the USSR, the number of women physicians has fallen. The number of women physicians in the Academy of Medicine, however, has always been exceedingly small (less than 10 percent).

The Psychological Milieu of Women Leaders

Let us consider the dynamics--intrapsychic, interpersonal and systemic--of women in medicine and particularly in leadership. While the compassionate and caretaking roles of the physician certainly do not inherently contradict "traditional" views of women and women's roles, the technological and instrumental aspects and the status of the physician appear to be at variance with these traditional views. We will explore the concerns of women as they pursue leadership positions, using as examples what we have learned in our roles as training directors in academic departments of psychiatry. We will share our experiences and those of others in similar kinds of positions to clarify and elucidate areas for further study and action.

Women aspiring to leadership roles are generally aware that unanticipated and even surprising reactions occur in response to gender, even from those who are manifestly egalitarian. Gender related distinctions, so ingrained in our culture and in our colleagues, male and female, change slowly. We have all grown up with internalized values, attitudes and expectations from our own past and from the collective past. Thus, greater uncertainty and resistance to change exist than is often appreciated early in one's career.

Milwid,[7] from a study of women leaders, including vice presidents and managers in male dominated fields (banking, law and architecture), recently reported that these "successful" women felt excluded from office networks, increased resistance to them in higher echelons and a sense of intractability of the male culture in their fields. They had all seen themselves involved in a revolution which seemed to have been won. They reported that during their graduate school days, gender was no longer assumed to be a limitation, and few had anticipated that it would be a factor affecting their professional lives. They all believed that hard work and merit would carry them along. One said, "I guess I didn't realize how male dominated the world is until I got out of law school. Although my class was only 25 percent female there were always a lot of women around the campus. It was surprising to me to end up in the courtroom with no other women."[8]

In 1977, Rosabeth Moss-Kanter[9] described the role of women in corporations in four ways: as mother, seductress, maiden aunt or kid sister. Milwid suggests a fifth category, the good daughter. The women she studied reported being deferential and careful to be non-threatening. She notes that "the psychological baggage women bring to masculine culture is packed with the need to be nice and to be liked." Thus, they experienced considerable anxiety and all of those interviewed indicated that they needed to learn how to be more assertive, firmer and more self-confident.

For these women, as well as for other women in leadership roles, the beginning of their careers brings an excitement borne of energy and enthusiasm for the future. Too often this is modulated by subsequent events, including the subtle nuances of disappointing interpersonal and transferential responses. In academia as well as in corporations, all new faculty and administrators, male and female, experience certain areas of difficulty, particularly as they become aware of the complexity of assuming positions which assign them more responsibility than authority. But for women there are often special conflicts accompanying the necessity for making unpopular decisions, defining priorities and making choices, particularly since these may constitute compromises with previously held values and beliefs. This occurs in part because of the internalized self-concept of most women which does not include roles of authority, assertiveness and leadership. In addition, women have been described as having greater needs for affiliation which determines their style of interacting.[10] This focus on relationships brings a greater sensitivity to being disliked and criticized and a need for approval which is reinforced by early learned patterns of dependence and passivity. Lack of peer support, mentors or models functioning in similar roles or assuming equivalent responsibilities adds a further complication. Thus, women must cope with their own and others' internal resistance to

assuming the attitudes and behaviors necessary for effective leadership. They must be alert to the manifestations of contradictory self-perceptions.

While obviously there are different styles of effective leadership, there are some common requirements for organizational ability, independence, decisiveness and assertiveness. Aspects of these are often unfamiliar to women.

As Moulton[11] indicates, women are accustomed to the "good girl" role. Bright industrious women often have achieved success by maintaining a self-effacing facade, avoiding situations of possible disapproval, relying on authoritative directives and not saying "no." They are unaccustomed to open rivalry or hard negotiation. Some research[12] suggests that women become more anxious after asserting themselves whereas men feel a sense of relief.

Assumption and projection of authority are problematic for many women who feel uncomfortable about abandoning the culturally assigned "feminine" traits of responsiveness, accommodation and nurturance or allowing the emergence of others which are often seen as "masculine" e.g. assertiveness, competitiveness, decisiveness. Because of ambivalence about these aspects of identity, women in positions of leadership experience conflict between their needs for competence and success and the comfort of a socially sanctioned role. Relinquishing familiar postures may be at the cost of reduction in self-esteem and loss of traditional affirmation.

The concept of androgyny[13,14] offers a conceptualization of personality traits that does not rely on the traditional polarizations of masculine and feminine. It hypothesizes that individual characteristics can operate independently of each other i.e., so-called masculine and feminine traits can co-exist in one person without conflicting. Indeed, the data indicate that those with more of both traits tend to be more adaptive and flexible in their functioning. While this perspective may point toward encouraging future directions, how it will translate into attitude and behavior is far from clear.

Beyond these psychological phenomena, cultural expectations also have substantial impact on women's leadership. As sociologists have shown, women's opinions spark negative and resistant responses and their credibility in positions of leadership is significantly less than men's, on the basis of their gender.[15] Since women are socialized to achieve vicariously and to measure their success by the success of individuals to whom they are related, with whom they identify, and to whose success they have contributed, direct acting on their own behalf is unfamiliar.[15] In positions of authority men lead predominantly men to whom they relate as peers and competitors; women lead predominantly men to whom they are socialized to be less assertive. Clearly these factors must influence the success of women in leadership roles.

The power of gender role expectations is illustrated by Mayes'[16] description of the analysis of a 17-month series of Tavistock group experiences held at a university undergoing major turmoil as the result of an effort by university women to gain greater access to positions of power and authority. The groups consisted of psychiatrists, nurses and graduate students. Mayes found significant and pervasive differences in behavior depending on the gender of the group leader. In female-led groups, male members were hostile and generally refused to cooperate, speaking and initiating conversation infrequently; or they were dependent, trying to gain the leader's approval by being "good boys" and expressing resentment about the lack of female closeness and fears about their masculinity. The men described feelings of loss of control because their ability to function "as males" was hampered. These men expressed great relief and a sense of "return to normalcy" when able to join male-led groups. Initially the women in female-led groups were assertive, instrumental and task-oriented. Over time they became "less assertive, less identified with the leader and sought to keep male attention in a traditional manner." Women who refused to relinquish their assertive roles received the majority of male and female anger and expressed confusion and fear about the future of relationships with these men. Groups with male leaders reported traditional sex-role patterns of behavior in both men and women.

Women as Leaders in Academic Departments: Training Directors

In examining issues of leadership for women physicians, we must recall that medical training and organization are deeply rooted in an achievement-oriented paternalistic model and that the profession enjoys a position of social approval,

esteem and success. As research from many fields describes male response patterns of testing or ignoring the reality of a female's authority, we may expect these tendencies to be intensified in a field structured as is medicine.

Women leaders, even those in major positions, e.g., college presidents and judges, report that in group discussions their ideas and opinions are often ignored, depreciated or trivialized. It is not unusual for these women to find that these same ideas are repeated by a male member of the group as his own and accorded acceptance. Research in areas as diverse as patterns of decision-making in families and sex-role differentiation in jury deliberations indicates that resistance to women's analyses and presentations creates serious obstacles to female organizational leadership.[15]

A response often reported by women in authority is the attempted sexualization of relationships by male colleagues, ranging from overt sexual advances to more veiled but transparent gestures. Women physicians report similar experiences beginning early in medical school, when, for instance, a male professor asking a woman medical student for a date may find her willing but only because she is aware of his potential power over her. Male fantasies of such encounters can be used to rationalize a woman's achievements, i.e., she is seen as successful not because of her own efforts or abilities, but because she is "sleeping with the right person."

While exact figures are difficult to obtain, it appears that in medical school departments of psychiatry, women are offered the position of director of medical student education with much greater frequency than that of residency director. Female membership in the Association of Directors of Medical Student Education in Psychiatry is 12-15 percent, while in the American Association of Directors of Psychiatry Residency Training it is less than 2 percent. Generally viewed as a lower status administrative post, the role of director of medical student programs is "almost tailor-made for the stereotypical view of a woman as soft, warm, compassionate, motherly, and only aggressive in the service of furthering the interests of her children."[17] Residency directorship or the inclusive "director of education," however, embodies significantly greater power and authority at all levels of departmental functioning.

The training director's role includes determination of the overall philosophy of training, acquisition of funds, administration of educational programs, decision-making about clinical and didactic educational content and resident recruitment and selection. The potential for conflict regarding power, control and leadership in these areas is apparent.

The training director also integrates various units of the program and in this role develops relationships with inpatient and outpatient services as well as with clinics and training sites off campus. This aspect of the job requires coordination, monitoring, allocation of resources, evaluation and priority setting, all of which can evoke negative responses for men as well as women. Responses can range from resentment to outright hostility when, for instance, the training director provides negative feedback about students' educational experiences to faculty colleagues or exercises appropriate administrative firmness about equitable assignment of trainees to a given service.

When the training director is female, general issues related to power are compounded by gender-role expectations. The leadership and authority of the training director tend to be elements incongruent with faculty and trainee internalized expectations of female behavior, and while the role itself embodies so-called feminine qualities, e.g. nurturance, caretaking, it is likely that anticipation of these responses is aroused more readily with a female training director than with a male. The substantial literature on women in managerial and administrative positions, including women in academic psychiatry,[18] highlights the problems inherent in assumption of power by a woman in a department where the major power is held by men. Lack of familiarity and comfort on the part of both men and women may evoke responses ranging from paternalistic reassuring to ignoring the reality of the female administrator's authority. The explicit exercise of authority by a woman can evoke regressive and demanding postures, petulance and fear of a loss of control to a woman. Outright resistance may be manifested by behaviors such as refusal to attend meetings or to participate in course reviews and going over her head for budgeting approval. An implicit expectation is that because she is a woman, the training director should be non-judgmental and supportive even in her administrative position.

Envy and competitiveness on the part of male colleagues may take the form of overt or subtle denigration of her "femininity" and minimization of her real accomplishments. When the training director is responsible for acquisition of increased curricular time or initiates and effects an affiliation with a new hospital she may find her colleagues attributing these successes to causes as variable as "systems factors" unrelated to her input or the assumption that some male capitulated to her out of "weakness" or in deference to her femaleness rather than because of her competence. On the other hand, successful negotiation may lead to acknowledgment of her political astuteness, with the implication that this trait diminishes her womanhood.

When she makes an error, the reaction of a male colleague may extend beyond the relief commonly experienced when anyone powerful fails. It may reinforce the underlying belief that women are weak and incompetent. As Brown and Klein note,[17] "If a woman acts in any manner that possibly could be seen as 'unprofessional,' it immediately feeds into a much more punitive mythology about her, whereas for a man, such actions might only serve to enhance his appeal."

The transference aspects of the education director's role manifest themselves with residents and students as well as with faculty. The power and authority of a woman-mother evoke fantasies of special care, at times manifested by expectations that she can make changes in night call schedules, requirements and even salaries. Alternately, she may be perceived not as the leader or the seat of authority, but rather in the attenuated and diminished position of liaison or handmaiden to the faculty, having no power of her own.

The good mother/terrible mother dichotomy described by Neumann[19] is reflected in interactions with trainees. The good mother is supposed to be nurturing, loving, and compassionate; the terrible mother is feared to be devouring, dangerous, and punitive. If expectations of the good mother are frustrated and she is not more sympathetic and understanding, overlooking infractions or mistakes, then she is likely to evoke more "primitive" fantasies, often still expressed in terms of "castration" threats. For women students and residents if she is not the "good" mother, association with a woman in authority can stimulate disavowal of identification, competitive feelings expressed as denigration of her accomplishments and even echoing of the stereotypic name-calling. These trainees are thus deprived of the role models and mentors they so clearly desire. A male education director in the same circumstance, who addresses issues directly, is seen as simply doing his job, being firm and consistent. Even if he does not meet demands, the anger evoked may not emerge from the same depth or be expressed with the same intensity. Likewise, constructive or disciplinary criticism from a woman may be experienced by a trainee as rejection rather than simply "being graded" for a specific task. A male specifying expectations and monitoring performance is experienced more often by trainees as appropriately setting limits. The woman in this situation may be interfering with the accepting, idealizing mother/child experience.

While everyone in a position of leadership is familiar with aggressive, competitive, hostile and demanding responses, the experience of women is unique because of these early maternal transference issues. The powerful and persistent affects aroused by the child's helpless dependency on the maternal figure include envy and rage. These may be defensively dealt with by depreciation and devaluation of women.[20] As Lerner indicates,[21] our gender definitions and sex-role stereotypes may reflect an attempt to reinstate and retain, in adult relations, the nurturing qualities of the so-called good mother without any element of dominance or control. They may take further shape from the need for revenge resulting from the profound narcissistic injuries inflicted on the infant by the omnipotent mother.[22]

We have looked at responses to the woman in authority, but what about her experience as an "authority." She may become demoralized and distance herself, intensifying the loneliness and isolation often experienced by the "solo woman in a group."[23] Role confusion and anxiety can lead to compromise in her functioning and ultimately to failure to achieve the educational objectives of the program. Women in senior positions who did not "grow up" with women peers find their expectations for sustenance and support for their achievements unmet. They often face even greater pain when their "daughters," the women students and residents, respond to the powerful terrible mother they may have become and are rejecting and dissatisfied. Drachman,[24] in her eloquent description of the history of the New England Hospital, clearly alludes to a similar phenomenon in the 19th century, and this is consonant with Chodorow's[20] delineation of the special mother-daughter tie and its implications for separation, as well as closeness.

Future Directions

Obviously, many complex dynamic constructs are operative in the interactions of men and women with women in authority. Understanding these allows us to predict some elements of the evolution in attitudes and behaviors which can lead to appropriate constructive change. We know that in all cultures gender-stereotypes are rooted in powerful psychological constellations related to deep-seated needs, expectations and fears. Since we have the legacy of our history to help us predict the future, we must face the likelihood that change will occur slowly and that gains made in one generation may be lost in the next.

Psychiatrists must seek increased awareness of the role of gender in the determination of attitude and response in all relationships. We must continue to educate ourselves and our students in these areas. There is much to do. As Lerner[21] points out, psychiatrists have tended to incorporate stereotypes into their concepts and language. Practitioners and theorists persist in using perjorative labels as they describe active displays of competitiveness, aggression and intellectual ambitiousness in women as "phallic" or "masculine" and similarly label manifestations of passivity, submission, malleability and dependency in men as "effeminate" or "feminine." As recently as 1965, a prominent American analytic writer commented, " . . . as much as women want to be good scientists or engineers, they want first and foremost to be womanly companions to men and to be mothers."[25] Have we progressed far from Freud's "dark continent" of femininity with its transference-laden tone of foreboding and sense of an alien, fearsome specialness of women? A small number of contemporary psychoanalytic writers (mostly women) have recognized the "intense cultural pressures that combine with intrapsychic factors to encourage women [to] accept neurotically dependent, self-effacing solutions in life."[26] But we as a field have not turned our attention to these writers, and systematically investigated gender issues. As Lederer[27] commented, " . . . of our fear and envy of women, we, the psychoanalytic-papers-writing men, have managed to maintain a dignified fraternal silence."[27]

The introduction into some residency programs and a few psychoanalytic institutes of courses in Women's Studies, the Psychology of Women, etc. heightens awareness that an issue exists. However, since the elements of transference determined by gender are significant and pervasive in all relationships, we must move this field from the status of a peripheral or special-interest topic to a central place in our thinking and education.

We must prepare the way for increasing numbers of women in leadership positions in psychiatry. The prior experience of many male psychiatrists does not include women as peers, colleagues and "chiefs." As the balance in departments of psychiatry shifts to more women, we must move toward assumption of roles based less on stereotype and more on full utilization of individual potential.

Women aspiring to leadership roles must learn the history of women and understand their own experience within that context. They must be prepared for more criticism and greater career uncertainty than male peers. They must plan to cope with powerful internal resistances to assuming some of the attitudes and behaviors which today will facilitate effective leadership. The combination of their "female" socialization and their "male" career aspirations may have produced confused and contradictory self-perceptions and self-concepts; women must be alert to their manifestations. Realizing that the discontent with and perplexity about their work situations will lessen only gradually, women must be prepared for the loss of time and energy spent thinking about and coping with gender related attitudes and realities. Informal networks have played a central role for men, as the counterpoint to formal organizational structure. The small numbers of women in each field require that women develop networks outside their own workplace with other professional women in positions of leadership. They will find the colleagueship supportive of their own emotional, social and intellectual needs and the contacts invaluable for career advancement and personal evolution.

References

[1] AAMC Data Files, personal communication, Kathleen Turner, December, 1985.

[2] Flexner A: Medical Education in the United States and Canada: A Report to the Carnegie Foundation for the Advancement of Teaching. New York: The Carnegie Foundation, 1910.

[3] Walsh MR: Doctors Wanted: No Women Need Apply. New Haven: Yale University Press, 1977, p. 186.

[4] Braslow JB, Heins M: Women in Medical Education: A Decade of Change. N Engl J Med 304 (19):1129-1135, 1981.

[5] AAMC, Kathleen Turner, personal communication, December, 1985.

[6] Rinke C: The economic and academic status of women physicians. JAMA 245(22):2305-2306, 1981.

[7] Milwid ME: Women in Male Dominated Professions: A Study of Bankers, Architects, and Lawyers. Doctoral dissertation, Wright Institute, Berkeley, CA, 1982.

[8] Milwid ME: as quoted in Bernikow L: We're Dancing As Fast As We Can. Savvy, 1984.

[9] Kanter RM: Men and Women of the Corporation. New York, Basic Books, Inc., 1977.

[10] Gilligan C: In A Different Voice. Cambridge, MA: Harvard University Press, 1982.

[11] Moulton R: Some Effects of the New Feminism. Am J Psychiatry 134:1-6, 1977.

[12] Dunbar C, Edwards V, Gede E, et al: Successful Coping Styles in Professional Women. Can J Psychiatry 24:43-46, 1979.

[13] Bem SL: Sex Role Adaptability: One Consequence of Psychological Androgyny. Journal of Personality and Social Psychology 5(3):260-267, 1967.

[14] Spence JT: Traits, roles and the concept of androgyny. In J.E. Gullahorn (ed), Psychology and Women: In Transition. Washington, D.C.: V.H. Winton & Sons, 1979.

[15] Lipman-Blumen J: Emerging Patterns of Female Leadership in Formal Organizations: Must the Female Leader Go Formal? in M Horner, C Nadelson, M Notman, (eds.) The Challenge of Change. New York: Plenum Press, 1983.

[16] Mays S: Women in Positions of Authority: A Case Study of Changing Sex Roles. Signs: Journal of Women in Culture and Society 4(3):556-568, 1979.

[17] Brown and Klein: Women-power in Medical Hierarchy. Journal of the American Medical Women's Association 37:155-164, 1982.

[18] Robinowitz C, Nadelson C, Notman M: Women in Academic Psychiatry: Politics and Progress. Am J Psychiatry 138:1357-1361, 1981.

[19] Newmann E: The Great Mother. Princeton, NJ:

Princeton University Press, 1955.

20 Chodorow N: The Reproduction of Mothering: Psychoanalysis and the Sociology of Gender. Berkeley: University of California Press, 1978.

21 Lerner H: Early Origins of Envy and Devaluation of Women. Bulletin of Menninger Clinic 28:538-553, 1974.

22 David CA: A Masculine Mythology of Femininity. In Chasseguet-Smirgel J, et al. Female Sexuality: New Psychoanalytic Views, Ann Arbor: University of Michigan Press, 1970, pp. 47-67.

23 Wolman C, Frank H: The Solo Woman in a Professional Peer Group. Am J Orthopsychiatry 45(1):164-171, 1975.

24 Drachman V: Hospital with a Heart. Ithaca, NY: Cornell University Press, 1984.

25 Bettelheim B: The Commitment Required of a Woman Entering a Scientific Profession in Present-Day American Society. In Women and the Scientific Professions: The M.I.T. Symposium of American Women in Science and Engineering, J.A. Mattfeld & C.G. Van Aken, eds. Cambridge, MA: M.I.T. Press, 1965, pp. 3-19.

26 Symonds A: Discussion (of Ruth Moulton's paper, "Psychoanalytic Reflections on Women's Liberation"). Contemp Psychoanal 8:224-228, 1971-72.

27 Lederer W: The Fear of Women. New York: Grune and Stratton, 1968.

31

_____

A Woman Associate
in the Dean's Office

_____

Leah J. Dickstein, M.D.

*Associate Dean for Student Affairs
and Associate Professor,
Department of Psychiatry and Behavioral Sciences,
University of Louisville School of Medicine,
Louisville, Kentucky*

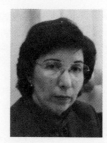

Leah J. Dickstein, M.D.

31

A Woman Associate
in the Dean's Office

I had not planned to include my own personal experiences in this biographical collection about the giants among women leaders in psychiatry. I consented to do so rationalizing that my evolution could balance these magnificent role models with one who is more like many competent readers of this book.

In late August 1981, at the time I accepted being catapulted into my present role as Associate Dean for Student Affairs at the Medical School, I had not planned it. However, through the benevolent and opportune efforts of one of the school's (and my) most respected and beloved teachers and colleagues, Dr. Mary Hilton, and the ready enthusiasm of Dean, Donald R. Kmetz, M.D., I began this new role. In addition to this serendipitous turn of events, a number of experiences and role models enabled me to actualize early fantasies of becoming a physician.

I grew up the older of two daughters in a working class family. My father, William Chernoble, is a high school graduate, now a retired linotypist, who read the New York Times daily. My mother, Sadye Engelman, was a formally educated, full-time home-maker. We lived in a walk-up apartment house which faced one of the largest city hospital complexes in Brooklyn: the Kingston Avenue Hospital and the Contagious Diseases Building of the 3,000 bed Kings County Hospital, now Downstate Medical Center. I can still vividly and poignantly recall the summer of 1947 when, at age 13, I heard the constant wailing of hundreds of children stricken during one of the last severe polio epidemics. I watched their parents file in and out of the Contagious Diseases Building looking distraught and helpless. Occasionally, I was invited to play with the Kingston Avenue Hospital physician-director's children on the hospital grounds where they lived. Brooklyn State (Psychiatric) Hospital was only two blocks away. I heard tales of what kinds of people were taken there and occasionally passed bathrobed patients on our street as they escaped.

Born on August 17, 1934, I experienced World War II from a number of vantage points. I listened to male air raid wardens direct that our apartment windows be draped in black, followed female teachers' directions to take cover under desks and in hallways in practice drills, and rolled and rerolled bandages I kept in an empty White Owl cigar box of my father's, which I turned into a first-aid kit. I saw my father drafted into the Navy and leave for the South Pacific on a light cruiser not to be heard from for months at a time.

My mother, a full-time homemaker after she married in 1932, became a volunteer and an immediate leader for a number of organizations--U.S. Bond Drives, Polio Mothers and Hadassah. The latter is a national Jewish Zionist organization whose women raised hundreds of thousands of dollars to help Holocaust survivors, particularly children, and Hadassah Hospital and Medical Organization in Jerusalem. She blossomed with enthusiasm through her creative and joint efforts with other women and worked with fervor and boundless, joyful energy to become president of

Maimonides, a local Hadassah chapter, as well as a regional leader. In addition to raising money and running all kinds of programs, she used her musical talents to write songs and skits, as well as play the piano and sing in these programs. Although she had graduated from Bushwick High School at 16, and from Brooklyn's Maxwell Training School for Teachers in 1929 at age 19, (one of 453 women and 22 men), she had not been able to obtain a teaching job in those Depression years. Instead she worked as she could, the longest period in a magazine publishing office. In her late 40's, she accepted an office job after I had left home, and once again I saw her genuine pleasure in accomplishment and collegiality along with more financial independence. I consciously vowed then to ensure that I would work outside my home even if I married and had children.

At the turn of the century, my maternal grandmother and grandfather, Gussie Finestein and Jacob Engelman, came to New York as teenagers with family members from Brest-Litovsk, Russia-Poland. They were also role models of volunteer-leaders, who worked for those less fortunate. My grandmother's efforts were with the Pioneer Women, a Jewish group of Zionists, and my grandfather's efforts were with the Labor Zionist Organization, the Farband, and with helping to organize a Jewish Folk School in Brooklyn in the 1930's. He also helped a young general practitioner build his practice, and this man, Mendel Klepper, our family doctor, impressed me with his quiet gentleness, skillful care and childlike spirit as he came to our home to treat earaches and sat on my bike and played the piano before he left.

I had the emotional luxury of a large and loving extended family, many within walking distance. I also enjoyed the Brooklyn public libraries, whose books, including *Arrowsmith, Marie Curie* and something about Freud, I flew through as I imitated my mother.

From my father's side, I formed the secret fantasy of becoming a physician as I heard about his mother's brothers who had become physicians in the Russian-Ukraine and in America. One of these great uncles had, so the story went, cleaned spitoons in Chicago's subway system while working his way successfully through medical school there. I met only one of these professionals, a dentist, who was loving and caring to his extended family.

In 7th and 8th grades I had leadership roles, including editorship of the school newspaper under the guidance of a male English teacher, Mr. Lewis. At Erasmus Hall High School, I struggled with algebra and with my father's help passed with honors, to continue on with advanced math classes and to later serve as vice president of the math honor society. I took only biology and a required general science course, as my mother had occasionally mentioned how hard she found physics.

Due to family finances, I felt my only option was to attend Brooklyn College, where I was told on matriculation in 1951 that my placement tests showed I had no scientific ability. I therefore took the safe way out, majored in elementary education, worked as much as I could at numerous tutoring jobs and in my Uncle Sam's printing plant as a proofreader-copyholder and office assistant in Manhattan by day, and at Brooklyn College's Student Affairs office at night, in fact seven days a week during my senior year. I graduated with honors, married and moved to Belgium to be with my husband as he completed medical school.

I was accepted as a non-matriculated student at the University of Ghent and passed the oral exams in Flemish for the year-long clinical psychiatry and criminology courses in the medical school in 1956. I was fascinated at lectures where patients were interviewed and when we visited psychiatric hospitals. I finally obtained a Belgian work permit, not an easy accomplishment for a foreigner, and was the only European representative for a New York-based girdle and bra company. Though I had no formal training, I actually obtained one order from the largest department store in Brussels! Fortunately I then secured a job for the next two and one-half years at a local Berlitz School as a professor of English. I also gave private lessons to a surgeon in his home clinic one night a week.

Upon returning to New York, I resumed teaching at a public elementary school, occasionally taught night English classes for foreigners and began to work toward a master's degree in education. I continued taking pre-medical science courses as my husband completed his pathology residency at Kings County, after obtaining my M.S. Then I met Dr. Carolyn Weber, a pathology resident who worked with my husband. We became friends, and I shared my dream with her.

She, he and other friends cheered from the sidelines as I completed the requirements and began the application process. The premedical adviser, tried to dissuade me from applying. By this time I was pregnant. After two years I gained acceptance to two U.S. schools, Meharry and Louisville. I chose Louisville because it appeared I would have some free time in the mornings to be with our two-year-old son, Stuart. I received one rejection the day after he was born with my application fee returned. The Admissions Dean of that school stated he had decided not to waste my $5 in presenting my application to the Committee because I was 32 with an unproven track record and a new child.

My years in medical school were happy, challenging and very satisfying. As the oldest, and one of the seven women in a class of 96 students, I felt accepted and energized. When I occasionally became discouraged with the workload, and conflicted about not being a full-time mother, my husband, Herb, would tease saying, "You're right; you have no scientific ability and probably should be home full-time." That always spurred me on.

At that time women could not join any of the medical fraternities. They were important because they provided a support network and access to old exams. On the wards the women students were often mistaken for nurses and dressed in nurses' uniforms in their dressing rooms. Sleeping accommodations for women were scarce. I can recall "sleeping" in a labor room with a patient in another bed, or on a stretcher on a ward. One midnight in an operating room, the surgeon demanded that I get an instrument. When I looked puzzled, the resident apologized to the attending, stating, "She's only a medical student, not a knowledgeable nurse!"

I received my M.D. degree in 1970 and tried pathology for my internship year. I learned a great deal, but I missed patient contact. My dream since age 8 was to become a psychiatrist. After taking six months off to be home with our second son, Daniel, I found a wonderful woman, to care for him. I began a psychiatry residency. Our last son, Steven, was born at the end of my second year in residency. Mrs. Forrester, our baby sitter, and my husband made it possible for me to devote my energies, in a less stressful manner, to becoming a psychiatrist.

To corroborate that I indeed was competent, I took the three boys to London, England for sev-

eral months during my last year with two social work students to help. I worked hard at the Maudsley Hospital and at the Tavistock Clinic. I also visited a number of world-reknowned facilities and returned with a new sense of professional confidence. For the first six months of my last year, I had enjoyed serving as chief resident.

As I planned to enter private practice, Dr. Edward Landis, professor of psychiatry and medical director of one of the Department's facilities, suggested I join the faculty. I accepted a newly available part-time position as psychiatrist at the University Health Service in 1975 and currently continue this work. Until 1981 I served as founder and director of the Mental Health Section of the Health Service, where we offered a variety of services to all students and training opportunities to psychiatry residents, medical students, psychology, social work and pastoral counseling trainees.

Through the encouragement of the Health Service Director, I became involved in the American College Health Association, eventually serving as chair of the mental health section in 1981-1982 and as president of the regional Mid-America College Health Association in 1980-1981. Through the encouragement of Dr. Harvey St. Clair, my first long-term supervisor during my residency, I became involved in the State Psychiatric Society, serving in all offices and eventually becoming the first woman president in 1981-1982. Dr. John Schwab, our department chair, encouraged and assisted in my initial attempts at research and in consistently supporting my attendance at national meetings.

I attended my first American Psychiatric Association meeting in 1976. On a shuttle bus, I introduced myself to Dr. Elissa Benedek, whose work I had read. Her sensitive welcome and ensuing encouragement, as well as role modeling of effective leadership, can still always be counted on. That initial encounter with Elissa was the beginning of a women's national network for me, which has been vital to my continued professional evolution and at times personal constructive coping.

I was asked to organize resident seminars in 1975 on the subject of the new psychology of women. I spent much of the year reading the literature and becoming a more conscious and informed feminist. These lively and well-received seminars for second year psychiatry residents continue and in recent years include the new psychology of men.

About 10 years ago with an interested cadre of students, I developed a support program, The Student Hour, for entering students after school commenced. I worked with Dr. Joel Elkes to develop The Health Awareness Workshop, a voluntary, educational and support program for entering students and their significant others, held the week before the onset of classes. The obvious usefulness and evident pleasure everyone participating has experienced have made all our efforts worthwhile. In fact my husband, Herb, himself an accomplished painter, organizes an evening's art exhibit, and my youngest son, Steven, and I wrote a children's workbook for the Workshop. It is evident that early small steps in leadership have meshed in what I clearly feel are useful and personally satisfying directions.

Four and a half years as associate dean have allowed me numerous opportunities to develop a variety of programs for the benefit of students and, hopefully, for the School. In the early 1980's, I began a voluntary freshman student-community clinician match which allowed students to watch clinicians in action on a one-to-one basis. I have continued to teach medical students and residents required, as well as a number of elective, courses I have developed, the most recent in the area of physicians and the arts. This course, in its third year, is one means of interesting students in developing constructive artistic outlets to cope with ongoing stress and responsibility.

All of these varied experiences have been extremely useful in my attempt to be an appropriate, available, useful and creative associate dean for Student Affairs. My research and teaching interests, as well as clinical experiences in dealing with current women's and men's issues, have definitely been of benefit to the Student Affairs Office's functioning. Currently, my serving as the only woman in administration in the dean's office has been enlightening, I suspect for everyone. In direct and subtle ways I have consistently tried to educate students and involve faculty about gender issues and alternative coping strategies.

I also served as first president of the local branch of the American Medical Women's Association. A few years later I became state director and I have just stepped into the role of Councilor for Professional Development at the national level. In the last several years I have enjoyed the privilege of serving as the University's women's

liaison officer to the Association of American Medical Colleges. I mention these offices to encourage others to begin gaining leadership experience and skills locally and in a variety of settings. These experiences with men and women colleagues have balanced the clinical responsibilities I have thoroughly enjoyed and have enabled me to feel connected to the greater psychiatric and medical community. In fact, I always refer to my time at meetings in both formal and informal sessions as my psychotherapy.

It seems clear to me that my ongoing enjoyment of the clinical practice of psychiatry is vital to my functioning as part of the Dean's office. The variety of activities and opportunities for creative functioning and interactions with colleagues in student affairs throughout the country enables me to look forward to the arrival of each new day with excitement. As an administrator I also want to acknowledge the steadfast support, patience and humor of my staff. I believe I have effectively awakened or strengthened their feminist and creative tendencies, also with humor, as they have enabled me to function competently.

My sons, who have attended meetings with me, have become feminists and assistants in various projects from videotaping women physicians for a book on the *History of Women Physicians of Kentucky*, to being part of The Health Awareness Workshop staff and assisting in Freshman Orientation each year. Their homemaker skills have enriched their coffers as they have relieved me. Herb has also joined me in several professional ventures, as well as household engineering roles, talking about our dual career family and being a panelist of physician-artists who encourage medical students to maintain or discover independent and artistic expressions as a way to decrease stress and enjoy the fruits of creativity.

Serving as associate dean for Student Affairs is a natural professional role for a psychiatrist and a parent, and not unexpectedly, a woman. Nurturing and encouraging young professionals' development are fun, especially with parallel opportunities to use power constructively and creatively, reaching across all medical school departments. I am pleased when women and men faculty and staff seek counsel about professional and personal matters. Three years ago I offered to counsel each of the juniors during the spring and summer regarding residency selection before writing their Dean's letters. Despite the often overwhelming time pressures, the task has allowed me access to many students I had not met through student government, The Health Awareness Workshop or academic and personal problems. In addition, being so visible and available can breakdown barriers and dispel myths about psychiatrists. My commitment to health promotion and prevention of impairment is well known. I am no longer surprised or amazed at the number of students in particular who come for consultation about family, medical and personal problems and I attempt to respond appropriately.

I have enjoyed my three committee assignments for the APA (American Psychiatric Association): Comprehensive Health Care Planning, Scientific Program Committee and Medical Student Education. Through each I have developed invaluable and rewarding professional contacts with men and women nationally and across our northern border. Most recently I have begun a term in the Assem-

bly representing the women's caucus. Encouraging students and residents to participate in their respective organizations and to attend medical meetings has been an important task. I have also gained satisfaction in helping young clinicians enter local leadership tracts. Serving as our branch's chair for the committee on women and, with colleagues' encouragement, as secretary to the recently organized Association for Women Psychiatrists have been among my most valued responsibilities and challenges.

What is apparent, but needs to be stated, is that I could not have achieved my childhood fantasy of becoming a physician nor fulfilled current, unexpected commitments, emergencies and programs as well as ongoing responsibilities, without the generous and sensitive support and sacrifices of my husband of 30 years, my numerous mentors and friends and my children.

32

Women in Psychiatry:
A Canadian Perspective

Judith H. Gold, M.D., F.R.C.P.(c)

*Private Practice and
Associate Professor,
Department of Psychiatry,
Dalhousie University,
Halifax, Nova Scotia, Canada*

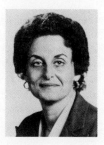

Judith H. Gold, M.D., F.R.C.P.(c)

32

Women in Psychiatry:
A Canadian Perspective

The role of women in Canadian psychiatry cannot be discussed without first briefly examining Canada's unique medical care system. The Canadian medical system is presently in a state of flux with considerable confrontation between physicians, their medical societies and the provincial governments. The disagreements center on payment methods which physicians fear will insidiously develop into salaries. They guard against encroachment on their freedom to practice as they please and dread income capping. These disputes have been ongoing for almost twenty years.

On July 1, 1968, the federal Canada Health Act introduced government paid medical care. Despite widespread protests about the lack of consultation with physicians and fears that the freedom of medical practice would be curtailed, medicare was established. Funded by a cost-sharing agreement between the federal government and the provinces, it provided Canadians with free health care. Earlier free hospitalization had already begun. Some variations already existed in different provinces, but essentially health care since 1968 has been financed by government rather than the individual.

The impact upon physicians and health care delivery has been considerable. Guaranteed fee-for-service payments meant increased income for most doctors, but negotiated fee schedules formalized inequalities between the various specialties and between specialists and general practitioners. Psychiatrists found themselves at the lower end of the scale, caught by time. Unable to increase the number of services offered in an hour, they could earn more only by working longer hours. Despite concerted efforts by every provincial medical association, psychiatry remains one of the lowest remunerated specialties along with pediatrics and followed only by general practitioners.

This is a definite dilemma for the profession. It further limits the attractiveness of the specialty to potential residents in psychiatry and continues the image of psychiatry as a less-valued branch of medicine. Even though fee scales vary interprovincially, psychiatry's financial position does not. Fees are adjusted annually through negotiations between each provincial medical association as "bargaining agent" and each provincial government department of health. Specialties are able to make representation only through their provincial medical association. The federal government is not involved in this aspect. The Canadian Psychiatric Association has been assisting the provincial psychiatric associations.

Psychiatry's low position in the fee scale has led many psychiatrists to opt out of the system particularly in provinces, such as Ontario, with especially poor remuneration. As a result Canadian medical practice patterns vary widely from area to area, often even within a province.

At present Canadian health care costs about 7.4 percent of the Gross National Product (GNP) and has varied little in the past decade. Physician costs are approximately 1 percent of the GNP and have been stable since 1975. Thus, despite the fuss over added billing by doctors, the greatest part of health costs remain administrative and technological. However, the medical profession generally does not receive favorable press coverage, and information about actual costs is often unreported or buried.

The government is also concerned about the growing supply of physicians in Canada. For the first time some doctors are receiving unemployment benefits. On the other hand, there is a shortage of psychiatrists throughout Canada except in a few large urban centers. At present just over 2,000 psychiatrists are registered with the Royal College of Physicians & Surgeons of Canada. The largest group is under 45 years of age, reflecting the slow increase of those going into the specialty. Obviously, 2,000 is a small number for a population of over 24 million. Even within the profession there is a further shortage of child psychiatrists, and few are psychoanalysts.

Like all medical specialty training, psychiatric training in Canada is overseen by the Royal College of Physicians & Surgeons of Canada. Four years of training after medical school are required with two of these being "core years." The remaining two years must include at least six months of chronic care experience. A rotating internship is preferred but most residency training programmes will accept straight internships in psychiatry. After two years of training acceptable to the College, the resident can sit a written examination and, upon completion of four years, an oral examination. Once certified as a psychiatrist by the College and possessing a licence to practice medicine in Canada, the physician can be registered as a specialist by the medical board of the province of residence. Such registration is a prerequisite before the medical care plan will reimburse the physician as a specialist.

The Task Force on Women of the Canadian Psychiatric Association (CPA) was established in response to the concerns of some women physicians that psychiatric training and practices were not attuned to the needs or the psychology of women. This Task Force arranged a symposium at each CPA Annual Meeting as well as frequent invited lecturers. In addition, it provided input into the training requirements developed by the Canadian Committee of Psychiatric Educators (COPE), which resulted in a section on gender-related issues. Members of the Task Force endeavored to convince their university training departments to include lectures, seminars and psychotherapy supervision which focused on the special problems of women. Despite much effort, only a few psychiatric departments in Canada have done so. However, the Task Force has provided a valuable support group for its members as well as encouragement to women residents.

Over the years the number of women in psychiatry has increased steadily. Of the 2,000 psychiatrists in Canada, 373 are female (February 1, 1984). Of these, 218 are under 45 years of age. This reflects the fact that, at present, about 50 percent of Canadian medical students are women. Practice patterns of these women psychiatrists have yet to be examined, but it can be assumed that, as in most professions, they will work slightly fewer hours and years than their male colleagues--for obvious reasons. Considering Canada's system of health care payments to psychiatrists, women psychiatrists will be among the physicians with the lowest incomes, which will clearly have an effect on recruitment in the field. However, the great demand for psychiatrists will compensate.

The Task Force on Women has now become a CPA Section with commensurate formal and permanent status. Women are still under-represented in elected offices of CPA at both national and provincial levels. This is, of course, partly due to the fact that so many women have become psychiatrists only within the past decade.

The Canadian Psychiatric Association was founded in 1951 with two women among the small group of charter members. However, since then, there have been only two women on the Executive Board of the Association and one woman president. There has been a slow increase in the number of women who are members of the CPA Board and Councils. The CPA is a national association whose members comprise about 85 percent of all psychiatrists in Canada. Every province has its own association and sends a predetermined number of elected members to sit on the national Board. The Association has had only two chief administrative officers since its foundation and both have been women.

The Canadian Psychiatric Association also publishes the *Canadian Journal of Psychiatry*. There has rarely been a woman member of the editorial board, but at present one associate editor is a woman psychiatrist.

As the number of women completing specialty

residencies has increased, the Royal College has made some attempt to appoint women as examiners. However, the ratio of women examiners reflects neither that of candidates nor of practitioners. The same problem is also apparent in the committees of the College. It is maintained that this is because few women hold academic positions in Canadian psychiatry but, certainly in the last decade, reflects the traditional male-oriented selection process. In addition, there has also been a notable absence of women as training program directors. At present only one woman psychiatrist holds such a position, although there are 16 training programs in Canada.

Because there are relatively few psychiatrists in Canada, it is possible for most to know each other, except in the large urban areas where it is easy to disappear into private practice, and many, especially women, have done so. A university appointment can help remove this anonymity, as can active membership in the local psychiatric association. Through these avenues women become involved in the wider psychiatric political and educational world. However, in the larger centers women must, of course, compete with male colleagues for the few available positions and generally lose out. Hopefully women will soon assume more appointments and elected offices by the sheer growth in their numbers as well as by their own increased willingness to become involved. The old struggle between career and family responsibilities continues for many women but is eased by the support now offered to each other in many places. Nevertheless traditional "old boy networks" remain and are difficult to change or remove.

However, some Canadian women have chosen another route by becoming active in their local American Psychiatric Association district branch. At present all three district branches in Canada have had a woman as president or president elect. On the other hand, only a few of the ten provincial psychiatric associations have ever had women presidents. This is a definite reflection of competition and existing bias.

History

The first Canadian woman to practice medicine in Canada was born in 1831. She was also the founder of the Canadian suffragette movement, and later in 1883 her daughter was the first woman graduate of a Canadian medical school. The medical colleges for women opened simultaneously in Toronto and Kingston, Ontario, in October 1883, and after a few years were absorbed into the University of Toronto. The early women physicians often became missionaries in India and in Africa, but many were involved in the care of the mentally retarded and, by the early 1900's, in psychiatry.

By 1920 one woman, Dr. Helen MacMurchy, had become head of the Division of Child Welfare in the federal government in Ottawa and was named one of the leading women physicians in the world. She was also prominent in the Canadian Medical Association and had considerable influence on federal policies regarding the health of mothers and children.

In 1931 another woman, Dr. Eliza Brison, became the psychiatrist for the province of Nova Scotia's Department of Health and Welfare, while another, Dr. Ella Hopgood, was appointed assistant superintendent of the Nova Scotia Mental Hospital in 1928. Meanwhile, Dr. Elizabeth Kilpatrick graduated from Dalhousie Medical School in 1915 and practiced psychiatry with Karen Horney in New York. Later she returned to Dalhousie and, upon her death, left her estate to benefit the residency training program of the psychiatry department at Dalhousie University.

A number of other women were also practicing psychiatry in Canada from the 1930's on, mostly in various cities in Ontario. Dr. Mary Jackson is the most prominent among these and was a founding member of the CPA. She was also responsible for the design of the presidential medal and seal of the association. These examples demonstrate that women have been active in Canadian psychiatry throughout the century but have generally remained in the background. They continued in a supportive traditional role even within their profession. This has been true not only in psychiatry but in all of medicine in Canada. One notable exception has been Dr. Bette Stephenson, who became the first and only female president of the Canadian Medical Association and later a cabinet minister in the Ontario provincial government.

More women are becoming physicians. In 1911, 2.6 percent of Canadian doctors were female; in 1964, 7 percent. Today 50 percent of medical students are women. Studies have shown that about 87 percent practice, and that this figure is only slightly lower than that of male graduates. Most women still enter pediatrics, anaesthesia and psychiatry, where regular hours allow more family time. This is also changing as women refuse to follow old patterns and assumptions. While this is encouraging for women in general, it is not indicative of a continuing increase in the number of women becoming psychiatrists.

The combination of the lower fee scale for psychiatrists and continuing secondary status of women within the psychiatric profession may still outweigh the inducements for women to enter psychiatry. Sheer numbers of graduates could increase trainee enrollment for a time, but as the other specialties become more attractive and welcoming, psychiatry may find itself struggling to attract residents. As more women graduate from medical schools, more programs will find that male residents are actually in the minority. Perhaps then the longstanding male networks will have to crumble, and women will have equal representation in both political and academic medical offices. It is unfortunate that this may be the only effective solution to overcome conservative attitudes in Canadian psychiatry.

As the first woman to become president of the Canadian Psychiatric Association, I experienced support as well as discouragement and resentment from both male and female colleagues. It continues to be necessary to remind psychiatrists to think of women as well as of men for offices and positions. Yet it is also necessary to encourage and push women forward, to ask them to go beyond their cultural reluctance to be involved in more of medicine than caring for patients. The strengths that allowed them to go to medical school and into residency years must be reorganized toward participation in the larger sphere of medical politics. After all, it is in that arena that policies are formulated and enacted.

It is conceded that women have avoided such involvement in Canada. I found it difficult to persuade women psychiatrists to become active in the CPA. They pleaded lack of time due to the demands of family and of practice. Some who agreed to participate initially did not carry out the responsibilities of the position they had accepted. On the other hand, some who wanted to do more were hindered by their male colleagues who often outmanoeuvered them in obtaining offices. Some women were impatient and unwilling to go through the steps necessary for *anyone* to advance.

They demanded immediate results, and their emotions obscured the obvious pathways.

A great deal is being written lately about the use of "networks" and "mentors." While the words may be tiresome by now, the concepts they embody are very real. Women are learning how to utilize both, despite the fact that this is not easy. Political networks and mentors are usually male, and women find it difficult to distinguish between offers of assistance and attempts at seduction. This is understandable, given the usual male-female interactions, and a suggestion to go for a drink and a chat may often be difficult to interpret correctly.

At the same time, women are not always comfortable with women mentors either. No doubt this is connected to the sexual competitiveness of our society, but also, must have links to unresolved conflicts with female siblings and with mother.

Whether trying to work with men or with other women, women are not accustomed to the purely rational approach. Sensitivity and intuition can overrule professional responses and hinder the formulation of strategy. We require much more training in the techniques of leadership.

Women are very gradually becoming more evident in the psychiatric hierarchy in Canada. However, the numbers are few and footsteps are allowed to grow cold and disappear. It is not just a matter of male domination, but also of permitting this to be so. Canada is a large country with a widespread population. Many women practice in isolation from other women but have not been able to advance with and through their male counterparts. They have yet to learn what the former mayor of Ottawa, Charlotte Whitton, meant, who when asked, "Is it true that women have to work twice as hard as men to obtain the same recognition?" replied, "Yes, but it's so easy."

Bibliography

Gray C: Few all-male bastions left in medical practice. CMA Journal 123:1046-1051, 1980.

Hacker C: The Indomitable Lady Doctors. Toronto: Clarke, Irwin and Company Limited, 1974.

Last JM: Sexual inequity in medical care. CMA Journal 123:834-838, 1980.

LeBourdais E: Is the noble experiment a failure? Canadian Doctor November: 50-56, 1984.

Penfold PS, Walker G: Women and the Psychiatric

Paradox. Montreal: Eden Press, 1983.

The Royal College of Physicians and Surgeons of Canada, Analysis of Fellows in Good Standing, Feb. 1, 1984.

Thompson MGG (Ed): Resident's Guide to Psy-chiatric Education. New York: Plenum Press, 1979.

Vincent MO: Female Physicians as Psychiatric Patients. Canadian Psychiatric Association Journal 21:461–465, 1976.

33

Women and Leadership
in Medicine in Australia

Beverley Raphael, A.M.M.D., FRANZCP, FRC

Professor and Chairperson,
Foundation Professor of Psychiatry,
University of Newcastle,
Australia

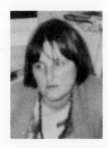

Beverley Raphael, A.M.M.D., FRANZCP, FRC

33

Women and Leadership in Medicine in Australia

To understand the leadership issues for women physicians in Australia it is necessary to understand the place women have held in Australian society and culture generally and the many changes that have occurred in recent years. The prototype of woman's role in Australia since European settlement commenced in 1788 has been that of "Colonial Eve," as one author has called it.[1] Women came to help and support their menfolk. The majority of the first women in this country were female convicts; later many women came as free settlers, with their husbands to help them establish lives in this new country. Many of the early convicts were condemned to the penal settlement for relatively minor or political crimes and there were, at various stages, many rebellious men and women amongst these, for example, the Irish. These early Australian women sometimes, when freed or free settlers, established themselves well in the new community, with its free standards and lack of rigid class structure. And some found minor leadership roles in business or in power in the early society. Yet, as elsewhere in the world, women's place was seen as ancillary to that of men.

Many Australian women in the early days of settlement lived lonely and isolated lives on sparsely populated outposts of civilization in the grey emptiness of the Australian bush. They often suffered and died in childbirth and saw many infants born yet few raised to adult life. Even from the early time this society developed a special closeness for men, and the concept of "mateship"

became a predominant theme in Australian life. By this is meant the closeness of men and their friendship and intense ties of loyalty, ties which often came ahead of any friendship between men and women, who may have seen little of each other and have had little to share except the pain and struggle for existence. Nevertheless, women early built their place in the various colonial states that would subsequently become the Australian nation.

From about the 1850's a new influx of colonial settlers occurred and the country expanded phenomenally. The gold rushes heralded this period of growth and development. There was extensive rural expansion with great sheep and cattle runs in the arid inland, expansion of the urban centers and growth of business and industry. Population growth was very rapid with the population more than trebling in the 40 years before 1900, its rate of increase in those years being the highest in the western world. This increase had significance for women because it was chiefly due to increased births with the large number of marriages of a young population. There was also a high life expectancy. This population growth had further significance in that it largely overcame the imbalance of the sexes since Australia had been a predominantly male country until that time.

Furthermore, although the population at that stage had developed largely from Anglo-Saxon origins, the rigidity of class structure did not become entrenched in the Australian social system. The need for self-reliance in the bush, as the Australian countryside is called, and the growth of business and commercial interests leading to wealth and power for the middle classes meant that there were opportunities for families that would not have existed in Britain. State control also existed to support the underprivileged, and this meant that more women had opportunities for work and for education.

Thus women gradually gained opportunity and access within a social system that did not have a rigid class structure. This was further reflected in the granting of voting privileges to all women over 21 by the Commonwealth in June 1902 and in several states before this time. This achievement occurred without a great deal of political agitation.

Thus in many ways it would seem that the political and social system was flexible and open to opportunities for women to rise through various levels of society to find their place in leadership roles. Yet subtle influences prevented this from happening. It is only in recent years that leadership roles in the fields of business, academic life, politics and administration have become occupied by women, and the numbers are still few. The subtle ethos of mateship, the loyalty of men to one another, and the traditional view of women as the helpmates to men in this rapidly developing society meant that women's position was often inflexibly fixed to traditional roles.

This is well exemplified by the early struggles of women to gain access to medical education and to the practice of medicine. The first medical faculty in Australia was established at the University of Melbourne in 1862. At that time the idea of women practicing in this field was considered absurd, and a visiting American woman surgeon was refused medical registration. In the 1870's and 1880's some women studied medicine overseas. It was not until 1887 that five young women succeeded in storming the bastions of tradition at Melbourne University to gain entry to the medical faculty, two years after the first woman had been admitted to Sydney University Medical Faculty in 1885. They were, when they graduated, however, as were women graduates from Sydney University, excluded from residency positions at the major teaching hospitals.

The first woman to practice medicine in Australia was Dr. Constance Stone, who had gained her qualifications in North America and England and returned to commence practice in 1889. She

and other Melbourne women graduates eventually banded together to develop first a clinic and subsequently a hospital for women. This hospital, the Queen Victoria, became the largest women's hospital, run by women, in the world. Later women doctors in Sydney were to develop a similar large women's hospital run by women doctors.

These early women in medicine were, by their very roles, pioneers and leaders. They had taken enormous steps against much resistance from the community and from men. For instance, Queen Victoria, head of the British Empire as it was in those days, vehemently stated: "Let women be what God intended, a help-mate for men." She wanted to do away with "The mad, wicked folly of women's rights"[2] which would "unsex" them. And the distinguished Dean of Medicine at the University of Sydney in opposing the decision of the Senate to admit women in 1881 said, "I think that the proper place for women is in the home, and the proper function for a woman is to be a man's wife, and for women to be the mothers of our future generation."

For the most part women who overcame these barriers had only been able to accomplish this from the background of privilege--they had been brought up in well-to-do and cultured families who had supported and encouraged them. In many instances they had especially been supported by their fathers.

Over the early years of the twentieth century, women continued to graduate from our medical schools, but their numbers were small by comparison to the numbers of their male classmates. They usually did well academically, and many succeeded in specialist fields such as obstetrics, gynecology and pediatrics. In the care of women and children they made major contributions to health care in Australia, and many were internationally recognized. Nevertheless, once again their numbers were small. Even though some of these distinguished women married and had families, many did not. The theme was one of devoting their lives, their love and their psychological investment to medical work in their chosen fields. It was usual for these to be the fields that related to women and children, and it was rare for women to rise to leadership roles in fields such as surgery.

This type of leadership development was well exemplified by Dr. Kate Campbell, who was responsible for the development of neonatal pediatrics and became the first person in Australia to be appointed to an academic post in this field in 1929. Almost four decades later in 1965, she became the first woman president of the Australian Pediatric Association. She acted to improve the care of the newborn in Australia, and although she was situated in Melbourne, her work had implications for pediatric care throughout the country.

There was a gradual increase in enrollment of women in medicine during and up to the Second World War. Greater opportunities arose during the war years because of the shortage of medical practitioners, and many women became involved in active medical work in the fields of general practice, obstetrics and anesthetics, as well as pediatrics. Women started to appear more frequently in specialties other than these, but their numbers were very few. Women also started to take some leadership roles in medical politics and in academic life, but there were very few opportunities for senior posts, and the women who did rise to these were unusual.

When the author commenced medical school at Sydney University in 1952, of the 450 or so first-year students, less than a tenth were women and a small proportion likewise appeared at graduation. There were some women academics who taught preclinical subjects as well as senior women physicians who taught in the clinical areas. Dr. Margaret Mulney, for instance, a distinguished gynecologist, was one of the few role models for women students in terms of a leadership role in medicine.

This picture of small numbers of women students and graduates reflected major and current elements of the Australian society and culture. A woman's place was still in the home. Girls were likely to be told that there was no point in doing medicine because they would only get married and have babies and never practice anyway. This strong imprint of women's helpmate and ancillary role was still powerfully operant in the fifties and even to some degree in the sixties, although many women graduated, often very well, and practiced as capably and as long as men.

The need for change in the perception of women and in their roles in Australian society as a whole became highlighted with the rise of the women's movement. It can be no accident that Australian society bred perhaps the most vocal and outspoken of the feminists, Germaine Greer,

whose 1971 book *The Female Eunuch* spoke of the state of women-kind not only in the world, but also in Australia. The feminist movement certainly raised the consciousness of Australian women generally, and of medical women as well, to the issues of their stereotyped and ultimately narrow place in the society of that day. Whether change was already in progress in those decades following world and nuclear war, and was simply voiced by such movements, or whether it was induced by them is still not totally clear--perhaps both things are true. Nevertheless these changes also laid foundations with women and their daughters for it to be increasingly likely that they might see themselves as occupying leadership roles and that this would be an acceptable to do.

Another change in Australian society following the 1940's was the massive migration which again led to rapid population growth. Australia changed from an essentially Anglo-Saxon community to a multicultural society. Melbourne, for instance, a city of three million, is the second largest Greek-speaking city in the world. In the cities of Australia large population groups of Italian, Spanish, Eastern Europeans and many others added to a rich cultural mix. More recently large numbers of Asian and South American migrants have further diversified society. Women coming from these countries tended to see themselves in more traditional roles or in basic occupations and so added little initially to the substrate that might promote leadership amongst women. However, from this group and from the reawakening Aboriginal leadership, a number of women political and community leaders arose.

It is likely with second and third generations of migrants, opportunities for women leaders in medicine and other fields will follow. But because most migrants have come from traditional cultures they have not readily seen their daughters becoming doctors. Nevertheless, these resourceful, independent, achieving, and upwardly mobile people have brought a richness and complexity to Australian life that is likely to add to flexibility and breadth, and thus provide fertile background from which women leaders will ultimately emerge.

In more recent years two issues confront women as they consider career streams in medicine. These are the question of family life and career obligations and the conflict that may in fantasy, belief, or reality arise between these. Such conflict is not readily resolved. Because there have not been many women leaders in medicine, there are few role models of women in leadership roles successfully combining family life and career. I find that I often have women students coming to my office, just to discuss, perhaps only briefly, the issue as to whether or not it can be done. Underlying this, however, is the fantasy, not easy to dispel, that it must be done perfectly. This conflict is not unique to Australian professional women, but must be seen in its Australian context. We have a strong, early tradition from the beginnings of our colonial life that women came as men's helpmates and had importance and survival value in how they fulfilled traditional female roles of wife, housekeeper and mother. Even with recent population expansion by migration, groups came with the same entrenched traditional values.

Thus women have felt that they could be truly successful only if they could be "superwomen," perfect wives and mothers and perfect doctors. There has been a reluctance to manage both less than completely, and women doctors have often opted for one or the other: a highly successful career life with little or no family obligations or a highly successful family role of wife and mother with part-time general practice. Both these choices may be very satisfying to some women, but those who would wish to move to leadership roles and have a full family life may not easily see others ahead of them who have done so.

One way in which this appears is in postgraduate career streaming. To gain professional qualifications as a specialist in any field the young woman is likely to face a further five years of detailed competitive work, stringent examinations, and then the need for further development to gain consultancies or seniority in this field. Should she graduate at 23 or 24 years of age, as she may do in this country, and then undertake one or two years of residency, then five years of specialist training, she is likely to be well into her thirties and she may have no wish to postpone child bearing to this stage. If she embarks on it earlier she may find difficulties with discontinuing training or few opportunities to carry it out part-time as the needs of her children may dictate. Psychiatric training provides special opportunities for women to carry out their postgraduate work part-time and makes allowance for child rearing, but it is only most recently that other specialist training bodies have given any acceptance of this option.

Still, with such prolonged time spans the young woman doctor may feel she does not want to add further stress or commitment of years that will be required to reach leadership roles.

Women may face stresses or subtle barriers to leadership roles in medicine not just from their own conflicts and internalizations, but also from the responses of others. Husbands may not find it easy to accept their wives in senior roles in medicine. Even if they believe they do, they may have underlying resentments that cloud the success and the relationship. Social forces may also still subtly operate so that the woman's fulfillment of such roles is not accepted: she is not seen as the most appropriate candidate for the leadership position, or if she gets it, she is seen as less able to fulfill it adequately.

It is from such a background that the future forces of women in medical leadership will arise. Women students are now equal in numbers with men students in most Australian medical schools by natural selection on grounds of ability. Equal opportunity and antidiscrimination legislation mean that positions will be open to them at many levels, including the top. Whether they will be able to make the commitment and sacrifice along the way remains to be established, although it seems likely that many will. And increasingly there will be role models to guide some of their career development in this way.

Academic leadership roles held by women clinicians are very important in this context, for they are a guide to what is possible for students. About the mid-1970's women started to be appointed to academic posts in the major medical schools. Professor Kincaid Smith, a leading nephrologist, was the first woman professor at the Melbourne Medical Faculty. Professor Narelle Lickiss was the first woman professor of community medicine at the Tasmanian Medical Faculty and Professor Tess Brophy was the first professor of anesthetics at Queensland University, to name a few. I was the first woman to hold an associate professorship in the medical faculty at Sydney University in the mid-seventies before becoming the first woman professor of psychiatry in Australia in 1978. Recently Professor Sue Dorsch has become the professor of pathology at Sydney University and Professor Ann Woolcock has held the first personal chair in medicine. For most of these women there has been a long-term dedication to their specialist field. There has been general acceptance of their ability and this had led to senior academic opportunities. However, it is safe to say that there are a great many other women of equal ability who have not had the opportunity to reach such positions, which they might well deserve. There is a great need to redress the imbalance with many more women in academic and senior academic roles in the medical schools of this country. In interaction with students they can provide the chance for women students to identify with some of the many leadership roles they, too, may come to fulfill.

Perhaps one of the most interesting leadership roles for an Australian medical woman has been that fulfilled by Dr. Helen Caldicott in the Peace Movement. It is clear that many students feel strongly attracted to such a role, projecting caring and leadership at an international level. In some instances leadership in spheres such as those outlined may reflect a model of caring, mothering qualities, alongside powerful leadership in a way that will be acceptable to many women.

Perhaps the most poignant and hopeful story with which I can conclude is one which speaks well for the processes of change and how they may eventually be reflected in women physicians' leadership. I had been working at a senior professorial level for a year when the new professor heading my department arrived. We arranged to entertain him and his family at dinner and my daughter, then aged three and one-half, met him at the front door. I carefully introduced her to Professor B. She turned around and said to me most seriously, a few moments later, "No, that's not right, Mummy. He cannot be a Professor, he's a man!" It is to be hoped that true complementary of leadership roles will develop for men and women in all branches of medical practice.

References

[1]Teale R (editor): Colonial Eve. Sources of Women in Australia 1778-1914. Oxford University Press. Oxford, Wellington, New York, 1978.
[2]Neve MH: This Mad Folly! The History of Australia's Pioneer Women Doctors. Library of Australian History, Sydney, 1980.

34

A Distant Dream Come True:
APA's First Woman President

Carol C. Nadelson, M.D.

President, American Psychiatric Association;
Professor and Vice-Chairman,
Associate Psychiatrist-in-Chief, and
Director, Training and Education,
Department of Psychiatry,
New England Medical Center,
Boston, Massachusetts

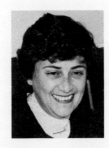

Carol C. Nadelson, M.D.

34

A Distant Dream Come True: APA's First Woman President

I often remind my residents that the excitement of beginning a career in psychiatry is to continue to explore new paths and open doors. It is never possible to know which one is "right" before beginning. We must approximate, take tentative steps, peer in and sometimes plunge. As long as we don't foreclose the future there is always adventure, excitement and new challenge.

When I finished my residency twenty years ago, I would never have dreamed that I'd find myself where I am now. I'm often puzzled when I consider how it all happened--not, I assure you, by deliberate design or careful plan, but rather with some prediction, some chance, some luck, and a lot of work, not always goal-directed. I have always loved new experience, not random or even the kind that takes some people up mountains or into the clouds. For me, experience has always been people--psychiatry was natural, although I didn't know it earlier in my life.

I didn't even hear about psychiatry until a college classmate had a "breakdown" and disappeared for a year. When she returned, there was silence. She was silent and I was silent. We both knew something had changed, but we didn't speak about it. I didn't understand what had happened until years later when, as a junior medical student on my psychiatry clerkship, I learned about her pain and how a rift had occurred between us.

At that time, I tentatively opened the door to psychiatry and tested. I went from being mystified, awestruck, and terrified, to being entranced and excited by this "new" field. As a second year student in my pyschopathology course I was cynical, disbelieving and even disdainful of those who "wasted" their "valuable" medical training. I had, after all, spent years determined to "save" lives, fantasizing about great discoveries and extraordinary efforts.

Early in my life I knew I would be a doctor! From the time I was in grade school I alternated between being a lawyer or a doctor as a future career. Despite a negative response from my family, I was undaunted. On reflection, my family always knew I was "stubborn."

I don't suppose there was any one factor that I could point to which led me here. There were no doctors in my family although there were some lawyers. I see it as a combination of events planned and serendipitous, personalities, and ambience and a number of circumstances which coalesced to make this all happen. I don't suppose I shall ever comprehend it all or cease looking back and wondering how it happened.

I was the elder of two daughters raised in the shadow of the "Depression." My parents were married in the early 1930's. One of my earliest memories involved discussion about those who had and those who did not have jobs. The toll of those Depression years was enormous. My father was never able to take a job risk after that time because he feared being left without resources.

Our Eastern European Jewish heritage was also terribly important. Although girls were not expected to achieve the status or education of boys, they were expected to obtain an education, to be able to contribute, "if necessary." My mother's perception of herself and her role were very important. She never attained the education that she would have liked because the money was "for the boys' education." Her brothers were well educated professionals but both the "girls" were not. They worked to support their brothers. She felt stifled, frustrated, and somewhat angry about not having had a chance. She was a bright, witty, competent person who did not work outside the home after she married. She repeatedly told me that in her generation good wives and mothers didn't work, they stayed home with their children. The question of what I was to do was never clear, always ambiguous and eternally met with ambivalence.

My educational supports came from my family. There was a hushed conspiracy. My grandfather always told me, when others were not within earshot, that he valued my achievement. I suspect he had some guilt about my mother. I spent a good deal of time with him, and adored him. My mother's brother, perhaps also returning past debt, was a lawyer who was a bachelor until his middle forties. He was a constant and incisive source of support, and at times even pressure. When I was a small child I spent a great deal of time with him. He was demanding, yet exciting and challenging. It was a treat to visit him and perhaps it contributed to a large degree to my ability to manage "difficult" styles. When my uncle married a woman who was a lawyer, I was enthralled. I had never met anyone like her. She continues to be a source of strength and humor.

My grandfather's death when I was 12 was perhaps the single most salient event in shaping my career. His terminal illness with cancer sparked a need to "rescue him" and also a commitment to fulfill myself, a promise I had made to him.

My adolescent years were filled with hard work and great fun. I enjoyed my double life as a student and as a participant in the sights and smells of New York. I had many friends although none who shared my particular goal. I had no choice about which college to attend: Brooklyn College was free so I went there. After my freshman year I realized that I actually could "do it." I was surprised when I found the work quite manageable. I let my family and friends know that I was serious about going to medical school. This decision was fueled by a "guidance counselor" who told me that science wasn't for me. I enjoyed my courses including science, and only

had difficulty, ironically, with writing and public speaking. My family worried about finances, and that motivated me even more. I knew I had to get a scholarship.

Although I consistently failed to think of myself as a leader, when I look back I "found" myself president of one organization or another, including the Pre-Medical Society, where I was in a distinct minority as a woman.

Applying to medical school was an ordeal that I look back on with the blinders lifted and cannot imagine how I contained my anger. I applied to 23 medical schools and was only accepted at one, despite substantial qualifications including election to Phi Beta Kappa. I assumed then that discrimination existed and that I had to face it and so I continued to grow more determined.

After marrying a classmate in a different medical school, I was able to transfer to the University of Rochester, which had initially rejected me. It was a pivotal life experience, since it was a new world with new people and places. It was exciting, rewarding, and I loved it. There were only two women in my class; the other is now a psychiatrist also. We plowed through difficult times and frequently the women in the school--all eight of us--found ourselves in the "ladies lounge," a pink locker room, sometimes in tears, sometimes exhausted and often sharing our joys and laughter. I always felt that I had to prove that they were right to allow me to transfer. It was not different than many of the women, who were "grateful" to be there.

Through this time my parents, although initially reluctant, were proud and supportive. I had known that they would be and counted on it despite their negative feelings initially. At the time my ambitions were in the direction of full-time private practice, the only model I knew, in family medicine or internal medicine.

The consolidation of my choice of psychiatry came when on graduation I won the prize in psychiatry, ironically the Benjamin Rush Award. I had already accepted an internship in medicine at Rochester after a devastating series of experiences interviewing around the country, despite honors and awards, including AOA.[1] My students continue to be incredulous when I tell them about my internship trip. I was told "we don't take women" and "when are you planning to have a baby," "perhaps you should go into pediatrics, dear." It was a relief that my medical school wanted me, so

I signed on.

After the first few months psychiatry became increasingly more appealing. I had a rotation in psychiatry during that first summer and although I loved medicine, I felt more at home with psychiatry.

Within a few months of coming to Boston for a residency in psychiatry, my marriage broke up. It was an extraordinarily difficult time and I counted on the support of my fellow residents, who were close and warm. They continue to be my good friends, my brothers. We shared our pains and joys, as well as cooking and taking care of each other. There were four women out of 24 residents, and that seemed "standard."

Despite the fact that the men in my group were continuing their discussions about career directions, I did not plan. Even when offered a chief residency I rejected the idea and decided to take my senior year to learn more about psychotherapy. My chief, Dr. Jack Ewalt, made it clear that he wasn't going to let me "cop out." I didn't know at the time what he had planned, but I subsequently learned that he had career visions that hadn't yet entered my mind. When he called me after my residency to say that he had nominated me to be a career teacher in psychiatry, I was elated. It had been a bargain we had made, yet it was unspoken until well on in my residency. I did not realize at the time what an extraordinary gift it was. It was a rewarding time and it set a career direction. During that fellowship I married Ted and began a family and also entered psychoanalytic training. As I look back it's not clear to me how I managed all of this, except that I certainly didn't sleep very much.

After the birth of my second child, a friend of mine, a plastic surgeon, inveigled me into writing a brief editorial in the Archives of Surgery on Women in Surgery. When he asked I was initially flattered and pleased, but somewhat overwhelmed since I thought back on my dismal attempts at writing in the past. My husband and friends rallied and pushed, and being a "good girl," I acceded.

I had just become stirred by the feminist movement as it was beginning to evolve and even more concretely, several female colleagues used to meet regularly in the hospital cafeteria to plan a day care center. After many frustrating attempts at obtaining good child care we decided that, as we had done in the past, we'd have to do it ourselves.

We accepted a challenge that was to take us through several years of trying meetings, confrontations, and disappointments. The experience was extraordinary: we were ignored, negated and second-guessed. Each frustration was fuel to our determination to succeed. We had all shared common experiences and obstacles and had banded together; and we were definitely not threatened by negativism. We even learned how to use our own authority; we became aware that we had some "clout" and that we could make it happen. For me it was an enormous and intense strain, and a triumph. We developed a cooperative day care center and I became its first president. This became the beginning for me of actually seeing myself in a more active sphere, overcoming a natural shyness, which most of my friends are hardly aware is there.

At this time I was also a young faculty member at Beth Israel Hospital and Harvard Medical School. With the help of my colleagues in the career teacher fellowship, I learned about academic politics. I discovered that I could take a clinical appointment and and be part-time or move toward a more academically oriented career. I don't remember making an active choice, but rather I see myself as having "fallen in." My personal psychoanalysis helped me emerge from the quiet, shy medical student who did not speak for the first two years of medical school, to a somewhat more assertive person.

One of my teachers and now colleague, Leston Havens, probably doesn't remember nominating me to be Secretary of the Massachusetts Psychiatric Society, then known as the Northern New England Psychiatric Society. Apparently the women's movement had raised consciousness in the group and when they realized that they had never had a woman officer, they decided to make some changes. In his unique and inimicable way he had exercised his marvelous ironic style, pushing a young woman into "the old boys' club."

That beginning led through several years of council and committee meetings, to my ultimate succession to the presidency of the Psychiatric Society as the first woman in 1974. When it was initially suggested that I continue to move ahead, I looked around to see who they meant. It seems obvious in retrospect that this path made sense. I was flattered, honored, and excited by the possibility. I also knew that I represented all women, and that I had to take this on, not necessarily for myself alone. I was also actually evolving an academic career--as a liaison psychiatrist for OB-GYN and then as Director of Medical Student Education.

Throughout, my husband remained my stalwart supporter, friend, and coach. My closest friends and colleagues listened and responded. Malkah Notman, with whom I had begun a writing career that would lead us through an intertwining of more than two decades of work together, was a source of strength and sharing that continues to be unique and very special. We wrote, we talked, and we worked. Mona Bennett, whose self-confidence and assertion touched a corner in me, was an endless source of ideas and directions.

After the Dallas Meeting in 1972 the Women's Caucus was born. Malkah and I had submitted a paper on women and medicine. In retrospect it's difficult to reconstruct what gave us the courage and the impetus. The support was enormous, and we found ourselves amidst a group of women who felt that time for change had come.

The next chapter is history. The Task Force on Women was formed, with Nancy Roeske chairing it. Subsequently we became a permanent committee. The APA, in a changing social climate was beginning to open up. The civil rights movement had catapulted minorities and women into medical schools in unprecedented numbers. It was clear that this was "an emerging issue," and there was active support from many of the male leadership. The atmosphere was exhilarating, albeit disquieting, at times.

Within two years of our beginning, each woman on the Task Force had attained a new leadership position, both at her local institution and in the APA. This was also the context of my assumption of the Massachusetts Psychiatric presidency. It also coincided with my decision to pursue my academic career and I learned ground rules for promotion. I had already taken the first step and pursued an appointment as Assistant Professor; now I felt confident to go on to the next step.

After my term on the Committee on Women I was appointed to the APA Committee on Medical Education--and this launched my new "component career." Forays into the world of NIMH[2] and other consulting activities as well as GAP,[3] for which my old supervisor, Henry Greenebaum, had nominated me helped me to move ahead. The excitement of new opportunities and openings pushed me and my career moved very rapidly

with writing, lecturing, and increasing APA involvement.

The next step was national leadership. I was asked to run for trustee-at-large at a time when there had been less than a handful of women who had achieved national office. It was an honor and an opportunity. I ran and lost. I really hadn't expected to win that time so I took it rather well. I learned about campaigning and about the "old boys' network." I was determined that the next time would be more successful. When I was asked to run for vice-president, I was delighted, surprised, and deeply honored.

I very rapidly had to learn how to develop a national campaign and although it was somewhat low key, it was a "massive" effort--my friends were heroic and my family, extraordinary. I surprised myself with my self-confidence. I really did expect to win this time, but I was prepared not to; my narcissism was not so fragile that I would feel reprimanded, unloved, undermined or ineffective if I didn't win. I was surprised by some of the responses to my candidacy by my colleagues. Some ignored it; others felt that I was being given special opportunities because I was a woman and were resentful. Most, however, were enthusiastic and volunteered to help. It was a difficult time--I knew that I had worked hard to earn this statement of trust, but it was clear that many would not accept it so readily.

From the time of that election, I began to hear comments about running for the presidency. Up until then it had not crossed my mind. I incorporated some of my naive and ingenuous "who me?" attitude. I took on the vice-presidency with enthusiasm and excitement. My family was proud and pleased. It wasn't as if we talked about it all the time. At home, it was still, "Mom, where are my shoes?" or "We don't have any milk in the house." Likewise, I'd hear, "Oh, where were you today?" after I had come back from Washington. I frequently commuted during the day so that I could be there in the morning and home at dinner. My children often were not aware of the extent of my schedule maneuvering.

We developed an informal women's phone network. There were often times when we talked together, and found support. Carolyn Robinowitz and Lisa Benedek were mainstays of my support and information center. I could turn to them for advice and comfort, and I still do.

In this period I had also changed jobs, and the

pressure around this, as well as the experience of loss and change, was far greater than I had ever anticipated. When Dick Shader became chairman, I moved to Tufts as the vice-chair and director of training and education. I recognize that I had to give up one entire self-image and take on another. I moved from the favorite daughter, peer, colleague and beloved teacher at "the best" to the maternal transference object--feared, envied, and ambivalently held. It was enormously difficult and painful to make this transition. Although it was necessary, as leaving home always is, it was never completely resolved. In this context I became the APA vice president. At Tufts few noticed.

The APA vice-presidency put me in touch in a more direct and concrete way with the organizational leadership. I was on the Board of Trustees, the heart of the organization. What was even better, there were other women on it, Martha Kirkpatrick and Lisa Benedek and then Naomi Goldstein. This was a new experience. Initially we began to get together during the course of the meetings for dinner, to share perceptions and views and to figure out "the agenda." We had to understand "the game-plan," which issues were the salient ones and how to make credible decisions about priorities and emphases. We learned about the political process within a power structure. It was a fascinating and exciting education. Our dinner groups and informal meetings expanded and we became an integral part of the Board.

It was somewhere during this term as vice president that I increasingly began to hear from people that I should consider running for president. I had never given it serious thought before, yet it was clear to many people that it was assumed that that was the next step. I also knew about the unofficial list of who was considering running. I was very encouraged by Mel Sabshin's enthusiasm and wisdom. I faced myself and recognized that I wanted to do it.

Friends and colleagues were overwhelmingly positive. I was touched and pleased by this. Indeed, when my name first came up I was very pleased but not surprised when I wasn't nominated. John Talbott, my close friend and colleague, was nominated. What was even more enlightening was that everybody assumed that I knew he was interested and that I was willing to run against him. It would never have occurred to me to do that.

Since I was no longer on the Board after my term, and there was support for my continued participation, George Tarjan, the president-elect, appointed me chair of the Council of National Affairs. I had been Board Liaison to that council for a year, and it was seen as a real challenge. The council consisted of diverse groups, addressing critical social and political issues, which needed direction and leadership. There was no question in my mind that this was a test of my effectiveness and mettle.

I found it exciting to take it on, particularly since I know it was a way of assessing me. It implied that I would need to move some of the committees toward putting their special issues into a context which addressed larger societal and APA issues. The impact of prospective payment on minority populations, and the mental health impact of AIDS were among the most immediate concerns.

Only a month after I took over, Bob Pasnau casually said to me, "I guess it will be you against me this time." I was quite surprised, since it hadn't occurred to me that I would be nominated so soon, or that I would run against him. Apparently the discussion had been occurring in the "locker rooms." Bob and I talked about it at some length over the next few months and decided that if we were to run against each other, we could maintain our relationship and "keep it clean." I felt reassured and relieved.

The summer was busy and I thought about the election only periodically. People asked if they could write letters for me and I agreed, but did not feel impelled to push. I tried to avoid thinking about the kind of opponent Bob would be. The pressure came to focus in September when Danny Friedman called me about the nomination and said, "I've left you alone all summer, and now the time has come. You've got to make a decision." I found myself in great conflict. On the one hand, it was a great honor and very exciting. The idea of being the first woman president of the APA was a distant dream come true. I remembered thinking, as a little girl, about being president, probably of the United States, in those days. Ted and my friends were cautious yet positive about my running. I decided to say yes.

I knew that many people thought that Bob couldn't be beaten. I also knew that if I said no I would be saying no perhaps for other women also, and perhaps I'd even be saying that women couldn't take it. I felt that I owed it to all of us to stand up and push to win. It meant rearranging my life and suddenly being catapulted into a major national campaign. This was a different dimension than the last one; the rules had changed and the stakes were different. Both men and women I had worked with over the years offered to help. I was particularly gratified by the enthusiasm among the male leaders of American psychiatry. Many felt that it was time to have a woman, that we were equal candidates, and that Bob would have a chance another time.

The campaign was a painful and difficult time, as well as being exciting, uplifting, and rewarding. I don't remember ever having been in such an ambiguous, dichotomous and exhilarating situation. It was hard to know whether I was exhausted or euphoric or some mixture of both. It was a time of reckoning, a time of learning who cared, who was ambivalent, who my real friends were and how to deal with competition, envy, and all of the affects and feelings that make relationships sometimes painful. People had to come forward and make decisions. Since nobody likes to back a loser, it was a tough time for many people. I was overjoyed and rewarded by the offers of help that continued to come and the unsolicited support which grew around me.

My life changed. For the next four and a half months I devoted myself almost entirely to the job ahead, the campaign. I met people, organized and learned. Everyone helped, including my family. My daughter was especially proud and pleased, albeit conflicted, as she folded envelopes. I became superwoman during this period, campaigning, helping Robert with college applications, Jenny with homework, taking care of my patients, my department, my residents and having time for Ted. He was incredibly generous and very loving.

I was on stage all the time. At times it was lonely and isolating. Staying with friends as I traveled around gave me a sense of being cared for. It was terribly important. I had never been so pressured before. From the moment the candidates were announced I was a different person in other people's eyes. Although I had experienced what so many women professionals report, that men often ignore their comments and attribute them to others, I found this happening with greater regularity. The transference complexities made it more difficult. Statements were misperceived and chal-

lenged more often than they had been even before. Since there were no funds which could be solicited, the financial pressures of campaigning were substantial. My department was excited, albeit ambivalent about my absences, and I felt eternally guilty about what I wasn't doing there.

I enjoyed members everywhere and I learned what it feels like to be a politician. At times I was like a wind-up toy, I worked ceaselessly, writing and rewriting talks, and perfecting them. I knew that my credibility depended upon being a reasonable, confident and knowledgeable person who was not nominated because of gender but because of leadership and expertise. It was clear that name recognition was a critical factor and my past academic record and involvement in the organization gave me that, but Bob had that also. Could the APA have a woman president?

There were a number of interesting issues related to women and leadership and to the dynamics of leadership that emerged. I was perceived as younger than I was and paternalism as well as maternalism emerged. People not only told me what to do, but they were also extraordinarily warm and concerned. There was competitiveness and even hostility from some. I guess it was, "Why her, why not me?" The statements of affirmation were everywhere and they were rejuvenating. I was relieved that so many people offered help, because I would not have been able to think about asking some of those who came forward.

I also learned that most of the women had little knowledge of "how to do it." It was also discouraging to recognize that there were only a few who would be "electable" in the APA. Women in psychiatry, as in other fields, are not often on lists as recognized leaders in areas that are not "women's issues." One looks at advertisements for conferences in Psych News,[4] or any place else and finds that those whom we think of as authorities are most often men. While the argument that women don't come forward and lead has often been repeated, it is clearly a more complex issue than that. Perhaps it's women's reluctance to be assertive, perhaps it's a lack of self-confidence. Perhaps women have other priorities. It is problematic because I doubt that change occurs in organizational structure or representation unless it's from within. In order to make them men's and women's worlds both partners must meet and renegotiate the rules.

I criss-crossed the country many times. I had to

be available, to listen, and to learn. I learned also that running for office as president is not related to being an officer in any other dimension. One is looked upon as a different person. Since the president represents American psychiatry, can a woman be that representative? Can a woman be seen as the person who is going to speak for American psychiatry? When we think of national leaders, we think of men who we see as strong and assertive. It is not easy to overcome that kind of stereotype and to look more complexly at the meaning of leadership. I wondered whether our members could see me in that kind of role.

I was challenged repeatedly. Everyone wanted what they thought was right. It was difficult for people to recognize the perspective of those who disagreed or even to accept the validity of another position. Was I being challenged even more because I was a woman? Did I really know enough, could I really do it? Men were assumed to have some expertise in a large number of the areas of major concern. As I went around from district branch to district branch, and from meeting to meeting, it was clear that those were the questions in people's minds. People perceived the role of president in a very different way than I understood it, with enormous power so that the president's decision alone could determine policy and direction. An organization structured like the APA is clearly different--it is really more democratic, but that did not change the fantasy.

As we entered January 1984, campaign activity escalated. There were more talks and trips than I could count. Wherever I went there were more and more people coming to listen to me. It became clear that I could also say a great many things that people wouldn't listen to from someone else. For example, I had men listening to my presentation on the psychology of women, when in the past that topic at grand rounds attracted the converted, and most of the audience were women.

I also learned a lot about local issues. There were many concerns that I had not known about. People were most interested in being heard. I knew that the ballots had gone out two weeks before and it was likely that most people would vote fairly quickly so early in February the campaign really ended. I was encouraged by the response and increasingly more confident, although my friends and family were cautiously optimistic,

wondering what a crash would be like for me. I felt prepared; there were times when it was extraordinarily stressful and depressing. I don't think I could have made it without Ted and my friends. I felt as if I were in a whirlwind and I was carried along, but I enjoyed the excitement and it energized me.

The beginning of March marked the end of my tenure as president of the Association for Academic Psychiatry (AAP). It had been an exciting year. I felt that I had moved the organization along and had learned a lot. It wasn't clear what I was going on to, but the end brought me mixed feelings. It was one experience of--what's next?-- a feeling I reexperience now in the middle of my term as APA president. Part of my dynamic is to constantly seek new challenges; relaxation for me is in excitement.

On the day I was to learn about the election results, our phone was broken. I was tense but confident. Robert was in Washington, but the rest of the family was there when Mel called. I had won by a large margin--58 percent of the vote.

I realized that I had scheduled a resident's party for that Friday night and I couldn't imagine how I would have tolerated it had I lost. It became a victory celebration, and the rest of the weekend was filled with victory celebrations!

The next few weeks were constant excitement and new learning. As the mail and calls came in, I faced a new dilemma. My travels around the country had made it abundantly clear that the members really wanted the president to be available, responsive and a participant. The challenge had really just begun, it was an honor and a responsibility. I had to fulfill two full-time jobs, each of which was 80 hours a week. I had to pave the way for future female leadership, and I was determined to enjoy the year--and what it brought for all of us.

Notes

[1] Alpha Omega Alpha, the National Honor Medical Society.
[2] National Institute for Mental Health.
[3] Group for the Advancement of Psychiatry.
[4] Psychiatric News.

35

_____

Women, Leadership, and Political Activism

_____

Nancy C. A. Roeske, M.D.

*Professor,
Director, Undergraduate Curriculum, and
Coordinator of Medical Education,
Department of Psychiatry,
Indiana University School of Medicine,
Indianapolis, Indiana*

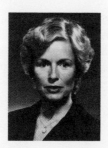

Nancy C. A. Roeske, M.D.

35

Women, Leadership, and Political Activism

For thousands of years women have been political activists according to the definition of politics in *Webster's Third New International Dictionary* (1965). Shrewd and prudent women have influenced policy affecting the lives of citizens. This influence has been primarily through traditional female roles; and therefore the influence in politics has been indirect. Until recently, women have avoided and been encouraged to avoid seeking power in government, public affairs, business, and the professions. Competition and adversary behaviors, traditionally considered non-feminine, are deemed necessary in seeking power, and most women do not meet these criteria. Within this perspective of a woman's place, the political power and leadership of women have usually been exercised through nurturing the family and secondarily through voluntary involvement in educational, cultural, social welfare, and health care institutions of the community. This situation is changing, particularly during the past 75 years, as more women have university undergraduate and graduate degrees.

The educated woman's recognition of the limitations of traditionally ascribed roles was skillfully depicted in *The Educated Woman*, published in 1960.[1] (See Figure 1.)

A woman assumes the burdens of the culture and is immobilized under their weight. Eventually she cracks and crumbles. A subsequent picture depicts the woman as an agent of change in the man's world. (See Figure 2.)

The woman forcefully exhibits her power by producing the intended effect of clearing the air and reorganizing the men's thinking. However, her power is indirect. By opening the window the woman produces an atmosphere for change; the wind does the job.

Two important questions for contemporary society are: 1) How should women compete, confront, or disagree with men in political situations? and 2) How do women define positions of leadership and administration?

In order to answer these questions it is necessary to understand how the terms leadership, administrator, and political power are defined and how women in medicine and women in government perceive and serve in these roles.

The purpose of this chapter is to examine the life experiences of politically active women in medicine and government and the economic, social, and psychological factors affecting their expression of leadership and political activism. My thesis is that all women who achieve leadership and administrative positions are political activists. Such women share many characteristics including early family life experiences, personality attributes, the process of achieving power, the focus of political interest, and some modification of the traditional definitions of leadership, administration, and political activism.

Leadership, Administration, and Political Power

Leadership is defined as that ingredient of personality which causes people to follow and involves an act, the essence of which is successful resolution of problems.[2] An administrator is one who has been appointed to manage or execute public affairs or who directs or superintends affairs as in a business, government, an organization or institution.[3]

The personality of the administrator is acknowledged as essential to success.[4-7] Leadership, imagination, and encouragement are the essential qualities. The good administrator possesses an extraordinary ability to conceive projects, work them through, and get them done. Other important attributes are good health, high energy and drive, physical endurance, maturity, a high capacity for concentration, the ability to appraise people without excessive sentiment, the capacity to encourage change and to tolerate disappointments with great resiliency, flexibility, and steadfast determination. The outstanding administrator

is able to delegate to subordinates and elicit their support. Greenblatt, and Barton and Barton have noted that the essential aspect of the administrative process is the ability to sense the organization as a whole and the total situation relevant to it. This attribute is also the essence of a good politician. The primary functions of the administrator are to influence the behavior of individuals so that they will work cooperatively in defining and accomplishing goals and to provide maximal personal satisfaction for each member of the group.

Greenblatt has written extensively about the relationship between leadership, administration, and power. He observes, "There is evidence that power holders tend to feel superior to others and to develop social distance. Sometimes in their exalted self-perception they assume they are exempt from common morality. Since the power holder is the recipient of much flattery and may

Figure 1

For more than a hundred years the Educated Woman has been an object of increasing concern to men. When we, the authors (who are women), first began our research into the subject, we were overwhelmed by the sheer weight and volume of masculine pronouncements, especially the baccalaureate addresses. We felt that our first object must be to portray, in some concrete form, the monumental image that had begun to emerge mistily from this mass of masculine specifications.

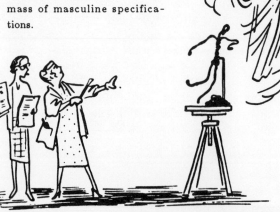
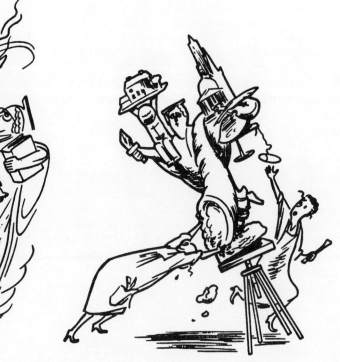

be protected by followers, the self-perception tends to become distorted."[8] An additional distortion occurs because those who work for the power holder must comply with his/her demands.

There are other problems that accrue from holding a power position which reflect people's perceptions and the power holder's responses. The problems include the person becoming a symbol, becoming famous, and becoming a lightning rod for anger and prejudice. First, a power holder may become a symbol rather than a person and thereby be further dehumanized. Second, there is an uneasy relationship between greatness and fame and the capacity of public attention in its idolatry of fame to destroy greatness. Greatness and fame are very different. Greatness is an inner quality, developed at the individual crossroads where talent and discipline meet high moral purpose and resolve. Fame is an outer thing thrown upon those whose abilities achieve visible results. Such intrusion into personal growth can undermine the ultimate contribution and power of the individual. Third, high visibility and high vulnerability are other aspects of the privilege of power. This fact may be especially true for

women because of the few who serve in public positions of power. In addition, a highly visible leader risks the progressive erosion of reputation. Since critical choices have to be made constantly, it is inevitable that some individuals and groups will be alienated, and as time goes on the coalescence of the alienated groups produces a sizable and hostile opposition.

Messner, a psychoanalyst who has served as an elected public official, notes that a special feature of the political arena is the constant shifting of alliances. Foes can suddenly become friends and friends foes.[9] Plaut discusses from a psychoanalytic perspective "the regressive pull of political power."[10] The first duty of a politician is not to convictions, principles, or the public weal but rather to getting votes. He concludes that the transitory nature of commitments with its undermining of trust and intimacy are powerful forces for the regressive coping behaviors of casual sex, alcohol, and the pursuit of money.

A person's need for power has been addressed from a variety of points of view by psychiatrists since 1900. Adler[11] believed that seeking power is an effort to overcome feelings of inferiority and

Figure 2

To the problems of practical politics...

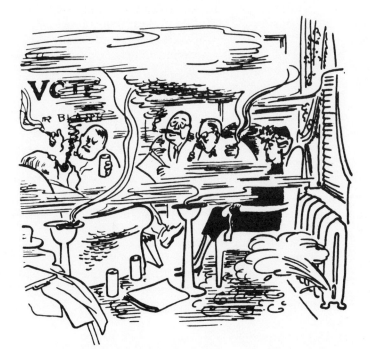

...she brings a fresh approach.

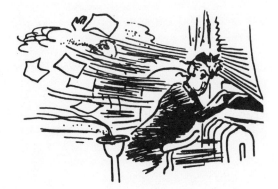

physical inadequacies which lead to aggressive behavior. He described "social feeling" as a basic counterforce to power and aggression. Social feelings can motivate an individual to strive towards superiority, perfection, and mastery with positive social consequences as opposed to striving merely for personal power. Writing in the early part of this century, he was sensitive to the inferior status of women which he perceived as resulting entirely from culturally determined influences. He believed that many of the troubles of our civilization could be traced to this unequal distribution of power. He thought education could correct a person's overwhelming desire for power and eliminate excessive dominance behavior and enhance social feelings.

Sullivan thought that feelings of competence or self-esteem are the most important drives in a person.[12] According to his theory, this basic feeling of self worth or power is necessary to overcome the helplessness, powerlessness, and dependency of the child. He writes of the valid use of power to pursue one's own creative development as opposed to a pathological use of power to seek dominance over others.

The only woman psychiatrist who has written extensively about power is Karen Horney.[13] She was convinced that anxiety is at the center of our psychodynamic life. The individual has available four mechanisms to protect himself/herself against anxiety. They are affection, submission, withdrawal, and power. Striving for power is reassurance against feelings of helplessness, humiliation, and destitution. Horney suggested that in our culture this basic anxiety leads to a striving for power, prestige, and possessions. In an extreme need for power there is a tendency to dominate, humiliate, and deprive--all of which express hostility.

Finally, Lasswell claims that deprivation experiences by politicians as children determine how they will use power as adults. He stated that "private motives displaced on public objects and rationalized as in the public interest equals political man."[14]

But power may not necessarily corrupt either those who have it or those who idolize the powerful. The responsibility of power can produce compassionate people by broadening and deepening their understanding of self and others. The rewards are many: the intellectual challenge, the joy of mastering new material, the broadening of

one's horizons, the possibility of doing a great deal of good, the honing of one's judgment, and the excitement of the demands upon one's personal capacities for performance and achievement.[4-7]

Women Psychiatrists' Perceptions of Leadership

Other authors of this volume, notably Spurlock, Chodorow, Miller, and Dickstein, have examined women's perceptions of leadership in a male dominated world, their methods of seeking self-expression, and the external constraints.

In her historical review of women in psychiatric administration, Spurlock reminds us that in some ways there have been few changes in attitudes over the past 100 years toward the role and value of having a woman physician as an administrator. Spurlock mentioned the characteristics of being "easy to keep," the woman's natural inclination to want to care for other women in the hospital and women employees, the woman physician's "salutary effect on the morals of the hospital" by cleaning up male speech and conduct, and finally "softening the insane and enforcing self-control." A strong belief in self and personal goals is a major theme according to Spurlock.

The women mentioned by Chodorow in her study of women psychoanalysts and many of the women described by Spurlock demonstrate a number of different interpretations of leadership. The female psychoanalysts' comments have a nurturing quality in the descriptions of the analysts' desire to pass on a craft through analytic supervision. The women administrators were devoted to the care of women in mental hospitals. Many of the women psychoanalysts did not write, become directors of institutions, or become politically active in the usual definition of the term, but they became extremely well-known and respected. They fulfilled a leadership role through their supervision. The ultimate women leaders in psychoanalysis were not administrators of clinics but theoretical giants, well-known to us all for their effects on the theory and practice of psychiatry.

The parturition of knowledge through teaching and serving as models of clinical skills has a core of traditional feminine qualities. Some of the women interviewed by Chodorow stated they preferred to leave the "dickering and bickering" to the men while they retained power through oral transmission of knowledge and insight, thereby shaping the care of patients and in considerable measure psychiatry.

Miller describes the woman administrator who uses herself as a conduit through which people can express their feelings and validate them. Her description of the process of administration is remarkably similar to that described by Greenblatt.[4,5,7] Miller also states that the woman's attitude toward being in charge of a family educates her to structure her administrative style in a manner to encourage individual self-discovery and contribution.

The Political Woman

Women physicians have worked on behalf of all women for over 100 years. During the past 75 years all professional women have become increasingly aware that American politics is a critical arena for societal changes. Women's involvement in changing laws and assuming leadership roles has become a major objective. Hence, I propose that women physicians must understand women politicians and work with them in order to maximize the efforts of everyone.

In the 1970's, a spate of research took place about women's power, past and present, in American politics.[15-27] A major finding was that most of the women who had held public office had not held a significant decision-making role nor had they wanted to hold such a position. Answers to the question of why women have not pursued a path of increasing responsibility can be found in an examination of the following factors: 1) the contemporary social and political system in a geographic area and its historical antecedents, 2) the urban and industrial demographics and employment patterns, 3) the social environment extending from birth through adult life within which the political personality develops including learned sex roles, and 4) the personality characteristics and coping styles.

An example of the impact of a local sociopolitical system is a study of state legislatures by Diamond.[21] She points out that the nature of the legislative job differs from state to state. Legislators differ in what is expected of them; therefore, they vary in their degree of professionalism. Like other researchers who examined women's participation in all areas of politics,[15,16,19,22-24] she found women were more likely than men to pursue a political life as an avocation and as a

source of fulfillment after children were grown up. Women were more likely than men to be asked to run for public office by male leaders of a political party, a community or state. The women saw this request as a natural sign of recognition because of volunteer involvement in the community including activities within the political party. Finally, women were more likely than men to seek office only after encouragement by the community and spouse.

The studies of state legislators and political party workers have found only 20 percent to 25 percent of the women to be interested in higher office.[15,21,28] In contrast, men were more apt to pursue greater political involvement and higher positions. Other evidence suggests that there are regional differences which reflect the local societal attitude toward women.[15,16,22,23] For example, in the south (Texas is an exception), it is generally thought unseemly for women to pursue a high official position.

Studies of the relationship between urbanization, industrialization, economics, and the pursuit of a political career have consistently found that politics is highly competitive and that women encounter the same forces at work as men.[16,23] The number of women in state and national legislatures resembles the employment curve. When times are good and public confidence is high, women stand a better chance in the political arena; in times of public unrest or anxiety, social pressure operates to keep women outside the political arena.

A 1981 study by Jones and Nelson found that there is a significant correlation between education, per capita income, industrialization, urbanization and women's representation in government.[29] In an analysis of these and other variables in 49 states they found that the highly industrialized states with a highly educated population of women provide the ideal milieu for the recruitment of women into government. The high correlation between the percentage of urban population of the state and women's representation in state government tends to confirm the general expectation that socio-economic conditions correlate with women's political roles within the state. A decade earlier Jaquette reviewed similar research in her introduction and found similar conclusions.[16]

Women who work at the local and state level of politics have a similar family background. They grew up in one community; in fact, they may live in the community where they grew up. They have had time to learn their way around, to learn information and rules by which the people in the community live, to internalize the norms of the community, to know the structure of power, and the identities of the incumbents. The women are less likely to come from a lower socio-economic class within the community than their male counterparts. Most women are likely to have a middle class or upper middle class origin but no class background is necessarily disabling. The woman and her husband are upwardly mobile.

As a child, the woman was encouraged by her father and mother to be involved in community activities. Most of the women grew up in homes where community activities and politics were a normal mode of adult behavior. The level of activities were many times higher than those found in the general public. Thus, the family's beliefs and values were repeatedly experienced during childhood and adolescence. Maternal aspirations are believed to be the most important motivator for the daughter's ambitions for success. Upward social mobility is a striking characteristic. The woman's social class is substantially higher than that of her parents and of her husband's parents.

Since the personality of a leader is of considerable importance in leadership and the political process, the personality characteristics of women who seek elected office should be considered. The studies reach the same conclusions.[15,20,21,24,25,30,31] Women politicians are more intelligent, more assertive, more adventuresome, more imaginative and unconventional, and more liberal in their attitudes than women in general. Other differences include sociability, optimism, willingness to take risks, and a sense of political efficacy. In addition, political women are warm, open, and sensitive to different kinds of people. They have a desire to find areas of agreement and opportunities for cooperation. They expect to do all of this in the absence of intimacy through understanding the use of cooperative personal relationships in working toward impersonal goals. Identification with a place, particularly a community and its people, is probably the most effective base for leadership because this identification subjectively links the fate of the community and the fate of the individual. Once this psychological link is forged, the woman feels the community's problems as personal concerns. As noted earlier

the woman usually has had years of connecting herself to community projects. In addition, as will be discussed subsequently, women may be more naturally inclined to this introjection than men.

Women political leaders have been noted to have high self-confidence, dominance, and achievement. In some ways they resemble their male colleagues. Their scores on a personality assessment inventory are very similar to those of their male colleagues. Compared with most other women they are more forceful, effective, ambitious, and socially sensitive. Most are strongly inner directed and have an unusual awareness of their values and the relationship of these values to their lives. They seem to believe what John Gardner called "the vital importance of renewal and continuity." He pointed out that the individual and society must be forever confronting change. The individual who matures has a framework out of which continuous innovation and renewal can occur. Renewal is not just innovation and change, it is also the process of bringing the results of change into line with personal purposes and values, thereby giving continuity to the process of change.[32]

The majority of women politicians serve in state legislatures, but there is increasing effort to have more women elected to Congress. Since these governmental bodies have enormous decision-making power it is crucial to understand the women who serve there.

A profile of an average woman legislator is a fairly attractive 48-year-old mother of two nearly grown children who has some college education. She may have worked outside of the home after the children became adolescents but it is more likely that she has volunteered in activities related to family life. The husband is reasonably financially successful and has encouraged her to run for office. Running for office was an extension of many years of community service. The decision to become a candidate is usually a desire to influence events, a belief in the possibility of influencing events, some knowledge of politics and politicians, and some base or potential base of community support. The woman who runs for political office is usually less politically informed and less skilled than a man in the same position.

Society at large does not support the woman politician's perspective of her ability to combine roles. In one study, Kirkpatrick found that 85 percent of women legislators disagree with the statement that it is almost impossible to be a good wife and mother and hold public office. In contrast, 67 percent of their male colleagues disagree and only 50 percent of men and women in general disagree that it is impossible to combine roles. Seventy-one percent of women legislators disagree with a statement that to be really active in politics women have to neglect their husbands and children; 41 percent of their male colleagues disagree and 41 percent of all women and 35 percent of all men disagree with the statement of neglect.[15] The importance of a strong character and a good relationship with spouse is stressed by Stoper[33] since women in political office are seen as deviant and as not being proper wives and mothers.

Women members of Congress have a background similar to women who are elected to municipal or state positions.[16,29,34] With rare exceptions, the majority of women who have been in Congress have been married. Gehlen's study of congressional women between 1916 and 1969[34] revealed that at the time of their initial election, two-thirds were widows and the majority were fulfilling a husband's term of office. This fact poses an interesting psychological phenomenon since it is through the loss of a husband and the function of replacing him as a congresswoman that the woman is expected to resolve her grief. The normal ambivalence, anxiety, and questions about taking over the job of a spouse are forced upon the woman within public view rather than the usual private resolution of these conflicts and feelings.

Currently, the preponderance of congressional women no longer wear widow's weeds. With law and business experiences they resemble congressional men. In addition, the length of time women serve in Congress has rapidly increased until now, despite their few numbers, women serve essentially the same average length of years as men (11-plus years). Law and business teach how to take an adversarial position. The use of these skills is critical in the hierarchy of and appointment to committees. However, in her study of women lawyers, Epstein found numerous examples of ways in which women lawyers face cross-pressures, are subject to double binds, and are manipulated through the use of rewards and punishments.[35] Women face disapproval for being aggressive; yet, not to do so is considered passive and inappropriate for the job. Epstein comments

that in the past male colleagues found women lawyers not tough enough; now they complain women lawyers are too tough.

Congress is the natural training ground for the higher offices of Vice President or President of the United States. Research regarding the percentage of men and women who would vote for a qualified woman to be President demonstrates that even among women there is considerable reluctance to support a woman for President.[17,36] Yet, there has been a shift in everyone's attitude over the past 50 years. The most rapid change occurred during the 1970's when support rose from 49 percent to 65 percent of the population saying they would vote for a qualified woman. A poll conducted in September 1984 regarding Ms. Ferraro's vice presidential candidacy highlighted current attitudes toward a woman in the Vice President's position. The NBC news survey found 29 percent of voters said they were less likely to vote Democratic because of the Ferraro candidacy. Only 18 percent said they were more likely to vote Democratic because of her candidacy. Fifty percent said a woman candidate did not influence their vote.[37]

The interaction and impact of all of these variables upon the 1984 congressional elections are unknown. The facts are that more women ran for Congress than ever before but there was no significant increase in the number elected.

Yet, changes within society are occurring with regard to electing women to office. The major changes have been at the municipal and state legislature levels. Over the past decade, the number of women legislators has doubled to 12 percent. The goal of the Center of The American Woman in Politics at Rutgers University for the next four years is to double this number again to 25 percent of the total members of state legislators.

In the past four years, this organization's surveys have noted the existence of a gender gap, a term defining the noticeable difference between women and men in political attitudes and voting behavior.[38] The Center's recently completed survey found a number of differences between female and male officeholders. First, differences exist in response to questions about economics, war and peace, the death penalty, and nuclear energy. The gender gap becomes even more pronounced in attitudes toward women's issues. Second, the differences are greater among those elected to higher levels of office. The gap between men and women is smallest at the municipal level, somewhat larger at the county level, and widest at the state legislative level. Third, black women holding elective office at all levels are the most liberal politicians when compared with the majority of women or with men serving at the same levels. Fourth, women politicians do not agree that the private sector could find ways to solve the nation's economic problems. Fifth, women are less likely than men to favor the death penalty. Sixth, women are far more supportive of the feminist position than are their male colleagues on an equal rights amendment and the legal right to have an abortion. Women in higher office are more likely than women in lower office to have a feminist viewpoint. The majority of women at all levels of office agree that the ERA should be ratified. Finally, women are considerably more likely than men to oppose the constitutional amendment to ban abortion.

In other ways the gender gap is widened by the fact that women are supporting other women through hiring other women, encouraging women to prepare and run for office, and speaking with groups of women stressing the importance of political involvement.

The reality of the gender gap is also the nidus for heightened conflict between men and women regarding the rules of society. The presence of more women in political office changes the content and process of every component. Their significant presence stimulates anxiety among men that institutional standards may no longer be familiar. In addition, the gender gap raises questions about the values of the previous decisions. Ultimately, the fear is of women's power in the world outside the home as well as within the home. If this change occurs, what are the issues in which men are the experts, and where are men to find sources of power?

Women in Medicine

The family background, personality characteristics, and support systems of women leaders in medicine are remarkably similar to those described by women in American politics.[39-42] The reports of women leaders have shown that these women physicians grew up in homes where parents were supportive, emotionally close, warm and attentive, and the parents shared with their daughters personal interests, activities, and

enthusiasms. Another essential family dynamic is the way that the family dealt with conflict that arose around sex role definitions. When schools or others tried to confine the girl's activities to traditional sex roles, the parental response was to support their daughter uniformly and at the same time either attempt to change the teacher's attitudes or the structural impediments or to seek an educational program that promoted the daughter's development. The positive family dynamics can be summarized as follows: 1) both parents highly valued femaleness, achievement, activity, and competitive success; 2) both parents valued each other highly and reinforced each other's role choices and behavior styles; 3) the daughter was treated by her family as a person who is female but who has available to her all roles and behavioral options of either sex, or the family constellation provided a secure base and source of personal reward, satisfaction, and reinforcement that allowed the daughter to overlook or to retreat from potential sex-role conflicts. At a very early age the daughter was allowed experiences of achievement, motivation, and action. Early experience of connecting achievement directly with self-esteem were of critical importance when the daughter became aware of sex-role taboos. Being denied these roles did not affect the desire for achievement or self-esteem; rather it directed anger towards ridiculous constraints on females.

A Comparison of Women Physicians and Women Politicians

Major differences between women politicians and women physicians are the education of parents, the role of father and other male mentors, and the age at which the woman decided to become a professional woman.

The composite picture presented by studies of women physicians is one of a highly self-reliant woman who seeks to balance demands upon her private life with available options for professional education and career. Like the woman in politics, the woman physician is more likely than non-physician women to have been raised in an urban community family. The woman physician is different from the woman in politics in some family experiences: the woman physician's father usually had a university education and was a professional and her mother was educated beyond secondary school and worked during the physician's childhood. The decision to become a physician was frequently made before or during adolescence. The conscious choice of wanting to be the boss and to run things is derived from psychodynamic factors. The theme of a close relationship with a strong father and male mentors is described in autobiographies.[40,41] Like women in politics, women physicians have a desire to help people. Unlike women in politics, they also have a high interest in biological sciences.

By and large, the personality characteristics of women physicians are also similar to those described for women politicians. Women physicians perceive their professional role as an extension of personal values, an opportunity for self-expression and for serving as a role model for other women.

Other similarities relate to the problems of combining professional and private life. Traditional attitudes are still common among men and women faculty.[43-45] Outside constraints are similar for both types of women. A significant number of men and women medical school faculty (47 percent men and 30 percent women) believe children are necessary for feeling fulfillment as a woman and are more important than a career.[43] Women medical students and women physicians think women should combine the two roles. However, they may be in conflict about which is more important. The woman politician who has fulfilled the role of mother prior to entering politics appears to have less conflict than the woman physician who is trying to do both and becomes a tired superwoman.

The answer to the question of whether women in medicine differ from women in American politics in assertiveness is unknown. Personal accounts of the former group indicate that like women politicians they have not sought advancement actively but rather have depended upon connections with male mentors to provide opportunities. However, the fatherly mentor is not limited to women. He is described as crucial for the development of the male administrator.[4]

A need for power by women physicians and women politicians, as described earlier in this chapter, has not been extensively studied to date. Nevertheless, it is of interest to note the similar life experiences of the three women who have been asked to be a candidate for Vice-President of the United States: Eleanor Roosevelt, India Edwards, and Geraldine Ferraro.[46-48] All had a number of childhood experiences which revolve

around loss: the loss of an intact family structure through the abandonment or death of the father; and the image of father's adoration maintained through either the memory of real experiences or through fantasy. None of these women had to confront what normally happens during adolescence between father and daughter. At the time the father reevaluates the daughter's intellectual accomplishments and the implications of her energy upon an adult traditional feminine role. A strong identification with a mother, or in Eleanor Roosevelt's case a mothering figure, who was self-reliant and able to support the daughter conveyed the inner strength of being a woman and her capacity to respond flexibly and resiliently to stress and deprivation. Each woman seemed to be constantly aware of and utilized the integration of contradictory psychological forces. A sense of helplessness and powerlessness fosters an identification with the disadvantaged. A belief in self-reliance and personal abilities supports intellectual curiosity and directs physical energy. The ever-present tensions between these factors combine to overcome personal losses. Eleanor Roosevelt acknowledged that she turned inner depression outward into actions on behalf of those who did not have the strength or opportunity to overcome a disadvantaged societal position.

Elsewhere in this volume, Dickstein's admirable survey of women in medical administration adds current evidence that personality characteristics, aspirations, and purposes of women in medical administration have not changed from earlier studies of women in science and medicine.[39,40] In addition, the descriptions of male psychiatrist administrators resemble the characteristics revealed by Dickstein's study. In essence, a key role is one of being a decision-maker. The evidence regarding women in American politics suggests that more women are seeking decision-making roles as mayors, chairpersons of committees, and other administrators.

As was pointed out at the beginning of this chapter, the requirements for good administration are characteristics which focus on a nurturing role, a role which is traditionally described as feminine. Yet, women may express this nurturing role in a way that is different from that of men. These differences have been described in detail by other authors of this volume.

A major source for the differences between men and women is undoubtedly the difference in the socialization process for males and females within our society. This process focuses on the male evolving a description of self as separate in relation to others and on the female defining self as interdependent with other people and responsible for their well being. The implications of the differences in childhood experiences upon the development of moral judgment has been thoroughly studied by Gilligan.[49] Her work sheds light on the gender gap in American politics and the different focus of men and women in American medicine. It is noteworthy that women are most likely to be in the specialties of pediatrics, family medicine, internal medicine, and psychiatry--medical specialties which require personal concern for the patient's well being. The areas of concern of women politicians likewise reflect a perspective of morality which is different from men. Gilligan believes that the differences in the experiences of male and female children affect moral development, i.e., how people come to construct experience in moral terms and how moral language, in turn, shapes and is changed by experiences of conflict and choice. In her research, she found women often spoke, not about matters of justice, the fair weighing and balancing of claims, but about care and problems of responsibility in relationships. In contrast, the men often spoke about right and wrong, rules and law, and whether the act was justified.

This different perspective of morality was also reflected in men's description of self as separate in relation to others and as independent. The men were more likely than the women to have a view of human relationships as rooted in impartiality and objectivity with the capacity to distance oneself and determine fair rules for mediating relationships. On the other hand, the women's view is rooted in the specific context of others, the ability to perceive people on their own terms and respond to their needs. Gilligan's work reflects a rapidly increasing interest by sociologists and social psychologists in the influence of feelings upon individual behavior and ultimately upon societal structure and goals.

In the final analysis, the seriousness of our societal problems requires that we learn to utilize creatively the tension between women and men that evolves from the differences in early attachment, separation experiences, and role socialization in a combined effort to solve our problems.

In conclusion, in our attempts to redefine the policies of government and the health care system, it is well to remember the healing balm of humor. For humor well used conveys a message, relieves tension, and expresses feelings. No one knew this better than Sojourner Truth. Born into slavery around 1795, Sojourner was active in both the abolitionist and women's rights movements. She tilled the soil like a man and bore 13 children, most of whom were sold off into slavery. Her insight and humorous wit are as alive today as they were in 1851 when she wrote, "If the first woman God ever made was strong enough to turn the whole world upside down all alone, these women together ought to be able to turn it back and get it right side up again. And now they is asking to do it, the men better let them."[50]

References

[1]Cleveland A, Anderson J: The Educated Woman. New York, EP Dutton & Co., 1960.
[2]Webster's Third New International Dictionary. New York, G & C Merriam Co, 1965, p. 1283.
[3]Webster's Third New International Dictionary. New York, G & C Merriam Co, 1965, p. 28.
[4]Greenblatt M, Rose SO: Illustrious psychiatric administrators. Am J Psychiatry 134:626-630, 1977.
[5]Greenblatt M: Psychopolitics. New York, Grune and Stratton, 1978.
[6]Barton W, Barton G: Mental Health Administration: Principles and Practice, vol 2. Science Press, 1983.
[7]Greenblatt M: The unique contributions of psychiatrists to leadership roles. Hosp Community Psychiatry 34:260-263, 1983.
[8]Greenblatt M: Psychopolitics. New York, Grune & Stratton, 1978, p. 225.
[9]Messner E: Coping with adversaries in elective public office. Am J Psychiatry 138:826-828, 1981.
[10]Plaut EA: The regressive pull of political power. American Journal of Social Psychiatry IV:19-24, 1984.
[11]Adler A: Understanding Human Nature. New York, Garden City Publishing Co, 1927.
[12]Sullivan HS: The Interpersonal Theory of Psychiatry. New York, WW Norton & Co, 1953.
[13]Horney K: The Collected Works of Karen Horney, vol 1. New York, WW Norton & Co, 1942.
[14]Lasswell HD: Psychopathology and Politics. New York, Viking Press, 1960, pp. 74-77.

[15]Kirkpatrick JJ: Political Woman. New York, Basic Books, Inc, 1974.

[16]Jaquett JS (ed): Women in Politics. New York, J Wiley & Sons, 1974.

[17]Morrow GR, Clarke WV, Merenda PF: Perception of role of the President: a nine-year follow-up. Percept Mot Skills 38:1259-1262, 1974.

[18]Welch S: Support among women for the issues of the women's movement. Sociological Quarterly 16:216-227, 1975.

[19]Bird AT: Women in politics--changing perceptions. J of the Assoc for the Study of Perception 10:1-9, 1975.

[20]Bachtold LM: Personality characteristics of women in distinction. Psychology of Women Quarterly 1:70-78, 1976.

[21]Diamond I: Sex Roles in the State House. New Haven, Yale Univ Press, 1977.

[22]McCourt K: Working Class Women and Grass-roots Politics. Bloomington, Indiana Univ Press, 1977.

[23]Githens M, Prestage JL (eds): A Portrait of Marginality, The Political Behavior of the American Woman. New York, David McKay Co, Inc, 1977.

[24]Kelly RM, Boutilier MA: Mothers, daughters, and the socialization of political women. Sex Roles 4:415-443, 1978.

[25]Chaney EM: Supermadre, Women in Politics in Latin America. Austin, The University of Texas Press, 1979.

[26]Laponce JA: Voting for X: of men, women, religion and politics. The use of an election experiment for the comparative analysis of conservative behavior. Social Science Information 19:955-969, 1980.

[27]Prince-Embury S, Deutchman I: Sphere of influence profile as a predictor of political behavior in women. Psychol Rep 48: 876-878, 1981.

[28]King EG: Women in Iowa legislative politics, in Portrait of Marginality. Edited by Githens M, Prestage JL. David McKay Co, Inc, 1977, pp. 284-303.

[29]Jones W, Nelson AJ: Correlates of women's representation in lower state legislative chambers. Social Behavior and Personality 9:9-15, 1981.

[30]Werner EE, Bachtold LM: Personality characteristics of women in American politics, in Women in Politics. Edited by Jaquette JS. J Wiley & Sons, 1974, pp. 75-84.

[31]Constantini E, Craik KH: Women as politicians: the social background, personality, and political careers of female party leaders, in A Portrait of Marginality. Edited by Githens M, Prestage JL. David McKay, Co, Inc, 1977, pp. 221-240.

[32]Gardner JW: Self-Renewal: The Individual and Innovative Society. New York, WW Norton & Co, 1965.

[33]Stoper E: Wife and politician: role strain among women in public office, in A Portrait of Marginality. Edited by Githens M, Prestage JL. David McKay Co, Inc, 1977, pp. 320-338.

[34]Gehlen FL: Women members of congress: a distinctive role, in A Portrait of Marginality. Edited by Githens M, Prestage JL. David McKay Co, Inc, 1977, pp. 304-319.

[35]Epstein CF: Women in Law. New York, Basic Books, 1981.

[36]Wells AS, Smeal EC: Women's attitudes toward women in Politics, in Women in Politics. Edited by Jaquette JS. J Wiley & Sons, 1974, pp. 54-72.

[37]Hume E: The Ferraro factor. The Wall Street Journal LXIV:241, Sept. 25, 1984.

[38]Houghton M: Women officeholders differ from men. Women's Political Times, July 1984.

[39]Lopate C: Women in Medicine. Baltimore, Johns Hopkins University Press, 1968.

[40]Kundsin RB (ed): Successful women in the sciences: an analysis of determinants. Ann NY Acad Sci 208:47-51, 1973.

[41]Roeske NCA: Women in psychiatry. Am J Psychiatry 133:365-372, 1976.

[42]Roeske NCA: Life stories as careers--careers as life stories. Perspect Biol Med 28:229-242, 1985.

[43]Rosen RAH: Occupational role innovators and sex role attitudes. J Med Educ 49:554-561, 1974.

[44]Heins M, Smock S, Jacobs J, et al: Productivity of women physicians. JAMA 236:1961-1964, 1976.

[45]Roeske NCA: Lake K: Role models for women medical students. J Med Educ 52:459-466, 1977.

[46]Hoff-Wilson J, Lightman M: Without Precedent: The Life and Career of Eleanor Roosevelt, Bloomington, Indiana Univ Press, 1984.

[47]Roeske NCA: Television interview, India Edwards. Symposium: Women in Politics. Texas Woman's University, Oct. 11, 1984.

[48]Roeske NCA: Personal letter from Geraldine Ferraro, Sept. 1984.

[49]Gilligan C: In A Different Voice. Cambridge,

Harvard Univ Press, 1982.

[50]Bernard J: Journey Toward Freedom--The Story of Sojourner Truth. New York, WW Norton & Co., 1967, p. 167.

Epilogue

"It was the best of times . . . it was the worst of times." Although Charles Dickens was speaking about the French Revolution, his comments hold well for the status of women in leadership positions. While opportunities and accomplishments have never seemed so great, there is a sense of concern or even disillusionment that the potential for women has not and may not be met.

Five years ago, a paper describing problems and progress for women in academic psychiatry noted optimistically that as the numbers of women in medicine increase, accommodations to particular needs and variations will become accepted as part of the system, and women's success will be self-perpetuating, proportional, and appropriate.[1]

If one examines the data, the recent increase of women in medicine has been phenomenal. Women were six percent of medical school entrants in 1960; by 1979, that figure had grown to 28 percent, leveling off at more than one-third of the entering first year class in 1985. Women have taken about 65 percent of the new places created in medical school since 1970, and their applications are still increasing.[2,3] Heins noted three major factors contributing to this growth. First was the enactment of federal antidiscrimination legislation, closely followed by the adoption in 1970, of a resolution on equal opportunity by the Association of American Medical Colleges. The third and most important was the change in women's attitudes and aspirations, as fostered by the women's liberation movement. While the first two factors lowered the barriers to entry, the change in social climate led to a change in women's aspirations and their seeking nontraditional education and careers.[4]

This change resulted in women's being able to choose specialty training in all areas of medicine, not just the traditional "women's fields," such that there are currently over 1300 women residents in surgery and the surgical specialties.[5]

Within the past two years, women have been elected president of two major national specialty societies (Obstetrics/Gynecology and Psychiatry); women are currently president of two ABMS member specialty boards (Pediatrics and Psychiatry); two women have been elected president of the 250,000 member Council of Medical Specialty Societies, and a woman attorney was recently appointed president of the American Hospital Association. Women are more visible in organized medicine and in positions of leadership. On the other hand, in the past five years, there has been a reduction of women chairing departments of psychiatry (from two to one), and following the early and tragic demise of Leah Lowenstein, no other women have been named medical school deans. None of the half dozen women on the 1985 ballot for elected positions at the American Medical Association was elected.

Although women outnumber men in the health care field, most women still work in low status and low paying jobs such as nursing. Women physicians are seen as less productive, working fewer hours and seeing fewer patients, although more recent data suggest that the productivity gap between male and female physicians is decreasing.[5] Yet, women physicians continue to earn less than their male colleagues for comparable work, even when taking into account factors of age and employment.[6] Women physicians still tend to be over-represented in the lower status positions-- generally those that are salaried or without much authority, while they are underrepresented in the higher ranks of organized medicine and academia.[1,7,8] In schools of medicine, only six percent of full professors are women, and the disparity between male and female faculty increases with age.[3]

Women in positions of authority face interpersonal and intrapsychic difficulties.[1] The socialization of males is seen as useful in management training. Boys are more independent and combative, and participate in team sports even with those they dislike, while girls tend to focus on quality of relationships, favoring compliance, and playing only with those whom they like.[9] To succeed as managers, women must be forceful and assertive, and their competence or success may lead to questions about their femininity. Role models and mentors are in short supply, and women entering a previously male system have many social as well as professional obstacles to surmount. As their numbers increase, they may lose the isolation that comes from being a "solo" woman, but an increase in female staff has, in many instances, led to anxiety and often pejorative statements by male colleagues that there are "enough" women.

Surveys and informal contacts with female colleagues document overt as well as covert examples of exclusion. Positions can be defined in ways that automatically exclude the female candidate (e.g., by defining an area of competence, expressing concern at a possible future change of location by her spouse, or limiting candidates to an age or experience group into which the woman candidate does not fall). Meetings are still held in all male clubs, and sexist or offensive after-dinner "jokes" are still told.

Thus, middle-aged physicians and leaders feel a conflict between their optimism and excitement at possibilities and what seems a painful reality. Women are in the mainstream, and are being accepted as competent leaders. At the same time, the hoped for equality and colleagueship is slower in unfolding. Will the bolus of women in the early stages of their careers provide the impetus to positive growth, or will they represent a potential threat to their male colleagues. Is it possible to "have it all"?

The authors of this volume have presented a comprehensive picture of the history and present status of women in leadership, as well as identified problems and prospects for the future. The women leaders through histories and self-portraits emphasize the energy, determination, and individuality as well as intellectual curiosity that has lead to their success. Thus, these chapters offer a brief "education" in leadership, bringing the issues to life, making these famous women and their successes and failures accessible to the reader who may not have been privileged to know or work

with them. These very real role models do much to ensure the survival of women as leaders and as contributors to equality in our society regardless of gender.

Carolyn B. Robinowitz, M.D.
Deputy Medical Director,
American Psychiatric Association

(Note: The opinions expressed here are those of the author and do not represent APA policy.)

References

[1]Robinowitz, CB, Nadelson, CC, Notman, MT: "Women in academic psychiatry: politics and progress." Am J Psychiatry 138:1357-1361, 1981.

[2]Braslow, JB, Heins, M: "Women in medical education: a decade of change." N Engl J Med 304:1129-1135, 1981.

[3]Personal Communication: Kathleen S. Turner, Special Assistant to the President. Washington, D.C., Association of American Medical Colleges, December, 1985.

[4]Heins, M: "Women in academic psychiatry." Unpublished paper presented at APA Conference: Women's Studies in Psychiatric Education, San Francisco, CA, 1983.

[5]"Today's Woman," Medica, pp 40-45, Fall, 1983.

[6]Holden, C: "Working women still segregated and underpaid." Science 231:449 January 31, 1986.

[7]Schapiro, R: "Women in medicine; the choices and challenges." The New Physician, March, 1984, pp 10-14

[8]Rinke, C: "The economic and academic status of women physicians." JAMA 245:2305-2306, 1981.

[9]Block, JH: "Psychological development of female children and adolescents." in Women: a developmental perspective. Berman, P, & Rainey, E: eds. Department of Health and Human Services, Public Health Service, National Institutes of Health, NIH Publ. #82-2298, 1982.

Conclusion

This volume on women physicians in leadership roles offers insights into the wonderful, creative experiences and achievements as well as the unnecessary hindrances and stereotypic barriers which were, and in some instances still are, part of the socio-cultural and political milieu for women in medicine.

The rich diversity of topics, which range from individual autobiography and biography to the general history of an era, a locale, a hospital, a specialty, subspeciality, and a national experience, attest to the vast body of knowledge heretofore nonexistent in collective form.

The power of this material will become evident to readers, whether they are female or male, researcher or clinician, interested adults, or students of all ages in any related discipline. We hope that this will provide greater understanding about aspects of leadership roles and the routes to their attainment for women.

An important general thread which runs throughout the book is the role of the family. Although concern about support from the family of origin and from current nuclear family or significant others exists for men in leadership roles also, for women these issues appear to be more emotionally fraught. Bearing and rearing children has been, and appears to continue to be, viewed differently by and for women. Many career women have felt the necessity to choose between having children and pursuing a career. Many mourned the sacrifices involved in either choice. Some still do, even when they choose to have both.

For the majority of women leaders, personal sacrifices have been an accepted part of professional success. We hope that continued research and changes in attitudes and practices will modify this unnecessarily painful and inappropriate experience for women leaders.

Women need to learn to view leadership roles as an expected part of their lives, if they choose them, rather than as an extraordinary option for only a few. From their earliest years this option must be part of their lives and experiences, if they are to develop and accept their own leadership skills and those of others. This will also enable them to be more astute about experiences of subtle discrimination against their assuming leadership roles and power and about having some, or none, or even losing power.

We regret the limits of time and space and our failure to include more women from the past, as well as from the present, who have made and continue to make unique contributions to the mental health field. We apologize to those we should have included in this volume. We view this as a beginning and we welcome suggestions for inclusion in a second volume.

Our hope is that, in the future, women leaders in medicine and other fields are offered the support and opportunity for the assumption of leadership roles. Women have much to offer to their patients and to the health care system.

Leah J. Dickstein, M.D.
Louisville, Kentucky

Carol C. Nadelson, M.D.
Boston, Massachusetts